S0-BUD-827

REVERSE SKIN AGING

THE MAGIC AND SCIENCE OF COPPER PEPTIDES

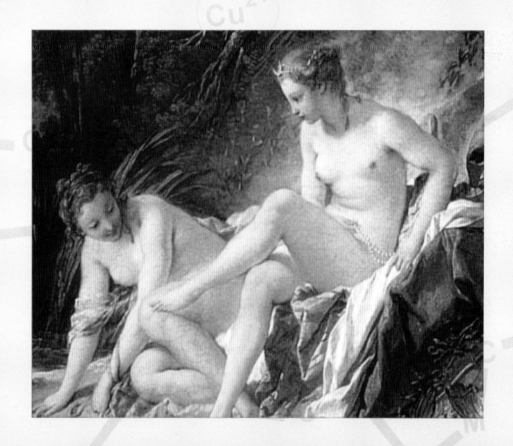

LOREN PICKART, PhD
IDELLE MUSIEK, MFA
ANNA MARGOLINA, PhD

Disclaimer and Cautions

The ideas, procedures, and suggestions contained in this book are intended to help improve health and are not intended to act as a substitute for regular medical care by a qualified health-care professional. Some individuals may have success with skin products not mentioned in this book. Skin Biology products are designed to improve skin health, but should not be used on broken or wounded skin. All products applied to the skin should be started cautiously since individuals may have unique allergies or sensitivities. If you develop sensitivity to any skin-care or hair-care product, discontinue its use immediately and consult your physician. If skin problems persist or worsen, consult a physician. Neither the author nor the publisher will be responsible for any loss, injury, or damage arising from any information or suggestion in this book. None of the statements in this book have been approved by the FDA. This book also suggests that moderate exposure to light has many health-enhancing virtues. However the FDA requires that we mention our products "do not contain a sunscreen and do not protect against sunburn. Repeated exposure of unprotected skin while tanning may increase skin aging, skin cancer, and other harmful effects to the skin even if you do not burn."

FIRST EDITION – JULY 2005
SECOND EDITION – DECEMBER 2011

Copyright © 2005, 2011 by Loren Pickart.

Published by
Cape San Juan Press
Summit Associates International
4122 Factoria Boulevard – Suite #200
Bellevue, WA 98006
425-644-0160
www.skinbiology.com

ISBN 978-0-9771853-0-6 (HB)
ISBN 978-0-9771853-1-3 (PB)
ISBN 978-0-9771853-2-0 (epub)

All rights reserved. This book, or parts thereof, may not be reproduced in any form without written permission of the copyright owner except for inclusion of quotations in a review.

Cartoon Scientist graphic used with the permission of Brad Fitzpatrick Illustration.

These products are trademarks of the following companies: Neova, Tricomin, Graftcyte (Procyte Corporation); Active Copper, Visibly Firm, Retin-A, Renova (Johnson & Johnson); Propecia (Merck Corporation); Rogaine (Pharmacia & Upjohn Consumer Healthcare).

In memory of my mother,
Grace Pickart,
who started all of this long ago
by taking me to see dinosaurs at museums.

— Loren Pickart

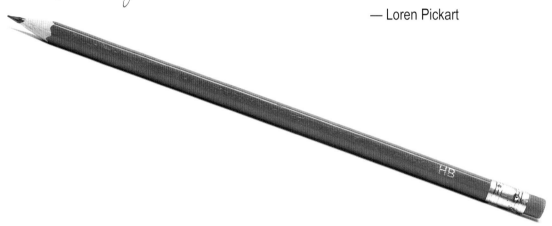

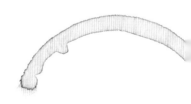

CONTENTS:

Forward / Acknowledgements / Introduction by Idelle Musiek 6-7

1   Reverse Skin Aging – The Magic and Science of Copper Peptides 8

2   Artificial & Unnatural Skin Treatments 16

3   Understanding Your Beautiful Skin 25

4   Six Magic Bullets to Beautify Skin 35

5   First and Second Generation SRCPs 49

6   Say Goodbye to Fine Lines & Wrinkles 55

7   Tighten Loose and Sagging Skin 69

8   The Balancing Act for Removing Scars and Blemishes 79

9   When Makeup Ravages the Skin 99

10   Caring for Sensitive and Extra Dry Skin 104

11   Keeping Your Skin Young and Beautiful 114

12   Healthy Hair Growth: Strengthen, Thicken, Lengthen from Root to Tip 132

13   Biology & Chemistry of Beautiful Hair 144

14   Nail Renewal: Restore Health for Nails that Grow Stronger 158

15   The Formula of Love 166

16   Glowing Good Health: Better Suntanning with Less Skin Damage 178

17   Nutrients that Turn Back the Clock – Bypassing Confusion and Food Wars 198

18   The Science Behind SRCPs 215

19   The Essentials of Copper: Your Body's Protective & Anti-Aging Metal 248

20   The Moral Need for Beauty 270

21   Resources: A Guide and Glossary 277

22   References 282

Index of Words 289

Forward and Acknowledgements

Loren Pickart, PhD

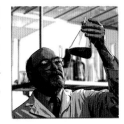

This book began over 49 years ago with my rather naive idea of finding a way to reverse human aging. Over the years, this quest led me to laboratories in Minneapolis, Santa Barbara, San Francisco, Seattle, and finally to my home on San Juan Island where I am writing today. During the course of this journey, I was more successful than I had ever imagined in discovering a human molecule that helps to turn back the clock on many types of aging.

Today this molecular gem, derived from copper peptides, can be found in many cosmetic and dermatological products. Copper truly rejuvenates damaged skin. But it took me until now to truly understand how the body's aging reversal system works. This book details my findings.

The topics explored on the following pages arose from the thousands of questions I have received from Skin Biology clients. Most of these individuals focused on their quest for healthier, more beautiful skin and hair.

However, clients have also asked me about a variety of topics such as pheromones, diets, supplements, suntanning, and the actual published science behind Skin Remodeling Copper Peptides (SRCPs), the skin's natural renewal signals. If you would like to quickly learn the best ways to benefit from SRCPs, read Chapters 3-9 and 11 which were written as "how-to" chapters.

I would like to thank my co-authors who helped bridge the gap between pedantic science and emotions (such as the thoughts that arise while sitting at a vanity table applying lip plumper).

And a special thanks to Cassia McClain who expertly formatted the manuscript and illustrated most of the graphics within the book.

I also would like to thank all of the scientists, clinicians, and veterinarians around the world whose work finally enabled a biochemical understanding of the mode of action of remodeling copper peptides.

Finally, a big thanks to my daughters Françoise and Genevieve for their comments and to my beautiful, gracious, and talented wife Charlene for all her help and support.

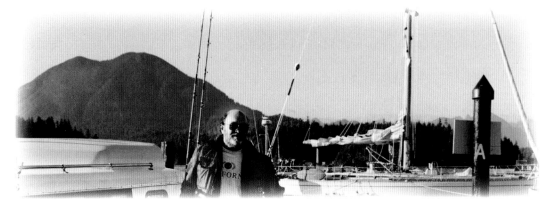

Idelle Musiek, MFA / Anna Margolina, PhD

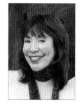

Like many of you, I am a beauty product junky with a singular quest. I seek sumptuous skin. For years my cosmetic quest led me to buy any product that would give me a boost, especially if it promised to reduce wrinkles and sag. I bought in to all the hype...hook, line and sinker as I went on fishing expeditions for skin elixirs in a jar. When I discovered Dr. Loren Pickart's copper peptide products five years ago, I was thrilled with the results and spent more than a few minutes gazing at my reflection. My skin glowed and my friends thought I looked years younger. I'm always inquisitive and suspicious of what I read online. I often feel that women fall prey to cosmetic deception. So I called Dr. Pickart with a laundry list of questions about skin care and the science behind his products. Although I'm not a biochemist, skin and health are my hobbies. I pride myself with the ability to research. Amazingly, Dr. Pickart took the time to address each and every question. He backed up his information with scientific data based on academic studies and his 30 years of research on copper peptides. No other owner of a cosmetic company, whether a dermatologist or chemist, had ever taken the time to respond so thoroughly. I truly believe that Dr. Pickart offers science and integrity. During one of my calls, I asked Dr. Pickart about a new product containing neuropeptides, which claims to reduce wrinkles. Dr. Pickart explained that neuropeptides are nerve inhibitors that make tissue dysfunctional and hence may damage the skin around the brain. I wrote him the following email in jest and was immediately embarrassed. You can't take back email!

> **"These nerve inhibitors are currently numbing my cute little brain. I think they are turning me into a Stepford Wife... But oh well, at least I'm wrinkle-free. Well, I guess I better go now. I have to get back to baking cookies and trying on my new lingerie and neuropeptides."**

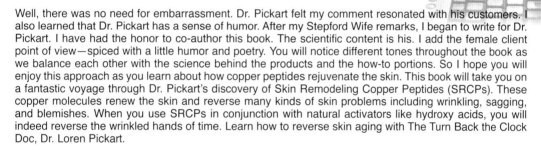

Well, there was no need for embarrassment. Dr. Pickart felt my comment resonated with his customers. I also learned that Dr. Pickart has a sense of humor. After my Stepford Wife remarks, I began to write for Dr. Pickart. I have had the honor to co-author this book. The scientific content is his. I add the female client point of view—spiced with a little humor and poetry. You will notice different tones throughout the book as we balance each other with the science behind the products and the how-to portions. So I hope you will enjoy this approach as you learn about how copper peptides rejuvenate the skin. This book will take you on a fantastic voyage through Dr. Pickart's discovery of Skin Remodeling Copper Peptides (SRCPs). These copper molecules renew the skin and reverse many kinds of skin problems including wrinkling, sagging, and blemishes. When you use SRCPs in conjunction with natural activators like hydroxy acids, you will indeed reverse the wrinkled hands of time. Learn how to reverse skin aging with The Turn Back the Clock Doc, Dr. Loren Pickart.

After being in the skin care industry for over 15 years, I can attest to the fact that despite a constant flow of commercials boasting "scientific breakthroughs in skin care", the vast majority of cosmetic ingredients have very little to do with real science. The copper peptide GHK is a wonderful exception. I became interested in cosmetic science soon after I graduated from the Russian Medical University with a major in biophysics. When I completed my graduate research on antioxidant enzymes and received my PhD in biology, I became a scientific editor for the Cosmetics & Medicine Journal (a publication aimed to Russian cosmetic chemists, dermatologists and skin care professionals). As I was constantly on lookout for good scientific materials, it was only a matter of time before I came across Dr. Pickart's articles. In 2001 I moved to Redmond, Washington. I was thrilled to learn that Dr. Pickart's office was only a short drive away. I decided it was time for me to meet him in person and prepare a detailed article about his groundbreaking research. Since then I have been fascinated with the GHK peptide and have kept myself updated on the most current research in this area.

I have also learned to pamper my skin with Skin Biology products and today credit them for my youthful and healthy skin. I was very excited when Dr. Pickart invited me to work on the second edition of the Reverse Skin Aging book, especially since recent years have brought so many new scientific discoveries on GHK's mode of action. Today we know that the wonderful effects that many women and men observe in their skin after using copper peptides are not accidental or miraculous—they are brought about by distinct biochemical actions of the GHK-Cu peptide, which now have become fully revealed by modern science. This book brings you the most comprehensive information on skin effects of GHK peptide, told in plain language. What's more, this is not just another dry scholastic theory, but living and breathing knowledge that you can immediately put into practical use to fight wrinkles and maintain the natural beauty of your skin for many years to come.

REVERSE SKIN AGING
The Magic and Science of Copper Peptides

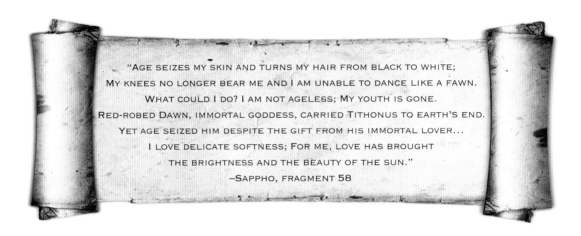

"AGE SEIZES MY SKIN AND TURNS MY HAIR FROM BLACK TO WHITE;
MY KNEES NO LONGER BEAR ME AND I AM UNABLE TO DANCE LIKE A FAWN.
WHAT COULD I DO? I AM NOT AGELESS; MY YOUTH IS GONE.
RED-ROBED DAWN, IMMORTAL GODDESS, CARRIED TITHONUS TO EARTH'S END.
YET AGE SEIZED HIM DESPITE THE GIFT FROM HIS IMMORTAL LOVER...
I LOVE DELICATE SOFTNESS; FOR ME, LOVE HAS BROUGHT
THE BRIGHTNESS AND THE BEAUTY OF THE SUN."
—SAPPHO, FRAGMENT 58

What causes aging? The most recent idea in aging research is that the primary cause of aging is a lack of signals to the tissues to start regeneration and repair. Secondary factors are tissue oxidation caused by free radicals, and the increased production of inflammatory proteins by our DNA and cancer promoting proteins. The interesting finding is that the regenerative copper peptides reverse all these negative effects. They have been proven to:

- Tighten loose skin and thicken older skin
- Repair protective skin barrier proteins
- Improve skin firmness
- Reduce fine lines and depth of wrinkles
- Smooth rough skin
- Improve overall appearance
- Act as anti-inflammatories
- Repair damaged DNA at cellular level
- Cause the differentiation of stem cells
- Reduce spots, photodamage and hyperpigmentation
- Help adult stem cells produce new skin cells
- Control or affect over 3,900 human genes
- Suppress numerous cancer metastasis genes

Causes of Wrinkles and Aging	Actions of Copper Peptides
Primary Cause:	
Lack of signals for tissue regeneration	Copper peptides increase regeneration of skin, hair follicles, the stomach lining, the intestinal lining, bony tissues, and activate adult stem cells
Secondary Causes:	
Tissue Oxidation	Copper peptides block tissue damage by reactive oxygen species and reactive carbonyl radicals
DNA produces more inflammatory proteins	Copper peptides suppress a broad array of inflammatory proteins
DNA produces more cancer promoting proteins	Copper peptides suppress cancer genes
Increased Infections	Copper peptides suppress infections

See Chapter 22: References

Very few "skin experts" are deep thinkers... Somehow this doesn't stop them from thinking that they know everything.

SKIN TRUTH: WHAT IS REALLY KNOWN?

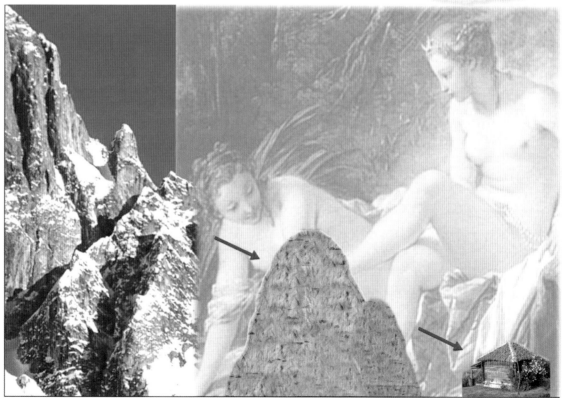

Mountain Ranges of Ignorance   Piles and Piles of Data   Actual Understanding

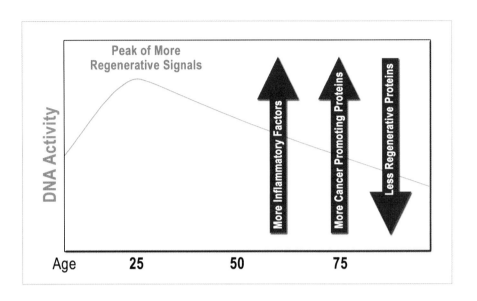

Would You Like to Know?

WHAT ARE COPPER PEPTIDES? Copper peptides are copper ions bound to small pieces of larger proteins. Not all copper peptides have positive actions.

In this book, we use copper peptides to mean a class of copper peptides that at a minimum, (1) speed skin repair, (2) have potent anti-inflammatory actions, and (3) increase hair follicle size. The best defined of such copper peptides is the one in your blood called GHK-Cu (glycyl-l-histidyl-l-lysine:copper 2+). The second generation copper peptides are less well defined but are approximately 10-fold more effective than GHK-Cu.

WHY AREN'T THEY BETTER KNOWN? The medical establishment often avidly preaches harmful health ideas for generations. The amazing spectrum of positive copper peptide actions was found by over 80 laboratories and published in journals.

But new ideas have a difficult time establishing themselves when trying to replace entrenched myths. Consider the following:

1. SMOKING. IN 1927, 12,745 PHYSICIANS ENDORSED SMOKING LUCKY STRIKE CIGARETTES AS A HEALTHFUL ACTIVITY. IN THE 1940S AND 1950S, THOUSANDS OF PROMINENT SURGEONS WERE USED IN NATIONAL CIGARETTE ADVERTISEMENTS TO REASSURE THE PUBLIC ABOUT THE SAFETY OF CIGARETTE SMOKING.

2. LOBOTOMIES. IN THE 1950'S, LOBOTOMIES WERE PROMOTED FOR MENTAL DISORDERS BUT PRODUCED NEAR-TOTALLY DYSFUNCTIONAL PEOPLE.

3. DIETARY FATS. IN THE 1960'S AND 1970'S, DIETS HIGH IN OMEGA-6 POLYUNSATURATED FATS AND PARTIALLY HYDROGENATED FATTY ACIDS SUCH AS SAFFLOWER OIL AND MARGARINE WERE RECOMMENDED TO REDUCE HEART DISEASE. HOWEVER, LONG TERM STUDIES FOUND THAT, WHILE SUCH DIETS AND MARGARINES (LOADED WITH TRANS-FATS) DECREASED HEART DISEASE, THEY INCREASED THE TOTAL DEATH RATE AND THE CANCER RATE.

4. SUDDEN INFANT DEATH SYNDROME (SIDS). BETWEEN 1943 AND 1988 PEDIATRICIANS TOLD MOTHERS TO FORCE THE BABY TO SLEEP ON THEIR STOMACH OR THEY WOULD DIE OF SUDDEN INFANT DEATH SYNDROME (SIDS). BABIES PREFER TO SLEEP ON THEIR BACKS AND DON'T WANT TO SLEEP ON THEIR STOMACHS, SO MOTHERS HAD TO USE BLANKET ROLLS OR SMALL PILLOWS TO KEEP THEM IN POSITION. IN THE PAST FEW YEARS, IT WAS REALIZED THAT BABIES WHO SLEPT ON THE BACKS HAD A MUCH LOWER INCIDENCE OF SIDS. CURRENT MEDICAL OPINION ADVISES LETTING THE BABIES BE NATURAL AND SLEEP ON THEIR BACKS. IT HAS BEEN ESTIMATED THAT THE SLEEP-ON-STOMACH ADVICE CAUSED OVER 50,000 EXCESSIVE INFANT DEATHS IN EUROPE, THE USA, AND AUSTRALIA. GILBERT R, SALANTI G, HARDEN M, SEE S. INT J EPIDEMIOL. 2005; 34:874-87.

5. SUNLIGHT ON SKIN. FOR OVER 50 YEARS DERMATOLOGISTS PREACHED ABOUT THE HORRORS OF SUNLIGHT EXPOSURE. SUPPOSEDLY, EVEN 45 SECONDS OF LIGHT COULD PERMANENTLY DAMAGE SKIN. THIS SURPRISED ME SINCE I GREW UP IN AN AREA OF MINNESOTA WITH VERY LIGHT SKINNED PEOPLE WHOSE ANCESTORS WERE PRIMARILY FROM SCANDINAVIA. AS KIDS, OUR MOTHERS WOULD SHOO US OUT OF THE HOMES IN SUMMER TO PLAY IN THE SUNLIGHT. WE OFTEN WOULD BE SUNBURNED, BUT AS TEENAGERS, OUR SKIN WAS BEAUTIFUL. FINALLY, EPIDEMIOLOGISTS DISCOVERED THAT PEOPLE WHO RECEIVED MORE SUNLIGHT WERE HEALTHIER AND HAD STRIKINGLY LOWER INCIDENCES OF AUTO-IMMUNE DISEASES AND CANCER. TAVERA-MENDOZA, LUZ E. AND WHITE, JOHN H. "CELL DEFENSES AND THE SUNSHINE VITAMIN." SCIENTIFIC AMERICAN, NOV 2007, 62-72.

• • • • • • • • • • • •

Ancient alchemists had three goals: turning base metals into gold, flying to the moon, and finding the elixir of eternal life. The first two have come to pass: lead can be turned into gold with an atomic accelerator and the moon bears human footprints. At long last, the final goal lies within our grasp as we journey through an exquisite elixir bursting with biochemical discoveries. We reside at a chemical crossroad, where we can reverse the signs of skin aging at a molecular level. So let us now discover how we can turn back the wrinkled hands of time.

For those of us over 35, we are all too aware that time takes a cruel toll on our skin. As we age, our skin becomes thinner and accumulates imperfections. The structural proteins are progressively damaged, causing collagen and elastin to lose resiliency. The skin's water-holding proteins and sugars diminish, the dermis and epidermis thin, the microcirculation becomes disorganized, and the subcutaneous fat cells diminish in number. Decades of exposure to ultraviolet rays, irritants, allergens, and various environmental toxins further intensify these effects. The result is wrinkled, dry, inelastic skin populated by unsightly lesions. See figure on following page.

Oily: 15% of skin lipids
are squalane/squalene

Skin is smooth
and blemish free

Thick acid mantle
Thick skin depth

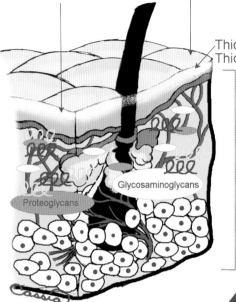

Glycosaminoglycans

Proteoglycans

Young Skin

Dense capillary beds, undamaged collagen
and elastin, ample water-holding proteins,
plus a thick layer of subcutaneous fat,
large follicles, and stem cells converted
into skin cells

ℓℓℓ : collagen

ℓℓℓ : elastin

Aging

Aging Reversal

Skin is wrinkled
and inelastic

Dry: 5% of skin lipids
are squalane/squalene

Thin acid mantle
Thin skin depth

Aged Skin

Fewer capillaries, fewer water-holding proteins,
damaged collagen and elastin, thinned
subcutaneous fat, diminished follicles,
fewer stem cells converted into skin cells,
and less inflammatory GHK

✶✶✶✶✶ : damaged
proteins

c Loren Pickart PhD

12

But have no fear. Why watch your skin's youthful glow fade without a fight? This book reveals practical ways to both prevent the harmful effects of aging and to reverse skin damage once it flares up. Most of the following methods, which are based on my research, led to my discovery of Skin Remodeling Copper Peptides, or SRCPs and the understanding of the Skin Renewal Cycle. So how do these age defying SRCPs do their beauty work? They send a signal in the body that helps trigger the skin's natural mechanism of renewal, restoring the skin to a biologically younger and healthier condition. Later chapters discuss how to reverse the effects of aging on other regions of the body, such as the scalp and hair.

What is Reverse Aging?

"Reverse aging" is a term you've probably seen before, perhaps on a vast array of miracle creams that promise to peel back the years. As you will learn later in this book, most beauty products not only fail to reverse aging, they may actually make you look older than your biological age. So what does "Reverse Aging" actually mean? Researchers will tell you that there are two types of aging: chronological aging and biological aging. To calculate our chronological age, we add up our birthdays in years, months and days that have passed since we were born, according to a steady clock that counts each circling of the earth around the sun as a year. But our bodies follow a different clock that measures biological age. This "biological clock" generally makes us look and feel older over time due to an inherent biological program that pushes us to age.

Now what if we could reverse our biological clock and take a youthful joy ride back to the past? After all, who wants to go "Back to the Future" to glimpse at our older selves? So here's the good news. Under some circumstances our biological clock can travel into "reverse mode" where parts of the body rejuvenate and in a sense they grow younger. Our bodies are lean mean chemical machines. In theory, most chemical reactions that occur with age are reversible. Physicists have claimed that some elementary particles actually go backwards in time. So the irony might be that as we travel back in time, we move into the future of age reversal.

We can take steps right now to slow down our biological clock. Many of these life style choices include regular exercise, a healthy diet, and a low level of stress. Studies show that in the United States, people live longest in small, idyllic towns where little changes other than the colors of each season. Conversely, noisy crowded cities, smoking, psychological stress, and medical conditions such as diabetes can accelerate our biological clock. In World War I, the severe stress of trench warfare could turn a young man's hair grey in two months. The next figure and table give examples of conditions that can alter the rate of biological aging in a hypothetical person.

AGING ACCELERATORS AND AGING REVERSERS

INCREASES AGING	SLOWS AGING
Smoking	Exercise
Fast Food	French and Italian Mediterranean Diets
Too Few Antioxidants	Supplements of: *Vitamin E, Alpha Lipoic Acid, Coenzyme Q-10, Chelated Copper-Ions*
Too Much Alcohol	Moderate Wine Consumption
Overeating	Fasting
Stressful Urban Area	Quiet Rural Area
Watching TV News	Gardening, Fishing, Reading Book
Hormone Shifts with Aging	Bioidentical Hormones
Solitary Life	Active Social Life
Stressful, Unrewarding Job	Vacations
Sun and Wind	Biological Oils, Skin Repair Products

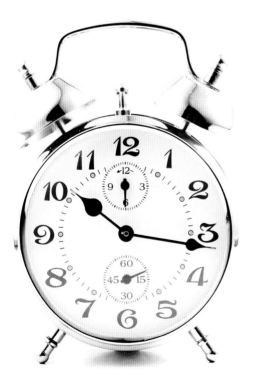

Keep In Mind:

This is not a definitive list of potential accelerators of aging. What affects one person adversely may not have the same effect for all...

Reverse Aging Is Within Your Grasp

We have taken a quantum leap beyond the anti-aging therapies of yesteryear. For decades experts have advised us to take antioxidants and consume a diet high in plants and low in calories. And clinical studies confirmed that many of these anti-aging therapies could indeed promote a healthy life style while reducing the risk of disease. The difference between anti-aging therapies of the past and aging reversal today is that we now have the capacity to turn back the clock on certain organs, returning to a biological state that more closely resembles our younger selves.

I'll bet some of you are thinking, "Reverse aging? Come on, Dr. Pickart, that sounds too good to be true." However, research doesn't lie. Drugs such as Proscar reverse prostate enlargement in men. A variety of anti-lipidemic drugs can reverse the aging elevation of blood lipids that cause vascular atherosclerosis. Alpha lipoic acid, taken as a supplement, can reverse the decline in mitochondrial energy production that occurs with time.

Just as we can reverse aging of internal organs, we can reverse skin aging, our largest external organ, in much the same way. It all starts with solid research on a molecular level. We have conducted numerous studies over the past 30 years. What arose from these studies on human aging and cell biology is truly remarkable. We discovered the biochemical signals for regeneration of skin and organs.

We know that skin is delicate, sensitive, and fragile. At times it must be "babied" back to health. Too often, we treat our skin like wood or leather. And this is where we depart from how traditional dermatology approaches skin aging. Supposed "skin experts" often burn it, poison it, and paint it, calling this the path to beauty (In fact, some skin products have been marketed because they are good for the leather of horse saddles). My bias is for the biological rather than the artificial; for slow, gentle, safe treatments. In my opinion, the only worthy products are those supported by credible, independent articles in scientific journals.

As such, many recommendations in this book are supported by published studies from more than 80 laboratories. Cosmetic products based on my inventions have proven effective in numerous controlled, published studies. They have been shown to reduce fine lines, coarse wrinkles, skin lesions, excess skin, and blotchiness (mottled hyperpigmentation). They improve overall appearance, skin elasticity, firmness, clarity, thickness, damage, skin tightness, and "glow". Recommendations for my new second-generation SRCPs (Skin Remodeling Copper Peptides) are based on more than experiments. We obtain reports from clients, estheticians, and dermatologists at clinics, spas and salons. So dear readers, when you see results, I hope you will drop me a line as well.

Throughout history, science has advanced through a mixture of astute observations and experimental studies. It is generally not realized that the successful theories of Newton, Einstein, and Darwin were built mainly on observation and thought. Like other scientific breakthroughs, the methods to reverse skin aging are accurately captured by a phrase from St. Paul: "We know in part, we prophecy in part..."

ARTIFICIAL & UNNATURAL SKIN TREATMENTS
ALIEN CHEMICALS, JUNK SCIENCE, CINDERELLA BECOMES COUNT DRACULA

Many years ago my mother and I gazed up to the trees to hear the chirping, warbling, whistling symphony of songbirds. These feathered singers filled the rolling hills and forests that surrounded our Minnesota farm with music. But then as years went by, the birds vanished. My mother would reminisce as the thousands of birds dwindled away and their music died. Then in 1962 Rachel Carson published Silent Spring, which examined how chemical pesticides such as DDT endangered plants and animals and how these chemicals killed bird populations. Often as I look at the list of ingredients in cosmetics, I reflect upon the songbirds.

After spending years in the laboratory raising skin cells, I learned just how fussy and finicky these skin cells can be about what they want. You can't just expose skin cells to any new compound. Yet chemical companies keep spewing out alien synthetic molecules for use in cosmetics, disregarding the fact that the body has difficulty handling chemicals that have never existed inside the skin before. These new chemicals are patented and then advertised as the newest "miracle" product to rejuvenate the skin. The true miracle is that companies can promise hype while padding their wallets. These hocus pocus potions are sold not because they make the skin look better and feel healthier, but because the new molecules are patented, and thus draw a premium price.

Many consumers don't realize how difficult it is to improve upon mother nature. In order to move forward on this global journey to rejuvenation, we need to respect the spirit of nature. It took 30 years of intensive research to develop effective anti-cholesterol drugs, and these medications are still far from perfect. Most manufactured chemicals achieve more harm than good. For example, I've seen women lose their eyebrows by the tender age of 40. Chemical dyes and metallic salts in eyebrow pencils rob women of their hair follicles. They then have no choice but to paint the meager brows that remain. In this way cosmetic companies prosper at the expense of women's health, beauty and finances.

Environmental hazards associated with DDT and PCBs took decades to surface. And these alien irritants still plague our environment today. I feel saddened to witness how toxic chemicals reduce the quality of life on earth. For years, I have spent time every summer fishing for salmon off San Juan Island, along with the local orca pod. These friendly and inquisitive whales always come over and check out the water around my boat, Regenerate, to see if I have found a school of big salmon. Today, these lovely creatures are plagued by toxic levels of PCBs that threaten their very survival.

Now what if I told you environmental toxins threaten the lives of adorable rodents scampering through your cabinets searching for cheese? You may say good riddance. Your cat's been asleep at the wheel anyway, purring over catnip. However, we humans are not immune to the toxins that plague rats. In fact humans and rats are similar at the DNA level. Many environmental toxins modify a mother's DNA by adding methyl groups—even though the DNA sequence remains the same. This mutation persists for about four generations in rats. Such changes fuel cancer and other disease, leading to early death in rats up to four generations later. As toxins move up the food chain, human survival may also be at risk.

QUOTABLE QUOTES: *Chuck a handful of weeds in the pot and you've got herbs – Terry Pratchett*

Speaking of survival, toxic chemicals also threaten the life of our skin. Color dyes in cosmetics such as blush, concealers and foundations, endanger the acid mantle. These products are brimming with a witch's brew of metallic salts, chemical dyes, optical diffusers, and alien synthetic chemicals. Now here's a bewitching fact. The average woman will absorb more than four pounds of this cosmetic brew into her body each year. Many of these chemicals lack a long track record of safety. I advise that you use as few color cosmetics as possible especially when they have a list of alien ingredients you can't even pronounce. Save the money you spend on these chemical dyes to treat yourself to fun fashions, jewelry, fragrances and pheromones instead. There are plenty of ways to attract attention without wreaking havoc on your skin.

Plant extracts also pose risks to skin. Just because a plant is natural, that doesn't mean it cannot kill you. Rattlesnakes and poison ivy are oh so natural and yet will sting

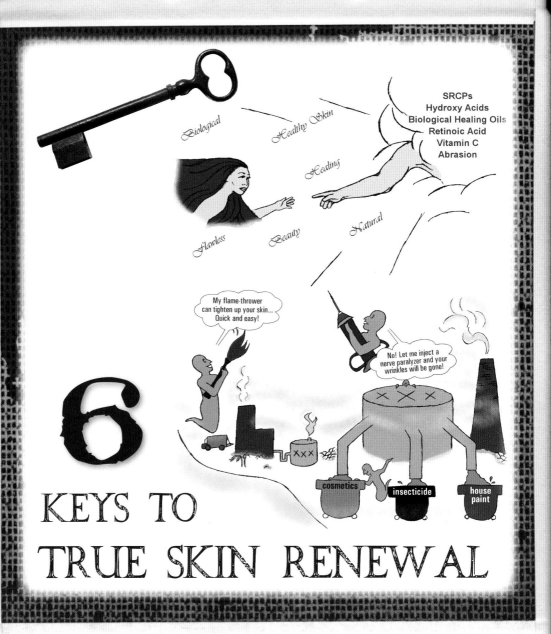

6 KEYS TO TRUE SKIN RENEWAL

FOR MORE INFORMATION SEE CHAPTER 4

- SRCPS
- BIOLOGICAL OILS
- RETINOIC ACID
- VITAMIN C
- ACIDS/ABRASION
- ANTIOXIDANTS

you with their venom. Nature protects poisonous plants by filling them with toxins and carcinogens so that they can ward off hungry animals. Safety tests demonstrate that most exotic flowers, stems, and leaves irritate the skin. Although many carcinogens enter our body from common foods, the gastrointestinal tract and liver detoxify the dangerous ingredients. The skin has no such protective system. Thus, you should only apply plant extracts and oils to your skin that are highly domesticated, and that have been used for at least a thousand years. Only a very few domesticated plants, such as aloe vera, have a positive effect on the skin.

Advertising Agency Science

Cosmetic companies harness the greatest collection of Junk Science on Planet Earth. Marketing tycoons control our cosmetic wallets by appealing to our vanity. These cosmetic hustlers reside in Dante's Ninth Circle (Realm of Compound Fraud) and are, consequently, beyond redemption.

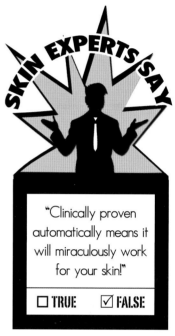

"Clinically proven automatically means it will miraculously work for your skin!"

☐ TRUE ☑ FALSE

The Advertising Agencies of the Cosmetic Cartel announce a new miracle product about every two years. Fifty years ago, the same beauty tycoons wooed our grandmothers with miracle elixirs that would both prevent and remove wrinkles. Do you remember how our grandmothers packed on the good old days-of-old cold creams? They smothered their faces with that pasty white gook. Rather than reducing wrinkles, cold cream increases lines because it prevents skin from rebuilding... so much for those good old "miracles."

The skin-care industry tries to appear scientific. But cosmetic companies peddle phrases that boast little meaning, such as "reduces the appearance of fine wrinkles." Any number of methods can diminish fine lines, none of which are "miraculous." Skin irritations such as bee stings, mild inflammation, excessive sunburn and infections can temporarily reduce wrinkles. I don't know about you but I would opt out on the bee sting wrinkle cure.

"Clinically proven" is another misleading phrase. Materials such as retinol, squalene, and Co-Q10 may have a positive effect on the skin when present at

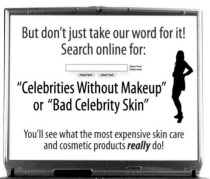

But don't just take our word for it! Search online for:

"Celebrities Without Makeup" or "Bad Celebrity Skin"

You'll see what the most expensive skin care and cosmetic products *really* do!

established concentrations. However, even when a product contains a microscopically small percentage, cosmetic companies often imply that the substance's presence offers the same benefit as a larger proven dose. Greed, not function feeds their bottom line. Manufacturers pump out products for the lowest possible cost with water ("the universal extender") and cheap chemicals.

Okay, I'm reading your mind friends. I'll bet you're asking, "If a product is clinically proven, isn't there a study to back up its claims?" Often in a "study," a clinician applies product to one side of a face with dry skin and nothing to the other side. Under such circumstances, even simple oils would appear to have an effect on dry skin.

We're talking about Junk Science here. These studies are funded by the meisters of junk science. Extremely few of these "clinical studies" ever make it into scientific journal articles. The cosmetic industry has yet to produce even one significant discovery that has enhanced skin health. All key discoveries have been produced by private dermatologists, estheticians, academic scientists, or pharmaceutical companies. Scientists in cosmetic companies have little influence. An executive at a very large cosmetic company once told me many years ago, "We pay our top model 20 times more than we pay our top scientist. You can guess who gets listened to the most."

If you were a fly on the wall at a cosmetic company, you would be shocked to discover how they make their wares. These companies order products from generic manufacturing plants that use standard formulas. Products with similar ingredients are given different fancy names such as Night Active Defense Cream, Anti-Gravity Skincare Lotion (this could save a fortune on airline fares if it worked), Cucumber Regenerative Tightening Gel, Natural Environmental Conditioner (how "natural" can it be with all the alien chemicals?), Stress-Reducing Lymphatic Drainage System, and so on. What links all of these products together is a lack of credible evidence that they do anything positive for the skin.

As one rather honest employee at a cosmetic company put it, "Our Anti-Wrinkle Night Cream is philosophically against wrinkles."

So just say no to junk science, to 99% of the beauty potions that promise hyped hope in a jar. Most beauty products lure you in with baited promises to turn back the clock. What they actually do is take you on a deceptive joy ride. You feel like Cinderella riding a slow coach until midnight. However, you wake up in the sunlight to see the same lines, the same sag. Cinderella's coach becomes a runaway train that speeds skin aging.

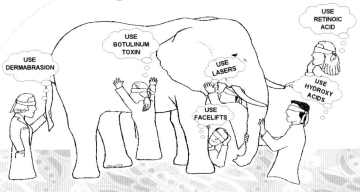

The Skin Experts Tell Us What to Do

Based on the Indian fable: "Six Blind Men and An Elephant"

Cinderella Becomes Count Dracula

Most cosmetics are designed to make you look dewy and youthful at the cosmetic counter so you will buy products. Wetting agents puff up the skin so that wrinkles and lines appear less noticeable. Then dyes and optical diffusers give skin a better color and "glow" and hide blemishes. So let's call these optical diffusers by their real names... optical confusers. And what about the plumpers? When products

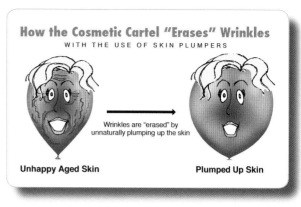

How the Cosmetic Cartel "Erases" Wrinkles
WITH THE USE OF SKIN PLUMPERS

Wrinkles are "erased" by unnaturally plumping up the skin

Unhappy Aged Skin   Plumped Up Skin

plump up the skin, the skin will ultimately deflate as if letting air out of a hot air balloon... and how apropos since much cosmetic hype is a lot of hot air.

All these hocus pocus potions make your skin glow like Cinderella at the store but wilt you into Count Dracula the next morning. This magic trick is not akin to skin health, and sadly, cosmetic voodoo has the opposite effect of slowly degrading the skin. Many skin products sell because they feel smooth and sensuous, but this does not relate to improving skin health. Cosmetic companies created the legend that skin "adapts" to good cosmetics and looks bad when you stop using them. But the truth is that as soon as the temporary effect is gone, you have to reapply the cosmetics. Moisturizers designed to plump up the skin by pushing water into the skin actually damage the skin barrier by breaking the water-resistant barrier of proteins and oils of the upper skin and wetting the proteins. This weakens the skin barrier and lets in more bacteria, viruses and allergens. Also by keeping the upper skin layers wet (hydrated), the lower skin layers fail to receive the proper signals to send new cells (keratinocytes) to the surface. The result is a weakened and leaky skin. The majority of cosmetic skin products are designed for long-term stability, that is, they can be frozen or thawed without change and have a long shelf-life, preferably years. But skin is a living tissue. Thus, effective products are more akin to perishable foods than perfectly stable creams or clear solutions. Remember, expensive wine has debris at the bottom of the bottle, while cheap wine is clear.

Truth…or Fiction?

By now you may wonder how the cosmetic industry rakes in bundles of riches while selling products that harm our skin. Unfortunately, the answer is deception.

Consider for a moment how many products claim to reduce wrinkles. Based on TV advertising and magazine ads, it would be easy to believe that every product on the market achieves a miraculous anti-wrinkle effect. But the cosmetic industry's main objective is to manufacture innocuous products that do not in any way irritate the skin. The cosmetic companies depend on advertising to create the illusion that their products benefit the skin. Many of these products employ unnatural and artificial methods to cause a sort of "skin renewal" or the appearance of skin renewal, but few are based on activating the skin's natural repair systems.

There Is No Quick Fix

While your doctor might advise you that lasers, microwaves, heating lights, and other popular methods of skin care induce collagen formation and, in turn, younger skin, this isn't that simple. At best, they inflict controlled skin damage in the hopes that it mounts a vigorous regenerative response. At worst, they cause temporal collagen tightening that is harmful in the long run. Even if at times these methods yield good results, they can lead to scarring and further damage. Are you willing to take the risk?

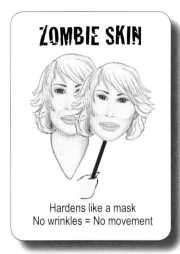

ZOMBIE SKIN

Hardens like a mask
No wrinkles = No movement

Some other methods such as nerve toxins and skin fillers can produce expressionless or a hardened "mask-like" face. Here is my zombie slogan: No wrinkles, no movement!

Surgical procedures, such as face lifts and implants, are followed by a long recovery period as scar lines fade and the skin adjusts to its new position. In addition, no one is sure what the future impact of such procedures will be. Remember, X-ray machines were once used to treat acne, but now, a few decades later, these patients are developing cancer from the treatment. And in the past, silicone injections were applied directly into women's faces and breasts. Later, many of these women found that the silicone slowly slid down inside their skin, necessitating surgical removal to avoid the consequence of disfigurement. The secret to beautiful skin can not be found in any of the multitudes of products or procedures you see in advertisements or hear about at the dermatology office. Rather, true beauty emerges from the idea that slower is better. Our bodies can only rebuild skin at a set pace. This is a slow process during which blemishes and damaged proteins are removed and replaced with more youthful skin. So let us now learn how to slowly and gently turn back mother time as we reverse the signs of skin aging at a cellular level.

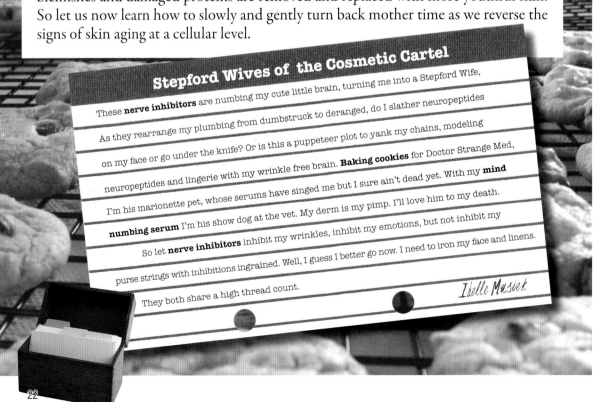

Stepford Wives of the Cosmetic Cartel

These **nerve inhibitors** are numbing my cute little brain, turning me into a Stepford Wife,

As they rearrange my plumbing from dumbstruck to deranged, do I slather neuropeptides

on my face or go under the knife? Or is this a puppeteer plot to yank my chains, modeling

neuropeptides and lingerie with my wrinkle free brain. **Baking cookies** for Doctor Strange Med,

I'm his marionette pet, whose serums have singed me but I sure ain't dead yet. With my **mind**

numbing serum I'm his show dog at the vet. My derm is my pimp. I'll love him to my death.

So let **nerve inhibitors** inhibit my wrinkles, inhibit my emotions, but not inhibit my

purse strings with inhibitions ingrained. Well, I guess I better go now. I need to iron my face and linens.

They both share a high thread count.

Idelle Musiek

Unnatural and Artificial Methods of Skin Renewal

METHOD	MECHANISM OF ACTION	RESULT	SIDE EFFECTS
Laser Resurfacing	CO_2 Lasers evaporate (ablate) the epidermis and cause heat damage to the dermal proteins. Deep damage brutally forces the skin into reparative response.	Immediate tightening of the skin due to skin protein denaturation. Works well for removing local skin lesions. Using lasers for larger areas increases the risk of side effects. If reparative process goes well, skin will look better with fewer wrinkles.	Redness and inflammation in post-treatment period, possibility of scarring, discoloration, hyperpigmentation, prolonged redness and a possibility of damage to skin's stem cells. Use SRCPs to promote healing and reduce side effects.
Deep Chemical Peels (phenol)	Chemical burning of the epidermis, possible damage to the dermis. Deep damage brutally forces the skin into reparative response.	If regenerative response goes well - improvement of wrinkles and skin elasticity, removal of pigmented spots.	Painful procedure (requires anesthesia), risk of heart failure (needs to be performed with heart monitor), redness, swelling and inflammation in post-treatment period, high risk of permanent skin discoloration and scarring, poisoning of skin cells. Permanent sensitivity to the UV-rays – no tanning allowed. Sharp contrast with the untreated skin may create an effect of a "clown mask".
Medium Chemical Peels (20-35% TCA, Jessner Chemical Peel)	Chemical burning of the epidermis with trichloroacetic acid. The skin is damaged and pushed into reparative response.	Reduces the depth of wrinkles, lightens pigmented spots.	Redness, swelling, possibility of hyper-pigmentation. Use SRCPs to promote healing and reduce side effects.
Deep Dermabrasion	Mechanical removal of epidermis. The skin is brutally forced into reparative response.	Improvement of wrinkles due to reparative process.	Infection, scarring, long-lasting redness, inflammation. Use SRCPs to promote healing and reduce side effects.
Fillers (Collagen, Hyaluronic Acids, Synthetic Gels)	The skin is injected with various alien substances – dissolvable such as bovine collagen, fat or hyaluronic acid, or permanent (various synthetic gels and combination of collagen with synthetic gels).	Typical fillers plump the skin, masking wrinkles or age-related degeneration of tissue. In some instances skin develops inflammation and surrounds the filling material with connective tissue, which produces tightening effect. No real rejuvenation is produced.	Can produce local hardening of skin. Some permanent fillers (synthetic gel) can produce disfigurement (bumps, depressions etc) if done incorrectly. Can cause chronic inflammation, speeding up aging.
Nerve Toxins	Block nerve stimulation of the skin's muscles, relaxing mimic wrinkles. Poison skin nerves and disturb their function.	Relaxation of "frown and smile" lines on your face. Does not stimulate skin remodeling.	Can travel in your brain causing long lasting headache or weird taste in your mouth, damage skin nerves, can get to the surrounding muscles producing drooling mouth, drooped eyelids etc. May create unnatural, emotionless expression.
Radiofrequency (RF) Non-ablative Technology (microwave)	Often promoted as safer alternative to lasers (does not evaporate upper layers of skin). In reality they just contract skin collagen like bacon in the microwave.	Immediate contraction of collagen creates an illusion of skin tightening. Does not make the skin younger, but on the contrary, adds more damage to its proteins.	May accelerate skin aging.
Infra-red (IF) Light Technology	Often promoted as safer alternative to lasers (does not evaporate upper layers of skin). Infra-red radiation passes into the dermis, causing heat damage.	Immediate contraction of skin proteins creates an effect of skin tightening. May stimulate mild skin repair in response to heat damage, but does not promote removal of damaged proteins.	May accelerate skin aging causing more damage.
Surgical Facelift	Surgical removal of loose skin, tightening of skin.	Gives good result with extensive sagging or lose skin. The skin doesn't get younger, it just gets tighter.	Painful, costly, with long healing period. Often create unnatural (tightened) look of the skin. Possibility of kelloid formation. Use SRCPs to promote healing and reduce side effects.
Biologically Active Peptides	Claim to stimulate skin renewal and collagen synthesis. But most of them never get below skin surface.	Only a few of them were tested in clinical studies.	Certain growth factors, such as TGF-beta produced scarring in wound healing studies.
Stem Cells (frozen or extracts)	Claim to stimulate skin renewal.	No published studies on the efficiency of any cosmetic treatment with frozen stem cells.	No clinical studies.
"Miracle" Ingredients	New miracle ingredients are launched and heavily promoted every several months. Claims are usually carefully formulated such as "visibly reduces appearance of wrinkles", "makes skin look younger" etc.	In most cases an effect is produced by other ingredients in the formulation that create temporary tightening or swelling of the skin (synthetic polymers, silicones, mild irritants etc). The effect is usually gone the next morning or when you stop using the product. Always ask for independent studies published in scientific journals.	

Although the Skin Renewal Cycle will rejuvenate your skin beautifully over time, some may prefer a quick fix. So in that case, I suggest in jest:

THE SKIN DISINTEGRATION CYCLE

The Cycle of Cosmetic Deception

Do you feel venom and malice when crows feet align your eyes?
So go take that venom inside from a feisty cobra that probes you.
Inject with a toxic disguise.
Hisssss Screech Sigh. Oh My!
Now let Botulism poison reside in your lines so that wrinkles fade away.
As your muscles grow dumb struck and numb from the junk, you say,
"My emotions are withered fray."
Void of expression and poisoned with deception, you yearn for the gentler days.
Bring back crows feet to dance upon your withered brow,
and prance upon on your flaccid face.
Now laugh your numbness away.
So what's another quick fix to shave years from your fears of old age?
Forget your lined eyes and wear shades.
Denial is currently the rage.
Now pucker up and harvest your lips.
Inject collagen for a thick wicked grin.
If that doesn't work, try lasers.
When your lips plump so much, that it's hard to eat lunch, whiten your teeth and wear blazers.

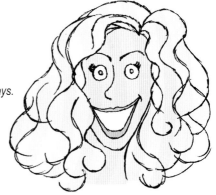

Idelle Musick

LINE REMOVERS FROZEN IN TIME

I'm freezing my face off so it won't grow old.
Like a petrified dummy, I'll put lines on hold.
Gluing my expression while numbing my mind,
I'm an Egyptian mummy all frozen in time

Let muscle numbing toxins
Box me right in
A facial glacier girdle
to tighten my skin.

I guess I look younger when I stand perfectly still
Relaxing my contours so that lines won't reveal
That muscles grow limp when
they can't move a stitch
Under iced shiny armour.
Now ain't that a bitch?

So bring on the line filling
Time chilling thrill
To look instantly younger
Not knowing what's real.

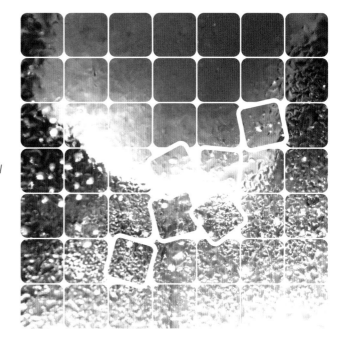

UNDERSTANDING YOUR BEAUTIFUL SKIN
How to Baby the Skin You Were Born With

ARM YOURSELF WITH KNOWLEDGE   Why do you need to know and understand your beautiful skin? Those who have knowledge are well armed. They won't be tricked by a smooth-talking salesperson and they won't buy a product only due to the fact that it is advertized in a glossy magazine or because its package looks pretty or because it is promoted by a glamorous model. They will ask questions such as, "How does it work?" or "Which ingredient is responsible for the promised result?" or even, "Who are you trying to fool?"

Being informed saves money. More important, it saves your skin. There are too many cosmetic products sold in cosmetic stores or over the internet, which can be dangerous to your skin. And the only reason they sell so well is because they often produce quick and impressive results at a cosmetic counter.

However, as you learned in the previous chapter, most products creating lustrous skin immediately after application can ruin your skin in the long run. Many surgical procedures that give such an amazing look to Hollywood stars can leave scars and discoloration when they are performed by a mainstream dermatologist without adequate examination and preparation. They may have side effects and can speed your aging. Even if you are willing to take the risk, do your homework first, because the knowledge will help you to avoid causing irreparable damage to your skin.

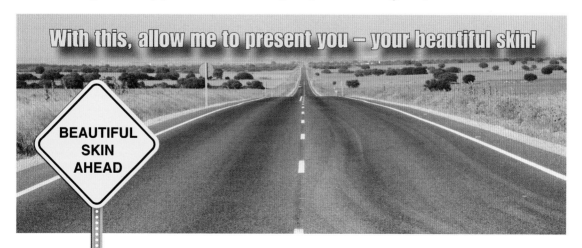

With this, allow me to present you – your beautiful skin!

BEAUTIFUL
SKIN
AHEAD

The First Frontier

The primary goal of our skin is to be a strong barrier that protects our tender inner organs from the harsh environment. It is not just more or less an attractive façade, nor is it just a pretty covering for our bodies. It is the first frontier that keeps away harmful microorganisms and toxins, shields us from UV-rays, and prevents our body from drying out in the dry air as well as from swelling from water like a sponge. It also allows us to experience the world around us through the many senses, as well as to interact with it. And finally, it allows us to interact with each other. It may even make other people fall in love with you.

Surprisingly, this vital barrier is very thin—from 0.03 mm on the eyelids to 1.3 mm on palms and soles. The secret why the skin can serve its protective function so well lies in its highly sophisticated structure, which is one of Nature's wonders. To know this structure is important because every wrinkle, every spot on our face that mar our beauty are not just superficial lesions, but correspond to the inner damage of the skin structure.

Human skin can be divided into three distinctive layers—**epidermis, dermis and subcutaneous fat** (see the picture). Each layer is important, and each contributes to both the skin's appearance and protective function.

THE LAYERS OF OUR SKIN

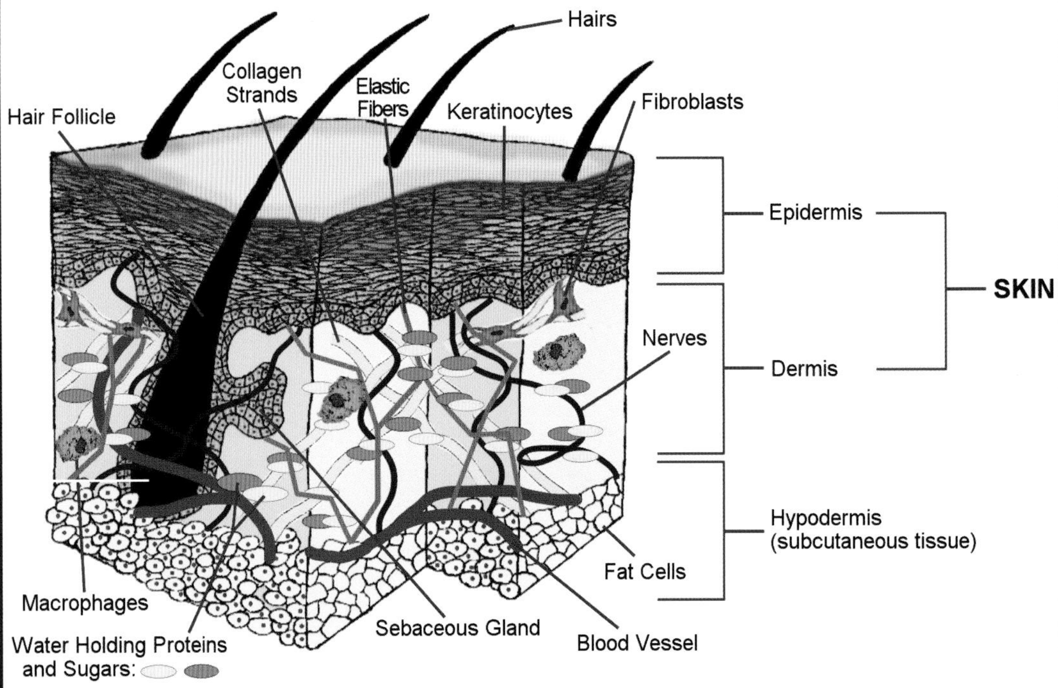

Hairs

Collagen Strands

Elastic Fibers

Keratinocytes

Fibroblasts

Hair Follicle

Epidermis

Nerves

Dermis

SKIN

Hypodermis (subcutaneous tissue)

Fat Cells

Macrophages

Sebaceous Gland

Blood Vessel

Water Holding Proteins and Sugars:

The Epidermis

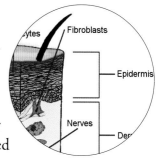

The outermost layer of skin is called the **epidermis**. Its thickness is only 0.03 mm in the eyelids and 1.3 mm in palms and soles. Since this layer has to withstand a significant amount of wear and tear, one may wonder how it manages this without getting worn out within a few months. In order to achieve this, Mother Nature devised a unique multilayered structure that continuously repairs and renovates itself.

The lower layer of the epidermis contains a **basement membrane**—something like a tightly woven mat that provides cell nourishment. The cells that reside on this mat are called the **stem cells**. They possess almost unlimited renovating power.

Approximately once every 24 hours, a stem cell divides producing two new cells: a stem cell and a committed cell.

All stem cells remain attached to the basement membrane, while every committed cell forms tight contacts with their neighbors and start moving up towards the skin's surface, hand in hand in a unified layer. This is a way to self-sacrifice, because as the cells move up, they fill themselves with hard, tough protein called **keratin**. The closer the cell gets to the surface, the tougher and harder it becomes, until it dies out and turns into a flat hard keratinous scale. These scales form a multilayered protective covering on the skin's surface called the **stratum corneum**.

Due to the fact that our skin is covered with a layer of tough, hard and quite dead scales, it can withstand all those insults coming from the hostile environment as well as from our own well-meaning attempts to "improve" it.

The stratum corneum is often compared to a "brick and mortar" wall, because of hard, protein-rich scales (bricks) that are held together with viscous lipids (mortar). Those lipids include ceramides, cholesterol and fatty acids and they contain a high amount of essential polyunsaturated omega 6 fatty acids. This protein-lipid structure is called the **epidermal barrier** and its main function is preventing water loss. If the epidermal barrier is damaged, the skin starts to lose water through excessive evaporation, which may cause it to become dry and wrinkled. A damaged barrier also opens a gate to swarms of invaders including viruses, bacteria and harmful chemicals. Since so many cosmetic products damage the skin barrier it is no surprise that dry skin, skin allergy and irritation are on the rise.

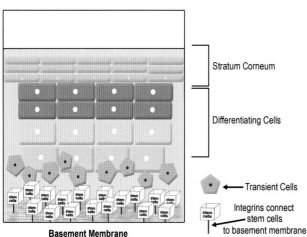

Stratum corneum not only prevents moisture loss from the skin, but it also can attract and bind water molecules thanks to the **Natural Moisturizing Factor (NMF)** — a complex of humectants that include certain amino acids, minerals, hyaluronic acid, urea etc. When NMF is washed away, skin became rough and dull looking.

When keratin scales are worn out or damaged, they are shed from the skin surface so the new scales can take their place.

As we age the rate of skin turnover goes down. At the age of 50 it usually takes 6-7 weeks to renew the epidermis. This leads to thinning out of the epidermis, thickening of the stratum corneum, gradual loss of NMF and epidermal lipids, roughening of the stratum corneum and moisture loss.

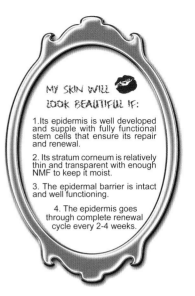

MY SKIN WILL LOOK BEAUTIFUL IF:

1. Its epidermis is well developed and supple with fully functional stem cells that ensure its repair and renewal.

2. Its stratum corneum is relatively thin and transparent with enough NMF to keep it moist.

3. The epidermal barrier is intact and well functioning.

4. The epidermis goes through complete renewal cycle every 2-4 weeks.

The Dermis

Dermis is a layer that cushions the epidermis, supplies it with water and nutrients as well as gives our skin its nice plump appearance and wonderful resilience. Dermis is only slightly thicker than the epidermis—0.03 mm on the eyelids and up to 3 mm on the back.

Dermis is somewhat like a mattress—it has "springs" or fibrous proteins that give it resilience and elasticity (they are called **collagen and elastin**) and the "filling" or water-binding gel made of large sugar based molecules (**proteoglycans and glycosaminoglycans**). The components of the dermis are produced by a special kind of cells—**fibroblasts**. These cells also play a key role in skin repair and renewal. The predominant protein of the dermis is collagen—it constitutes up to 75% of dry weight.

Glycosaminoglycan gel in the dermis attracts and binds water creating skin's turgor, while collagen and elastin give it an ability to stretch and to keep its shape.

Although the dermis does not have layers and does not seem to go through such a distinctive renovation process as the epidermis, it has its own renewal circle as well. All through the life, the dermal fibroblasts break down worn and aged skin proteins and sugars, replacing them with new ones. Unfortunately, this process slows down with aging as well, which leads to the accumulation of damaged, non-functioning proteins, sagging, loose skin, wrinkles and other imperfections.

MY SKIN WILL LOOK BEAUTIFUL IF:

1. Dermal fibroblasts are fully functional and active.

2. Dermis is thick and has enough collagen, elastin and glycosaminoglycans.

3. Dermal proteins have proper structure.

4. Dermis renews itself at a proper rate.

The Subcutaneous Fat

The **subcutaneous fat** insulates the body and gives it an additional cushioning, making it less painful for us to bump into a sharp corner. It also gives our faces and bodies their pleasant and alluring shape. When at old age fat cells start to deplete, it has devastating effect on our appearance. So when all those slimming ads in fashion magazines urge you to declare a war on your fat, just think what would happen if it goes away completely. The truth is that your skin needs subcutaneous fat—it is nothing less but a foundation of your beauty.

Today it is known that fat cells can produce female hormones, estrogens, supporting hormonal health of the skin during pre-menopause. Subcutaneous fat also contains stem cells that produce cytokines and growth factors activating wound healing and fibroblasts function. Therefore skin fat appears to be even more important than just a soft cushion underneath our skin.

Fat Cells

MY SKIN WILL LOOK BEAUTIFUL IF:

1. It has an appropriately developed, not too thick, not too thin, layer of sub-cutaneous fat.

2. Skin fat is evenly distributed without forming bulges, depressions and fat pockets.

Oil Glands and Hair Follicles

The entire surface of our skin is covered with **hair follicles**. But only in certain parts of the body such as on the head, armpits and in the genital area do hair follicles produce full grown terminal hair. The rest of the hair follicles produce so called vellus hair —thin and short. These vellus hair follicles are very important, because they, just like epidermis and subcutaneous fat, contain the stem cells. Hair follicle's stem cells play a key role in skin repair.

Sebaceous Gland

Closely associated with hair follicles are the **oil glands** that produce **sebum** or skin oil. Although for many people sebum is a nuisance, it plays an important protective role, containing antimicrobial and antioxidant substances. It smoothens up the skin surface and reduces water loss.

The oil glands open on the skin's surface as the skin **pores**. The upper part of the skin pore is covered with stratum corneum and therefore contains dead skin scales. Excessive production of skin sebum leads to a pore enlargement. A pore also can get clogged by a mixture of dead skin cells and sebum thus forming a comedone.

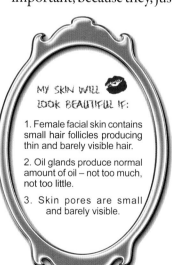

MY SKIN WILL LOOK BEAUTIFUL IF:

1. Female facial skin contains small hair follicles producing thin and barely visible hair.

2. Oil glands produce normal amount of oil – not too much, not too little.

3. Skin pores are small and barely visible.

The activity of oil glands is governed by hormones—male hormones androgens increase it and female hormones estrogens reduce it.

Blood Vessels, Nerves and Muscles

Epidermis does not have **blood vessels**, but the dermis does and so does subcutaneous fat. It is because of dermal blood vessels, that skin has a healthy rosy glow and can blush from emotions. Since the epidermis does not have blood vessels, it depends on dermal blood flow to supply it with water and nutrients. Therefore proper circulation in the dermis is absolutely essential for skin health and beauty. Certain diseases, excessive consumption of alcohol and age related inflammation can damage blood vessels, creating spider veins and red spots.

The skin has a rich **neuronal network**. Most important, **skin nerves** are closely linked with its immune and endocrine system. Skin nerves not only transmit various sensations from the skin surface receptors (touch, temperature etc), not only allow us to express different emotions, but they also can release signal molecules that regulate immune reactions, stress response and hormonal activity. For example, pleasant sensation in our skin is accompanied by production of endorphins—natural anti-stress and pain relieving hormones.

Skin muscles lie beneath the skin. Their unique feature is that they are connected together by a layer of connective tissue—SMAS (superficial aponeurotic system). This muscle layer is attached to the skin, forming something like a mask, and allowing us to create unlimited numbers of facial expressions. When we are young, the skin stretches and restores its shape without difficulties. But as we age, the skin loses elasticity and cannot fully restore its shape after stretching. As a result our emotions eventually leave traces on our skin, creating individual expression and distinct personality.... and yes, wrinkles as well.

PROTECTIVE SYSTEMS OF THE SKIN
Do you like gardening? How about playing outdoor sports? Going to a petting zoo? How often do you shake hands? All those activities shower your skin with myriads of microorganisms—viruses, bacteria, fungi. And yet, most of the time we are just fine, even when we are forgetting to wash our hands.

You also know that sun can be damaging to your skin. But how many hours did you spend in the sun when you were a kid? And yet, your skin remained smooth, rosy and beautiful for many years.

All of this is possible because our skin has such powerful reparative and protective systems. Without them, we would be doomed. We would have to live in sterilized, protective cocoons and could never touch the beach sand or the garden soil. Shaking hands would be suicide.

HOW DOES YOUR SKIN'S PROTECTIVE SYSTEMS WORK?

First of all, our skin is protected by the **acid mantle**—an emulsified mixture of sweat and skin oil. It contains noticeable amount of lactic acid and has acidic pH of about 4.7-5.5 (neutral pH is 7.0 and above it is alkaline). In addition, the acid mantle contains **antimicrobial peptides** that kill bacteria and fungi. The skin oil repels water and softens our skin. It also is rich in antioxidants, protecting skin from UV-radiation. Too frequent washing with harsh alkaline soaps can strip the skin from its acid mantle and increase a chance of drying and bacterial invasion.

Many of you will be shocked to learn that despite this acid mantle and anti-microbial peptides, not mentioning your frequent hand washing habit, our skin is always covered with bacteria. These bacteria have lived on our skin for so long that they formed mutually beneficial relationship with it—they don't harm our skin and they keep away many pathogenic invaders, especially fungi. One of the common side effects of antibiotic overuse is Candida infections—a fungi overgrowth in the absence of residential microorganisms.

The stratum corneum provides a mechanic barrier—if it is damaged, skin can get infected. In the epidermis there are special kinds of cells called **Langerhans cells** that are octopus-like cells that spread their "arms" to the skin surface. If they detect invaders, they launch immune response calling to arms other immune cells.

And finally the dermis contains blood vessels that can supply immune warriors such as lymphocytes, macrophages and mast cells. This system is normally activated when the skin is wounded and blood vessels are damaged. However, immune cells can also respond to irritants and allergens if they manage to get past the first line of defense.

When the acid mantle and the epidermal barrier function well, all alien chemicals and pathogenic bacteria are stopped before entering the skin, and therefore there is no need to launch an inflammatory immune response. But any breach in this defense can bring the fight inside the skin, where it would be accompanied by inflammation.

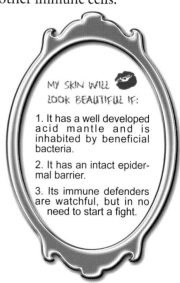

MY SKIN WILL LOOK BEAUTIFUL IF:

1. It has a well developed acid mantle and is inhabited by beneficial bacteria.

2. It has an intact epidermal barrier.

3. Its immune defenders are watchful, but in no need to start a fight.

WHY WE LOOK OLDER?

A number of changes sabotage skin as it ages. These include:

1 Cells replace themselves at a reduced rate, producing a thinner, more fragile skin. Skin replaces itself every three weeks at age 20 but only every nine weeks by age 70.

2 Antioxidants lose their ability to protect the skin by 80 percent between ages 15 and 60.

3 Protein damage accumulates and ages the skin as a result of scars, sun damage, oxidative damage, or the cross-linking of skin proteins by sugars.

4 The skin's oil producing sebaceous glands produce less sebum or "oil." Thus although we develop less acne, our skin grows drier. This drop in oil emerges at around age 25 and dramatically slows down after age 45.

5 Collagen and elastin break down causing our skin to wrinkle and sag. At the same time, water-holding proteins decrease, resulting in drier skin. We begin to form wrinkles and lose elasticity by age 25. The problem intensifies with passing years.

6 Vellus hair follicles diminish in size and efficiency. This colorless fine hair covers most of our body. Since these follicles supply new stem cells for skin repair, a loss of follicles damages the skin.

Can we battle skin damage by trying to avoid it? Not if we want to win the war on aging! While taking steps to protect your skin from ultraviolet light, allergens, detergents, damaging soaps, irritants, acne scars, airborne pollutants, chemical sunscreens, and so on will reduce some types of skin damage, this is only one piece of a much larger puzzle. You can hide from the sun until you evolve into a mole, but this will not keep your skin young.

	Effect of Aging	Effect of Skin Remodeling
SKIN	Thinner, more fragile skin	Thickened skin dermis and epidermis
	Less elastic skin	Rebuilt new collagen and elastin
	Less keratinocyte replacement for skin's surface	Increases keratinocyte flow to surface and replaces damaged old skin components with new material
	Less subcutaneous fat ("baby fat")	Increased subcutaneous fat
	More skin lesions, imperfections, blotchiness	Activate scar removal system that removes lesions and scars
	Poor blood capillary networks	Rebuilt capillary networks for better tissue nutrition
	Flabby, less firm skin	Increased synthesis of water-holding proteins
	Inflammation	Anti-Inflammation
HAIR	Less hair growth	Increased hair growth
	Smaller hair follicle size	Increased follicle size
	Thinner hair shafts	Thicker hair shafts
	More breakage of hair shafts and split ends	Thicker, more break resistant hair shafts

The Holy Grail of Skin Care:

The Skin's Natural Renewal Systems and Protectants

Natural Skin Enhancers
Copper-Peptides
Acids / Abrasion
Retinoic Acid / Retinol
Biological Healing Oils
Antioxidants
Vitamin C

How would you like to baby your skin back into the soft, supple, luscious skin you were born with? What if, like a child, your skin could repair itself from scars and other damage within a week or two? The good news is that young glowing skin is within reach. You can flash skin "soft as a baby's bottom" if you learn methods to remodel and rejuvenate this largest organ in your body. When we remodel our skin, we repair and replace old skin. So it's out with the old and in with the new. The remodeling process, which removes children's scars and damaged skin, also repairs adult wounds. Thus wound healing, like skin remodeling, repairs and rejuvenates skin. When our skin repairs itself, we emerge with a new blemish-free complexion. This restoration works beautifully for children. However, as we age, adult skin remodels far more slowly.

When children get sunburned or injure their skin, they do not develop wrinkles or blemishes. Their skin repairs quickly. So in order to win the war against wrinkles, it makes sense to arm ourselves with the secret to youthful adult skin. Our victory lies in enhancing the skin remodeling process.

When cosmetic products produce skin remodeling, they triumph as the Holy Grail of skin care. According to legend, the Holy Grail possessed the magical power to heal all wounds. And when we remodel skin with potent potions that heal us from wicked wrinkles, the result is pure magic.

Not all Remodeling Techniques are Created Equal

There is a multitude of remodeling options. However most have drawbacks. Retinoic acid slowly remodels skin, but at the price of chronic irritation and redness. It also increases the production of TGF-ß-1, the inflammatory scar-forming protein. Certain peptides, melatonin, and topical vitamin C increase collagen. However, the skin needs to rebuild its elastin (an elastic protein that helps tissues to resume their shape after being stretched, poked or pinched), its water holding molecules (proteoglycans that are proteins with chains of sugar molecules attached and glycosaminoglycans that are chains of sugar molecules, uronic acid, sulfate groups), its microcirculation of blood vessels that carry oxygen and nutrients to the skin, and its nerves that provide feeling and muscle control.

A class of peptides that functions like TGF-ß-1, the inflammatory scar-forming growth factor, increases the skin's extracellular matrix proteins. TGF-ß-1 was extensively tested in the 1990's for wound healing. Unfortunately, these peptides produce unacceptable skin thickening and scarring because they do not adequately remove older pre-existing proteins.

Lasers, chemical peels, and dermabrasion work well only if there is a vigorous post-therapy regenerative response from the damaged skin. There are also many ways in which the cosmetic industry can make you think that your skin got younger and prettier, while in fact very little has been done to it. The sales in the cosmetic business are driven by the first impression, by an emotional rather than rational response. This is why it is so easy to deceive people with a quick, but temporary result. Some cosmetic products contain a minute amount of "remodeling" ingredients, while achieving actual results with synthetic polymers that form a film that visually tightens the skin. Others disrupt an epidermal barrier with detergents and puff skin's protein with water, creating temporal swelling on the surface. Many anti-cellulite creams contain topical irritants that produce dermal swelling, temporarily masking the appearance of "orange peel skin" on the thighs. In this ocean of deception it is very difficult to tell apart truth from fiction.

Fortunately, I will present some safe and effective breakthroughs that can remodel you back to a new youthful you.

THE SKIN'S NATURAL RENEWAL SYSTEMS AND PROTECTANTS
230 Million Years of Skin Renewal

Over the past 230 million years, skin renewal has depended on only a small number of biological compounds. Dinosaurs and reptiles used similar molecules to heal their skin. Although their ancestors diverged during the Triassic Period, the wound healing process has evolved minimally over time. If the skin has not changed much over 230 million years, it certainly does not alter its biochemistry every few years.

However cosmetic companies launch new miracles about every two years that promise to renew skin back to youthful levels. Advertising campaigns use 18 to 25-year old models because these new products really do nothing to rejuvenate the skin.

Have you heard the expression, "tough skinned" women? Today, ladies are tough skinned and strong as they cry out, "I am woman. Hear me roar." Yet they also choose to retain their softness and feminity. What women don't want is a tough complexion. The journey of skin takes us on a dermal time trek from crotchety crocodiles, fossils of our leathery ancestors, to soft skinned vixens, today's powerful goddesses.

Our skin has reemerged with the power and resilience to renew itself, to remove blemishes, scars and tighten the skin. The goal of skin remodeling is to tap the natural activators within us. In the next chapter we will explore natural renewal molecules that I like to call the magic bullets of skin renewal.

SIX MAGIC BULLETS TO BEAUTIFY SKIN
The 3 R's of Skin Renewal - Rebuild, Remodel, and Renew

As we discussed in the previous chapters, there is no quick fix when it comes to skin aging reversal. If we really want to get rid of age-related damage, we have to do it properly. Step by step, your skin has to be remodeled, rebuilt and renewed. These three "Rs" are absolutely essential.

For example, many modern cosmetic products claim stimulation of collagen synthesis. But if we just stimulate synthesis of new collagen without getting rid of the old and worn out proteins, the skin will continue accumulating damage and with it—wrinkles, spots and other imperfection. Other products may contain substances that remove damaged skin layers. But without proper rebuilding, there will be no rejuvenation.

Only by diligently following the path of Mother Nature (by remodeling, rebuilding and renewing the skin at the same time) can we win the battle against aging and restore our beautiful skin to its youthful glory. It may not be as fast as we want it, but trust me—there is no shortcut.

we shall now explore six magic bullets that synergize with explosive beauty as they target skin renewal:

1. Skin Remodeling Copper Peptides (SRCPs) are key players in dermal restoration. SRCPs work by helping your skin to get rid of damaged and worn out proteins, while orchestrating and facilitating skin repair and renewal. They are clinically proven to reduce wrinkles, increase thickness of your skin, lessen sagging and produce other age defying changes.

2. Exfoliating Hydroxy Acids such as alpha hydroxy acids (AHAs) and beta hydroxy acids (BHAs). These molecules increase the effects of Copper Peptides by loosening and exfoliating old and worn out layers of skin, so that newer layers rebuild more quickly and completely. Also physical methods of **Abrasion** and skin needling further breakup scar tissue and damaged skin to aid in remodeling.

3. Biological Healing Oils (such as emu oil) compensate the age related depletion of natural skin oil, moisturizing the skin, helping it to rebuild a protective barrier and speeding up the repair process.

4. Retinoids —members of vitamin A family. Just like AHAs and BHAs, retinoids work with SRCPs to rebuild the skin. Trans-retinoic acid (tretinoin, Retin-A) and cis-retinoic acid (isotretinoin) are prescription drugs that are used to treat acne and sun damaged skin, while retinaldehyde, retinol, and retinyl esters are used in cosmetics for the same purpose.

5. Vitamin C (ascorbic acid)—an antioxidant vitamin that works together with vitamin E to protect your skin from damaging free radicals. When taken internally, it works with copper to help new collagen synthesis. However, to achieve the effect of aging reversal, vitamin C has to be combined with SRCPs to ensure skin remodeling.

6. Protective Antioxidants are natural compounds that scavenge and remove skin damaging free radicals.

SKIN REMODELING COPPER-PEPTIDES (SRCPS) TARGET SKIN REPAIR

How do SRCPs hit their magic mark? These miraculous molecules are the number one remodelers essential for renewing and restoring youthful skin. Exceptionally safe and exceptionally gentle... there is nothing else quite like SRCPs in the human body. However, be aware that not all copper peptides are created equal. Not all are SRCPs. I have analyzed and tested several other types of copper peptides and found little or no activity. And some copper peptides can even be toxic to the skin.

As I described in Chapter 1, SRCPs help trigger the natural mechanism of renewal and restore the skin to a biologically younger and healthier condition. We have learned a great deal about SRCPs in the past three decades. The first SRCP that I discovered and used for remodeling consisted of a small peptide-copper complex, present in human blood, saliva, and urine. This blue colored molecule, technically called GHK-Cu (glycyl-l-histidyl-l-lysine:copper(II)), reversed certain effects of aging in human and animal experiments. In 1984, a few colleagues and I created a company, Procyte (Latin "for the cell"), to develop GHK-Cu into useful products.

It is now used in cosmetics and hair-care and applied after clinical skin renewal procedures such as chemical peels, laser resurfacing, and dermabrasion to improve post-treatment skin recovery.

The GHK-Cu Breakthrough: Call Me Mr. Blue

As we discussed, many copper peptide products are inept at renewal. So as with all cosmetics in the market place, it's consumer beware. However, years ago as I began my skin renewal journey, I discovered the uniqueness of GHK-Cu, this blue jewel of a molecule with the power to heal. Thus I embarked upon my pilot study with 20 women in 1989. I investigated the wound healing and anti-inflammatory actions of GHK-Cu. To my delight, I discovered that skin creams containing GHK-Cu increased the thickness of the dermis and epidermis, enhanced elasticity, reduced wrinkles, and resulted in the removal of imperfections, such as blotchiness and sun damage, while producing a significant increase in subcutaneous fat cells.

I used my discovery to obtain patents on the cosmetic uses of GHK-Cu. Unfortunately, these observations languished for another 10 years. Most skin-care researchers found it difficult to accept that a single biochemical compound could both heal and beautify the skin.

Today the situation has changed significantly. First of all, numerous studies have established GHK-Cu's capacity to heal wounds and remodel the skin in experimental animals. We also learned a great deal about molecular actions of GHK-Cu, such as its ability to stimulate production of skin's proteins, increase level of antioxidants and other natural protectors such as decorin, restore function of damaged skin cells, and to revive skin's stem cells. It turned out that GHK-Cu even possesses anti-tumor properties and is able to block the spreading of certain cancers.

Finally, between 2002 and 2005, leading dermatologists published nine placebo-controlled studies confirming GHK-Cu's ability to reverse human skin aging. At long last, an increasing number of researchers are beginning to see the light at the end of the blue GHK-Cu tunnel. They now realize that one SRCP can both heal broken and damaged skin and improve the quality of intact undamaged dermis. (See references in Chapter 22).

Proof in the Cosmetic Pudding

GHK-Cu clinical studies have demonstrated that SRCPs produce the following cosmetic actions on human skin as shown in the graphic:

Reducing fine lines
Smoothing rough skin
Improving skin firmness
Improving overall appearance
Improving skin clarity and "glow"
Calming irritated and reddened skin
Reducing the depth of deep wrinkles
Tightening loose skin and improving elasticity
Tightening the protective skin barrier proteins
Reducing spots, photodamage, and hyperpigmentation

Second-Generation SRCPs Cosmetic Breakthrough

Just when it appears that we have developed the perfect cosmetic, it gets even better with the advent of a second generation of copper products. Although the original GHK-Cu performed well in many studies, especially around the eyes, its mildness makes it best suited for sensitive skin. GHK is a gentle molecule which feels both soothing and elegant. However for those who seek stronger products, my search continued.

Cosmetic products that contain GHK-Cu include lines such as Super GHK-Copper® by Skin Biology, Visibly Firm® by Neutrogena, and Neova®

Therefore, in 1994, I started Skin Biology to develop improved second-generation SRCPs with enhanced potency, breakdown resistance, and high adherence to the skin. GHK is quickly destroyed by certain types of enzymes that breakdown peptides (carboxypeptidases). So I isolated peptide fragments from soy protein digests that possessed the desired qualities when bound to copper(II). Such peptides do not cause allergic reactions and have a long history of safe use in cosmetic products.

These new products outperform prior SRCPs in their ability to heal wounds. In my tests, the second-generation of SRCPs have proven to be even more effective than the first. In veterinary studies, creams made from the new SRCPs produced rapid and scar-free healing in dogs and horses. At the *University of California, San Francisco*, Howard Maibach and colleagues tested these new copper peptides in four small, placebo-controlled human studies. They found that creams made from the new complexes produced significantly faster healing and reduced redness and inflammation after mild skin injuries.

This truly is a cosmetic breakthrough. Our work on the new SRCPs had an unexpected result. Somewhat accidentally, women and men began using these products for cosmetic purposes and reported improved skin condition and hair vitality. They found that when they combined breakdown-resistant SRCPs with hydroxy acids, the two products removed many types of blemishes and scars from the skin. Soon thereafter, many clients reported that the products reduced wrinkles, tightened skin, and improved their hair growth and its condition.

Recent studies by Lipotec, the *Barcelona Bioinorganic Chemistry Institute*, and the *University of Milan* examined this mixed soy peptides I first used at Skin Biology. They found that such peptides increased the synthesis of collagen-3 by 300% in fibroblasts. At age four, 90% of human skin collagen is collagen-3. This declines to less than 10% at age 50. So if more collagen-3 is produced in the skin, then our adult collagen should become more like the collagen in children (See Chapter 18). And we would all love to travel back to our young lush collagen rich skin.

SRCPs and Wound Healing

As we discussed earlier, baby skin remodels its rosy glow in one to two weeks. However, that rejuvenation halts to a snail's pace over time. So here's where the SRCP magic bullet hits its mark. SRCPs accelerate the pace of wound healing. And the process of remodeling uninjured skin appears similar to how skin remodels itself after wounding. Numerous studies have demonstrated that SRCPs accelerate the healing of wounds and damaged skin and also cause strong remodeling of intact, undamaged skin (For more details see Chapter 18).

Our bodies use the same biochemical mechanisms for closely related purposes. Many dermatological techniques used for skin remodeling (such as lasers, dermabrasion, and chemical peels) actually induce a mild wounding to trigger the remodeling process.

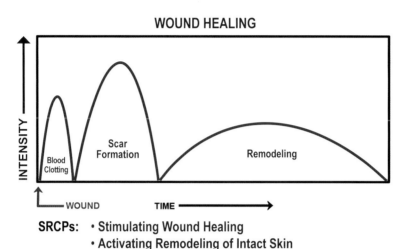

WOUND HEALING

SRCPs: • Stimulating Wound Healing
• Activating Remodeling of Intact Skin
(Not all copper-peptides and copper complexes are SRCPs, some used in cosmetics actually inhibit skin repair)

EXCITINGLY, RESEARCH SHOWS THAT THIS SAME MECHANISM CAN BE USED TO REDUCE WRINKLES

Example of Reversing Skin Aging by Skin Remodeling

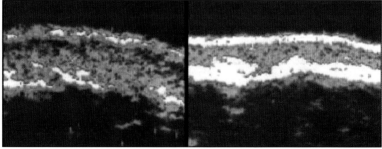

SRCPS REALLY WORK! When we apply SRCP complexes to our skin, these wondrous blue molecules create an environment that helps the skin tighten its barrier and increase its collagen production and elastin density. The above photos show ultrasound scans of a 59 year old woman before (left) and after (right) one month of treatment with SRCPs. The white-yellow colored areas illustrate the ultrasonic reflection in denser areas resulting from closer cellular binding and increased amounts of collagen and elastin. This creates the opposite effect from the usual thinning and loosening of skin produced by aging.

WHAT IS THE SKIN RENEWAL CYCLE? Why is it important? For the first time in the history of skin renewal and wound healing, the Skin Renewal Cycle offers a scientific explanation for how skin repairs itself. This cycle illustrates the biochemistry and cell biology involved with skin repair and remodeling. These mechanisms are based on the many reported actions of the human tripeptides GHK and GHK-Cu from stem cells which lead to the replacement of damaged skin. From these actions, we can predict practical actions that will help skin building. For a more detailed explanation, see Chapter 18.

The Skin Renewal Cycle Suggests That...

1 A certain amount of skin damage is needed to activate the early stages of rebuilding. Such damage could be induced by physical abrasion or by acid peels. Even destructive actions, such as burning (as with lasers or heating devices), can trigger some of these early stages of renewal.

2 A mild oxidation always accompanies tissue damage as neutrophils (white cells that arrive after injury and help kill bacteria) and macrophages (white cells that remove cellular debris and pathogens, and then secrete various growth factors) plus toxic oxygen radicals kill bacteria after wounding. This explains some of the skin healing actions of mild hydrogen peroxide.

3 SRCPs (Skin Remodeling Copper Peptides) are essential for the later stage of repair where inflammation is suppressed and skin remodeling begins. This requires adequate copper in the tissue.

4 Abnormal skin conditions such as psoriasis and the slow removal of skin scars and lesions may result from inadequate amounts of SRCPs in the skin.

5 SRCPs have multiple and powerful anti-inflammatory actions that protect skin.

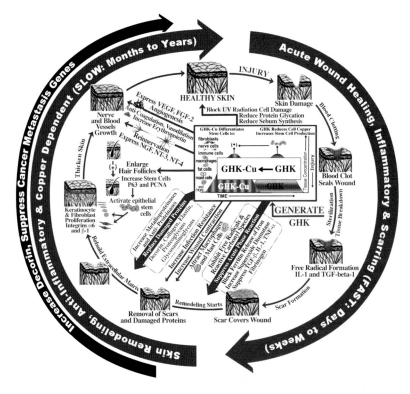

NATURAL ACTIVATORS	CELL BIOLOGY AND BIOCHEMISTRY	COMMENTS
Skin Remodeling Copper Peptides (SRCPs) **Used in human body** **Exist in tissues, plasma and saliva**	1. Anti-inflammatory: Increases Super-oxide Dismutase. Blocks Interleukin-1, TGF-beta-1, and release of oxidizing iron. Detoxifies free radicals and reactive carbonyl species. 2. Activates removal of damaged proteins, scars, and blemishes. 3. Helps synthesis of new collagen, elastin, and water-holding molecules for firmer, more elastic skin. 4. Helps rebuild microcirculation for better skin nutrition and youthful "glow". 5. Helps tighten collagen strands and loose skin. 6. Repairs skin barrier to be more protective against viruses and bacteria, and lose less moisture. 7. May increase production of stem cells for the skin. 8. SRCPs without copper increase stem cell production / SRCPs with copper differentiate stem cells into cells used for rebuilding skin. 9. Increases proliferation of fibroblasts and keratinocytes. 10. Protects keratinocytes from UV radiation. 11. Reduces protein glycation. 12. Activates epithelial (adult) stem cells and slows aging throughout the body by increasing p63. 13. Suppresses cancer metastasis genes.	Very safe.
Exfoliating Hydroxy Acids	Normally on and in skin. Lactic acid and salicylic acid are normally on the skin.	Irritating if used excessively.
Biological Healing Oils	Emu oil is similar to human skin oils. Squalane is normally in the skin.	Emu oil and squalane have proven healing effects.
Retinoic Acid	Normally in skin. Proven to remodel skin but may act by irritation and exfoliation. Role in skin appears to help differentiate stem cells into skin cells.	Often used with SRCPs for better effects with less irritation.
Vitamin C	Normally in skin. Acts with copper(II) to tighten collagen strands.	Best if taken as a supplement (500 mg - 1 g daily)
Protective Antioxidants	Naturally occur in our skin, but are depleted as we age. Prevent free radical damage to skin proteins and skin barrier.	Only natural antioxidants are protective. Avoid artificial and exotic antioxidants.

ALPHA HYDROXY ACIDS (AHAs) FOR SKIN RENEWAL

The origin of Alpha Hydroxy Acids traces back thousands of years to the days of Cleopatra. In the ancient book *Beautification*, Cleopatra described how she applied fruit acids, sour wine, and sour milk (all of which contain AHAs) to renew and beautify the skin. The book was on the Egyptian "best-seller" list for 200 years.

In 1974 doctors Ruey Yu and Eugene Van Scott investigated skin effects of alpha hydroxy acids (AHAs). It took another 15 years of research until these compounds made their way in cosmetic products. Today AHAs are proven to speed up skin turnover, remove skin lesions, and restore the skin's firmness, elasticity, and internal moisture-holding properties.

AHAs work by loosening dead cells in the skin's outer layers, helping to remove old and worn out layers. They also create an acid environment that stimulates skin's own exfoliating enzymes, speeding up natural skin renewal process. As a result, the newer skin rebuilds more quickly and completely. However, a word of caution before you rush to buy AHA products—just as any truly active ingredients they have to be present in certain concentration in order to produce effect. Consumer cosmetic products should contain at least 10% AHA, while estheticians in beauty salons can use 20-30% solutions. Up to 50-70% concentration is sometimes used by dermatologists, however at such concentrations AHAs lose their gentleness and may inflict too much damage to the skin.

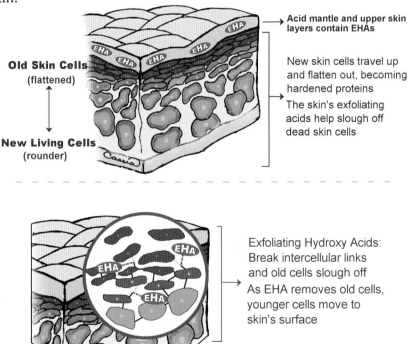

Acid mantle and upper skin layers contain EHAs

Old Skin Cells (flattened)

New skin cells travel up and flatten out, becoming hardened proteins

The skin's exfoliating acids help slough off dead skin cells

New Living Cells (rounder)

Exfoliating Hydroxy Acids: Break intercellular links and old cells slough off

As EHA removes old cells, younger cells move to skin's surface

Since at working concentrations AHAs may be irritating, many cosmetic products contain minute amounts of these acids and consequently offer no benefit to skin.

Similar to AHAs are BHAs (beta-hydroxy acids) such as salicylic acid. Initially they were used by medical doctors in high concentration for removal of pigmented spots and in low concentration for their anti-inflammatory and antibacterial action in acne treatment. In today's cosmetic products BHAs are used for gentle exfoliation of oily and acne prone skin.

AHAs work best on the skin surface, while BHAs can travel into the oil glands, which makes them really helpful for people with oily skin and acne. The most natural AHA is lactic acid which is naturally present in skin. Salicylic acid (BHA) is present in skin and in certain plants (e.g. raspberry, willow tree bark).

AHAs and BHAs work synergistically with SRCPs, removing upper layers of worn and damaged cells, speeding up skin renewal and improving SRCPs intake in the skin.

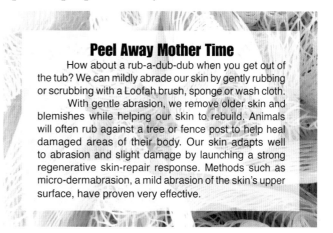

Peel Away Mother Time

How about a rub-a-dub-dub when you get out of the tub? We can mildly abrade our skin by gently rubbing or scrubbing with a Loofah brush, sponge or wash cloth.

With gentle abrasion, we remove older skin and blemishes while helping our skin to rebuild. Animals will often rub against a tree or fence post to help heal damaged areas of their body. Our skin adapts well to abrasion and slight damage by launching a strong regenerative skin-repair response. Methods such as micro-dermabrasion, a mild abrasion of the skin's upper surface, have proven very effective.

BIOLOGICAL HEALING OILS (BHO) BABY YOUR SKIN

Biological Healing Oils contain fats or lipids that exist naturally in the epidermis and on skin's surface. Skin surface is covered with sebum which is a special mixture of neutral fat and fatty acids (60%), waxes (25%), cholesterol and its esters (3%), and squalene (12%). The stratum corneum contains so called epidermal lipids which is a mixture of ceramides (approximately 25%), fatty acids (approximately 26%), cholesterol and its esters (approximately 22%).

Today we know that skin needs good oils to stay moist and supple, but for quite a long time there was a discussion on whether the skin needs oil or just more water to be soft, plump and smooth. The first scientist who proposed using oils to heal skin was Albert Kligman in the 1960s. He also coined the term "corneotherapy"—a method to correct skin's disorders by treating its stratum corneum.

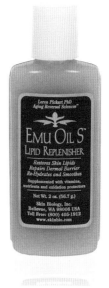

It has been established that oils that are similar to skin's oils help beautify our skin by protecting its barrier. They waterproof the skin. The oils also help repair the skin barrier by acting as glue that binds the outer proteins together, keeping them relatively dry, hard and protective. If you were to visualize these proteins as bricks in a wall, the BHOs would act as concrete holding them together. BHOs also moisturize the skin by blocking excessive water loss. Unfortunately, these naturally occurring oils lessen as we age.

We can apply these oils to our skin to modify the level of SRCP absorption. Depending on how we layer these oils with SRCPs, BHOs will either increase or reduce SRCP effects. For example if we apply BHOs over an SRCP product (such as Skin Biology's CP Serum), the oil then pushes more SRCPs into the skin or hair follicle, thus increasing its effects. However to reduce SRCP effects on irritated skin, we can apply BHOs before SRCPs. This reduces the uptake of SRCPs and thereby produces a milder reaction. Emu oil (such as Skin Biology's Emu Oil-S) contains a molecular structure similar to natural skin oils. Australian native peoples have used this amazing oil to moisturize and heal for thousands of years.

A word of warning: since natural oils may feel a bit greasy on your skin and not so easily incorporated into cosmetic formulations, many modern cosmetic products that claim to soften and moisturize your skin contain no natural oils whatsoever or very little of them. Instead they achieve the illusion of nourishment and moisturizing by adding artificial oil-like substances such as silicones and fatty acid esters. These ingredients are very different from natural skin lipids and may damage your barrier structures. They also can be comedogenic—that is they can clog the pores creating blackheads.

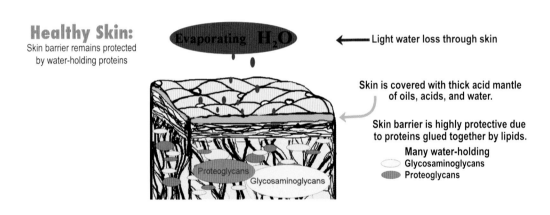

Healthy Skin:
Skin barrier remains protected by water-holding proteins

Evaporating H₂O

← Light water loss through skin

Skin is covered with thick acid mantle of oils, acids, and water.

Skin barrier is highly protective due to proteins glued together by lipids.

Many water-holding
◯ Glycosaminoglycans
▨ Proteoglycans

Proteoglycans

Glycosaminoglycans

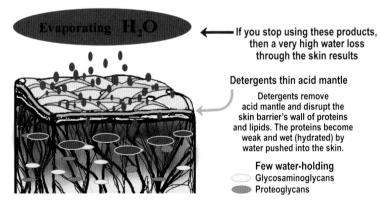

False Cosmetic Moisturizers:
Product quickly makes skin attractive at cosmetic sales counter, but slowly damages the skin inhibiting normal skin renewal and producing a daily moisturizer need somewhat like a drug addition

Evaporating H₂O

← If you stop using these products, then a very high water loss through the skin results

Detergents thin acid mantle

Detergents remove acid mantle and disrupt the skin barrier's wall of proteins and lipids. The proteins become weak and wet (hydrated) by water pushed into the skin.

Few water-holding
◯ Glycosaminoglycans
▨ Proteoglycans

The wetness of the upper skin layers stops the signals to the lower layers to produce more skin cells to move to the surface and reduces the production of water holding molecules in the skin.

RETINOIDS—MAGNIFY THE POWER OF SRCPS

Even before its official discovery vitamin A was used for centuries for its skin benefits. In Ancient Greece doctors used raw liver (rich in vitamin A) to cure certain skin diseases. During World War I, it was observed that a deficiency of vitamin A leads to extreme skin dryness (xerosis) and thickening of the stratum corneum (hyperkeratosis). Initially, cod liver oil was used in cosmetics as a source of vitamin A, however, not everybody appreciated its strong fishy smell.

In 1830s, H.W.F. Wackenroder isolated beta-carotene—a plant precursor of vitamin A. In 1930s, a highly active, but still impure form of vitamin A was isolated. In 1942, J.G. Baxter isolated pure vitamin A, and in 1947 A. van Dorp succeeded in synthesis of vitamin A. In 1968 pharmaceutical company Hoffmann-La-Roche began research on retinoids—chemical compounds that have structures and effects similar to vitamin A. In 1979, they were able to develop the first anti-acne products with retinoids.

Today's retinoid family includes vitamin A (retinol), retinoic acid, retinaldehyde, retinyl esters, as well as their synthetic derivatives. Today it is known that vitamin A is a natural gene regulator that is closely involved in cell growth and differentiation as well as in many other biological processes. In the skin, retinoids increase skin thickness, speed up cell turnover, stimulate glycosaminoglycans synthesis, and reduce oiliness and inflammation.

Trans-Retinoic acid (tretinoin) was first developed to treat acne. In 1984, dermatologist Albert Kligman proposed it for treatment of sun damaged skin. In 1986 Kligman and colleagues conducted the first clinical placebo controlled study in which they applied 0.05% tretinoin on the photoaged skin of volunteers for 3–12 months. Tretinoin improved photoaged skin, increasing dermal collagen formation (type I and III) and blood vessels in the dermis. Since then numerous clinical studies confirmed the efficiency of retinoic acid in treatment of photoaged skin. The effective concentration ranged from 0.025 to 0.1% with stronger solutions producing more skin irritation.

In 1993 Kligman et al conducted a clinical study of the tretinoin effect on chronologically aged skin. Although they observed some improvement in skin elasticity, complexion and thickness, the effect was less prominent than with photoaged skin.

Cis-retinoic acid (isotretinoin) has more prominent effect on acne compared to tretinoin, reducing skin oiliness and inflammation.

Cosmetic products may contain retinol, retinaldehyde or retinyl esters.

Retinol is somewhat less effective than retinoic acid (approximately 20 times less effective) and it requires conversion into retinoic acid in the skin in order to combat age related changes. However, if taken in high enough concentration (about 1%) retinol can also improve aging skin by increasing dermal thickness and new protein synthesis. Unfortunately, its skin irritating potential also increases with concentration. It also can give the product yellowish color that many consumers find unpleasant. This is why a majority of cosmetic products on the market contain very low concentrations of retinol, and therefore, are pretty useless.

More stable retinol esters such as retinyl acetate, retinyl propionate, and retinyl palmitate are often used in cosmetic products instead of retinol, however their efficiency hasn't been satisfactorily proven and in some studies they produced no effect.

Retinyl aldehyde has demonstrated efficiency in clinical studies and produced low irritation. It increases dermal thickness and collagen synthesis. Just as retinol it needs to be converted into retinoic acid in the skin in order to produce effect. It also has to be present in certain concentration (no less than 0.05%).

Many people use SRCPs and retinoic acid products together and report better results with less irritation. Retinoic acid can function in a similar manner to AHAs by helping SRCPs speed up skin renewal.

So why use retinol cream? For older women with dry skin, retinol adds skin oil which moisturizes the skin. I have found that products require only a low level of retinol to increase skin oils and work beautifully for women over 40. However, retinol can increase acne for those between 18 and 30 years of age. Paradoxically, clients between ages 25 and 40 often report that these creams help with chronic cystic acne. When using retinol cream, it is best to start slowly and work up to a higher dose.

Many women have asked me to clarify how the effects of retinoic acid and retinol differ. Cosmetic companies often foster confusion regarding these two products in order to promote their merchandise.

Retinoic acid, contained in various commercial products, helps remodel skin. Retinoic acid requires a prescription. Retinol, a weaker form of vitamin A sold by cosmetic companies, does not require a prescription. Although retinol offers many benefits, it does not remodel skin.

The following chart highlights the differences between the two:

	Retinoic Acid	Retinol
Chemical Name	Retinoic Acid	Retinyl alcohol
Common Name	Vitamin A acid	Vitamin A
Prescription Drugs	Retin-A	Not a drug
Effect on skin oil	Reduces skin oil	Increases skin oil
Effect on wrinkles	Strong wrinkle reduction	Mild effect on reduction of fine lines

VITAMIN C (ASCORBIC ACID) TIGHTENS YOUR SKIN

Vitamin C was discovered in 1932 as a factor in lemon juice that prevents scurvy—a potentially fatal disease manifesting with bleeding gums, loose teeth, hemorrhages and connective tissue fragility. Today it is known that scurvy is not the first, but the last and final symptom of vitamin C deficiency, since many more less noticeable but important deleterious changes occur in earlier stages of vitamin C deficiency. Many of them involve skin.

Our tissue cells use vitamin C and a copper enzyme called lysyl oxidase to cross-link and tighten collagen. It also serves as a powerful antioxidant that together with vitamin E scavengers and detoxifies harmful free radicals. In order to reap skin tightening benefits of vitamin C, your system requires adequate amounts of both copper(II) and vitamin C. Since ascorbic acid is very unstable in cosmetic formulations and cannot penetrate the skin well enough, it is best to put the copper products on the skin and to raise your vitamin C levels with oral supplements. You can take 500 mg to 1 gram daily since increased vitamin C is easily tolerated.

We need about 20 milligrams of vitamin C daily to stay alive. However, based on natural diets of other primates, studies suggest that 5 grams per day would be a better dosage for humans. Our ancestors evolved on a diet very high in vitamin C. The diet of primates such as gorillas, chimpanzees and monkeys contains high levels of vitamin C that would be comparable to ingesting 5 grams daily in humans.

Protective Antioxidants

In 1937, after several years of research, Olcott and Emerson established that vitamin E (alpha, beta and gamma tocopherols and some relative substances) are effective antioxidants in fatty liquids such as milk. But although it was known that the human body contains many fatty substances too, for a long time many researchers would not accept the idea that the same oxidative reactions that occur in milk and fatty solutions may be important in biological systems too. It took decades of research before the physiological role of natural antioxidants was established and their role as protectors against aging was proved. Now it is known that the human body and in particular the skin have an elaborate antioxidant system that includes vitamins such as vitamins A, E and C, low-weight molecular substances such as co-enzyme Q10 and alpha-lipoic acid, and antioxidant enzymes such as superoxide dismutase (SOD), catalase and glutathione peroxidase. Also our body makes use of many antioxidants present in food such as lycopene, lutein, flavonoids and others. Taken together all those antioxidants control free radicals in our body, protecting it from aging. Unfortunately, antioxidant defense weakens as we age. SRCPs were proven to increase the level of natural antioxidants in our skin, prolonging skin youth.

Antioxidants are often added to cosmetics to protect skin against free radicals caused by too much UV radiation and environmental pollutants (but stick to ingredients normally used in the body which include the vitamin E family, tocotrienols, lutein, lycopene, CoQ-10 and alpha-lipoic acid). Our body has learned what it needs over several hundred million years. Exotic antioxidants that the body chose not to use in the past, can harm us today. So just say no to artificial compounds advertised as more potent than the body's natural antioxidants. Remember also that many heavily advertised natural antioxidants are present in fruits and vegetables and work better when taken internally. For example, instead of buying an expensive cream with grape seed extract containing a potent antioxidant resveratrol, you can just as well indulge yourself with a glass of red wine.

While free radicals can damage skin and other tissues, we need a certain amount of them for many key reactions within the body. For example, immune cells require free radicals in order to kill bacteria, viruses, and cancer cells. Mitochondria use free radicals to produce energy. Artificial antioxidants are so powerful that they cause tissue damage by shutting down key reactions. Some have even produced cancer.

It's all about maintaining a delicate balance. Too much or too little of a good thing can create ill health. Artificial antioxidants cause havoc. Only when we nourish the body with what it needs, can we renew and revitalize our largest organ... the skin.

IN CONCLUSION The six magic bullets of skin rejuvenation—SRCPs, exfoliating hydroxy acids, healing bio-oils, retinoids, vitamin C and protective antioxidants—have earned their badges of honor. It took decades of research in many scientific laboratories before their molecular actions were investigated, their skin effects proven and their safety well established. From these examples you can see what it really takes to develop a true scientifically based cosmetic ingredient—the one that truly works without hurting the skin. Now I hope it will make you a bit suspicious when you are offered a new miracle anti-aging cure that no one has heard about just a month or so ago.

However, out of these six powerful tools of skin rejuvenation, only SRCPs provide the most complete spectrum of skin age reversal activity such as remodeling, rebuilding and renewal (three "Rs" of skin rejuvenation), while all of the remaining five bullets work as the trusty side-kicks intensifying and enhancing SRCPs action. In the following chapters, you will learn how to use synergistic action of SRCPs and other scientifically proven age reversal agents to solve various skin problems.

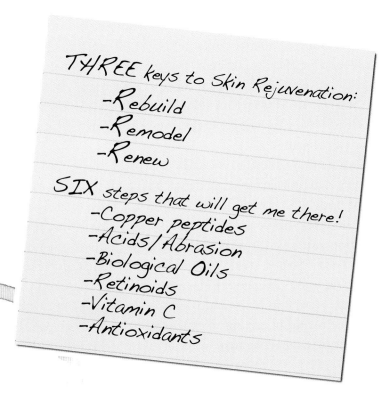

THREE keys to Skin Rejuvenation:
- Rebuild
- Remodel
- Renew

SIX steps that will get me there!
- Copper peptides
- Acids/Abrasion
- Biological Oils
- Retinoids
- Vitamin C
- Antioxidants

5

1ST AND 2ND GENERATION SRCPs
MY TRUE SCIENCE APPROACH TO SKIN PRODUCTS

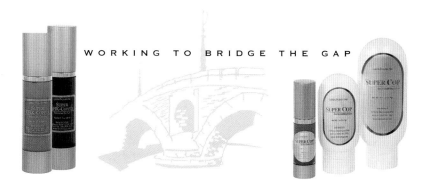

WORKING TO BRIDGE THE GAP

The Cosmetic Cartel has only one thing to sell...the fountain of deception, not youth. You become their marionettes... the Stepford Wives that nurture their bank accounts. The sad truth is that the cosmetic industry does not hold your best interests at heart. The good news is that SRCPs really do work without taking you to the poor house. SRCPs provide the key to younger-looking, healthier skin. In this chapter, you will discover the most effective methods for natural skin renewal and the recommended Skin Biology products. So let us now embark upon a journey to turn back the wrinkled hands of time.

One note: I give only general recommendations for the use of Skin Biology products because, like everything in life, you have to experiment to discover what works best for your individual skin. Each of us is unique. You could have an identical twin with the same DNA and yet react differently to equivalent products because of variations in diet, stress level, the condition of your skin, and previous exposure to dermal allergens. I advise that you keep experimenting until you find the combination of products that works best for you.

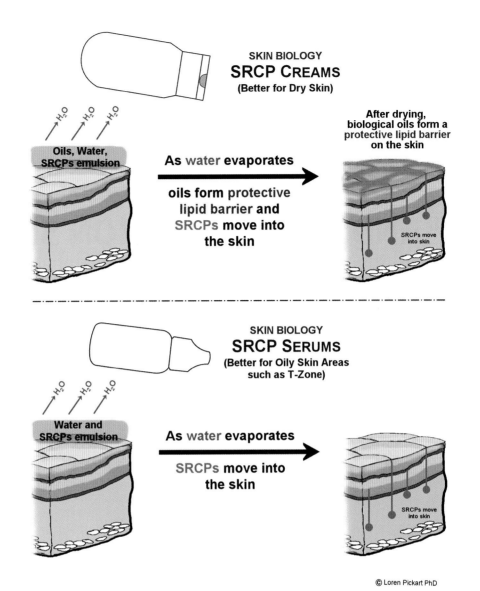

© Loren Pickart PhD

Damaged Skin Must Be Babied Back To Health

As your skin barrier repairs and rebuilds, it will strengthen and grow to shield itself. As a result, fewer materials, including SRCPs, will be able to penetrate it. The area surrounding our eyes is especially thin and delicate. You need to baby it back to health. Many women have reeked havoc on this fragile skin after years of applying harsh color cosmetics and make-up removers. So as you start with milder SRCPs, your skin will have an opportunity to adjust. You can then transition to stronger products if this sensitive area needs a more intensive rebuilding. So remember the Golden Rule and baby your skin.

The Golden Rule of SRCPs:

Start lightly and increase gradually

The following chart describes the relative strength of SRCPs in Skin Biology products and their various uses. Many people start with CP Serum, and then as their skin becomes stronger, progress on to Super CP Serum, and finally on to Super Cop.

Relative Strength of Skin Biology Products

STRENGTH	PRODUCTS	INTENDED USE
Very Mild	CP Night Eyes Premier	For under eye area use
Very Mild	Super GHK-Copper Cream / Super GHK-Copper Serum	Sensitive skin & under eye area
Mild	CP Night Eyes Regular	For under eye area use
Mild	Protect & Restore Day Cover	For face - fortified with UV reflector & anti-oxidants
Moderate	Protect & Restore Body Lotion	For body skin
Moderate	CP Serum	Good on oily skin
Moderate	Copper Sun—Tanning & Firming Lotion	For body skin - fortified with UV reflector
Moderate	Protect & Restore BND Cream	Breasts, Nipples, Decolletage (also good on the neck area)
Moderate	Protect & Restore Classic	Facial cream for under age 35
Moderate	Protect & Restore with Retinol	Facial cream for dry skin over 35
Moderate	Les Pieds Doux	Foot cream for skin repair
Moderate	BioHeal	Good on sensitive or irritated skin
Strong	Skin Signals Cream	Strong cream for skin tightening
Strong	Skin Signals Solution	Strong serum for skin tightening
Strong	Super CP Serum	Strong remodeling system
Strong	TriReduction Cream with Retinol	Better on dry skin
Very Strong	Super Cop Cream	Strong remodeling system
Very Strong	Super Cop Cream 2X - Extra Strength	Strongest remodeling system
Strong	Folligen Cream	Good for hairline and eyebrows
Strong	Folligen Lotion	Good for irritated scalp
Strong	Folligen Spray	Use on non-irritated scalp
Strong	Hair Signals Therapy Cream	Use on non-irritated scalp
Strong	Hair Signals Therapy Solution	Use on non-irritated scalp

NOTE: It is best to start with a milder product and slowly progress to a stronger product if needed.

The Signs of SRCPs at Work

As your skin adjusts to the SRCPs (particularly when combined with hydroxy acids), you may experience a brief two week period of skin loosening before it tightens. Damaged skin can behave somewhat like hard scar tissue since its toughness holds everything in place. As SRCPs help remove damage, your skin may briefly slacken. Skin fibroblasts then begin the rebuilding process by first producing collagen and elastin, after which they slowly pull the protein strands together and tighten the skin.

You might also notice the exposure of deeply buried scar tissue. Normal scar tissue often covers old wounds and blemishes, thereby concealing them. As an example, cystic acne can form hard blemishes under the skin, which are later covered by superficial skin cells. As the skin exfoliates, these old lesions can grow visible. When you apply SRCPs and hydroxy acids over the problem areas, this helps to remove the buried damage.

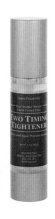

If your skin becomes loose, or puffy, I advise that you temporarily take a rest from SCRPs to ease your skin through its transition. During this time, I recommend you use only biological oils such as Emu Oil-S or Squalane. You might also apply a light DMAE (dimethylaminoethanol) serum. Skin Biology recently introduced **Two Timing Tightener** to help tighten skin. This product combines DMAE and algae polysaccharides that act to temporarily tighten, firm, and tone skin. After your complexion has calmed, you can slowly return to the use of the SRCPs. Many people tell me that when they rest from SRCPs in this manner, they find it an effective way to transition back into skin renewal.

Tips for Natural Skin Renewal
The following products and methods will help optimize your results.

If you have sensitive skin and want to decrease the activity of SRCPs, start by applying a biological healing oil (BHO). When you apply a BHO, such as Emu Oil-S (supplemented with the skin's natural antioxidants) or Squalane, before SRCPs, you reduce the effect. These healing oils penetrate the skin and form an oil barrier that slows the SRCP uptake into your skin. Women often use this method for irritated or sensitive skin, such as after laser burns or deep peels.

After you have used Skin Biology products for a while, you may want to step up the remodeling. To increase the activity of SRCPs, follow the product application with a biological healing oil. When you apply a BHO such as Emu Oil-S or Squalane after SRCPs, you increase the effect because the oil pushes more SRCPs into the skin. Women often use this method around the delicate eye area. These biological oils not only enhance SRCPs, they make great eye make up removers. Emu Oil-S and Squalane are much kinder to your skin than the make-up removers manufactured by cosmetic companies.

In addition to biological oils, we use exfoliating hydroxy acids (EHAs) to increase remodeling. EHAs can help rebuild and loosen older skin and scar tissue. Hydroxy acids exist naturally on the skin's surface and work synergistically with SRCPs. Lactic and salicylic acids are the most natural exfoliators. Normally we use one product in the morning and the other at night. Stronger hydroxy acids work faster, but overuse can irritate the skin. Some people use SRCPs and hydroxy acids on alternate days. Skin Biology offers exfoliating serums and creams. Exfol Serum contains salicylic acid plus antioxidants that work best for oily skin areas. Exfol Cream also contains salicylic acid plus protective lipids, such as squalane and octyl-palmitate, and works best for dry skin.

Now how about a fun way to remodel our skin? When we scrub our skin with a loofah, we can have fun fun fun in the tub while washing away our woes. Not only that, abrasion can help remove lesions. Various types of abrasion inflict mild damage that stimulate removal of scars and older skin. Abrasive methods, whether applied at the doctor's office or at home, remove damaged skin. Dermatologists offer dermabrasion, which helps remove elevated and flat scars and lesions; and needling (subcision), which removes and loosens scar tissue in depressed scars and pitted acne. At-home abrasion methods include microdermabrasion units, files, pumice stones and good old loofahs and brushes.

My True Science Approach to Skin Products:

1. All of our products are designed to help improve skin health. However, many cosmetics slowly degrade skin. Our approach emphasizes natural activators of renewal and remodeling: SRCPs, hydroxy acids, biological oils that occur naturally in the skin, abrasion, needling, retinoic acid, and vitamin C (this is best taken internally). It takes a rather narrow list of natural products to trigger the skin's renewal responses.

2. Our basic SRCP products have been tested by independent laboratories. They are classified as non-irritants, non-allergens, non-carcinogenic, and non-poisonous. Skin Biology water/oil creams contain no detergents or quasi-detergents (synthetic molecules not called "detergents" but which act like detergents). Thus, our products are more fragile than traditional cosmetics and may break up into a water and oil phase. They do not open and damage the dermal barrier. There are many published studies on the positive actions of SRCPs. Four of these published studies found they increase the skin barrier strength.

3. The selection of ingredients and formulations that improve skin health are based on published studies in reputable science journals by ourselves and many others.

4. We select ingredients from the FDA's GRAS (Generally Recognized As Safe) list of food ingredients and cosmetic ingredients with a long history of product safety. The FDA states that safety information exists on only 11 percent of the 10,500 cosmetic ingredients cataloged by the FDA.

5. FDA requirements call for the use of formulations that resist bacterial growth. We use preservatives with long records of safety in cosmetic products.

6. We avoid the following:

6.1 Formulations and moisturizers designed to push water into the skin, wet the outer proteins, and "puff up" the skin to make wrinkles and creases less obvious. The problem occurs because such products loosen and wet the skin: they damage the skin barrier and permit easier access by bacteria, viruses, and allergens. The chronic wetness also inhibits the signals that tell the skin to send more keratinocytes to the surface.

6.2 "New chemical entities", that is, synthetic molecules that the human body has never been exposed to in our history. It requires decades to determine the safety of such molecules, such as in the case of PCBs and DDT.

6.3 Most plant extracts are alien to human skin and, in time, may cause rashes and allergic reactions. However a few plants, such as Aloe Vera, can benefit the skin. Aloe Vera soothes while posing no allergic response.

6.4 Types of collagen-inducing peptides that act like Transforming Factor Beta-1, a protein that causes normal cells to grow like cancer cells. Concerns have been raised that such molecules may speed the spread of cancers and cause kidney failure.

6.5 Hyaluronic acid (hyaluronan), and other water attractors, because it wets the outer skin proteins. This damages the skin barrier and allows bacteria and viruses to pass into the skin. It also plays a critical role in the spread of cancer cells.

6.6 Ingredients used as nerve inhibitors, such as neuropeptides, which claim to relax muscles and thus reduce wrinkles. These inhibitors may migrate into the brain and possibly turn you into a clueless bimbo. Long term cosmetic use of such ingredients may inhibit nerve function in the brain (possibly lowering your intelligence or emotional responses) and other areas of the body.

6.7 Dyes and coloring agents.

6.8 Chemical sunscreen oils (See Chapter 16).

THE ADVENT OF OTHER PEPTIDES?

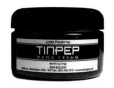

The outer layers of the skin are made of a protein called keratin. High levels of synthetic detergents found in many soaps (or other factors such as dry skin conditions) can strip away the skin mantle and loosen protective keratin proteins.

We have found that tin-peptides (a complex of ionic tin (2+) and hydrolyzed soy proteins) increase the production of keratinocytes that form the outer skin covering resulting in a softer, smoother surface.

Tin-peptides may lack the wound healing properties of copper peptides, but they should not be overlooked. They actually seem to be more effective at producing keratin, the major protein in nails and hair. Clients report that tin-peptides make their hands appear younger, smoother, and repair damage caused by harsh detergents and sun exposure. For more information see Chapter 14.

Our TINPEP Hand Cream is a unique combination of tin-peptides, anti-oxidants and biological moisturizers designed to remodel and smooth dry skin. Initial trials of this cream have produced very positive responses from users.

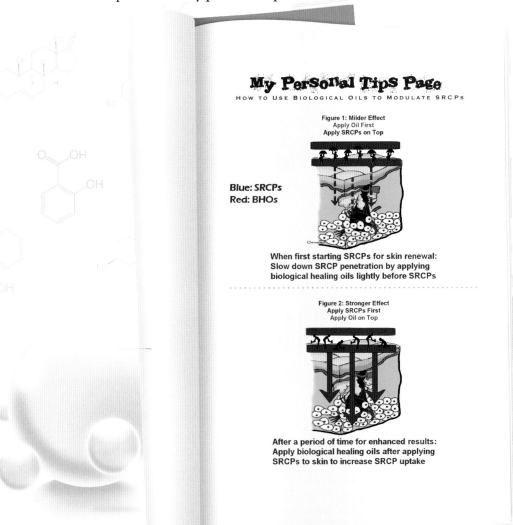

My Personal Tips Page

HOW TO USE BIOLOGICAL OILS TO MODULATE SRCPS

Figure 1: Milder Effect
Apply Oil First
Apply SRCPs on Top

Blue: SRCPs
Red: BHOs

When first starting SRCPs for skin renewal:
Slow down SRCP penetration by applying
biological healing oils lightly before SRCPs

Figure 2: Stronger Effect
Apply SRCPs First
Apply Oil on Top

After a period of time for enhanced results:
Apply biological healing oils after applying
SRCPs to skin to increase SRCP uptake

6

SAY GOODBYE TO FINE LINES & WRINKLES
Activating Your Body's Wrinkle Removal System

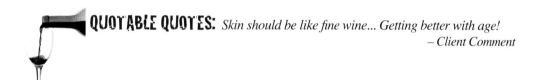

QUOTABLE QUOTES: *Skin should be like fine wine... Getting better with age!*
– Client Comment

What do you suppose the difference is between fine lines and fine wine? Many of us believe that our lines and wrinkles lay bare the inevitable sign of aging, kind of like a wrinkled badge of honor for living a long robust life. Of course, fine wine, unlike wrinkled skin, ages well. And wine even contains ingredients like hydroxy acids that may reduce wrinkles. We can talk more about the merits of wine later. However, for now, pour yourself a glass of wine if you wish and enjoy this chapter as you discover how you can erase your wrinkles and reclaim your youthful skin.

To understand how SRCPs work, it helps to know how a wrinkle develops.

Fine Lines

Not all wrinkles are created equal. Some wrinkles appear from the lack of adequate moisture in our skin, just like those wrinkles that develop on the skin of a dried up apple. Those wrinkles are very easy to remove, at least temporarily—all you have to do is swell your skin with water. And this is exactly what a majority of so called "anti-aging" creams do. The result is fast and amazing—it pleases our hearts to see that just a few seconds after we applied this seductive smelling and soft to the touch cream to our face, our skin becomes noticeably younger. Unfortunately, such fast swelling of the skin is not a good sign. It means that your skin barrier is compromised and water is pushed through it. This is not anti-aging, this is aging acceleration.

To truly get rid of this type of wrinkle, you need to gradually restore your skin barrier and increase the amount of water holding molecules in your dermis. SRCPs have been clinically proven to strengthen the skin's barrier and to increase the production of glycosaminoglycans and proteoglycans in the skin. Therefore, they are able to restore natural skin's capacity to bind and hold moisture eliminating those fine lines without inflicting any damage to your skin.

Mimic Wrinkles

Mimic wrinkles appear on our forehead, around the eyes and at the sides of the mouth (often called "smile and frown" lines). Although they are called mimic wrinkles and develop in places where our mimic muscles stretch our skin, their primary cause is actually loss of skin elasticity.

When you stroke a child's skin, you will notice that it feels tight and elastic, like the surface of a balloon. This is why children can laugh, cry and make faces and still have smooth and beautiful skin. Unfortunately as we age, our skin thins and becomes loose and inelastic. Over time, muscle tension in the face becomes stronger than the skin's elasticity, and muscle contractions begin to create wrinkles. That is why when dermatologists inject nerve toxins such as botulinum toxin, the muscles paralyze, relaxing muscle tension which gives the appearance of elastic skin. As a result muscle relaxers "reduce" or "remove" wrinkles.

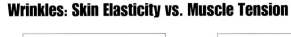

Wrinkles: Skin Elasticity vs. Muscle Tension

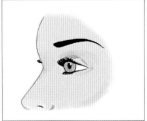

Skin elasticity pulls in
all directions
(like surface of a balloon)

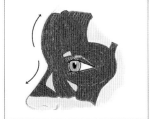

Muscle fibers pull along
axis of muscle fibers

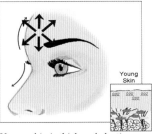

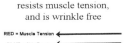

Young skin is thick and elastic,
resists muscle tension,
and is wrinkle free

RED = Muscle Tension ◄———
BLUE = Skin Tension ◄———

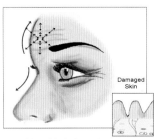

Older skin is less elastic
and cannot resist muscle wrinkling,
producing brow lines & "crows feet"

© Loren Pickart PhD

56

However, those who are injected with the toxin still have biologically old skin. The only difference is that their muscles are now paralyzed. This is not aging reversal. In fact, these toxins may actually age our faces in the long run by causing the muscles to atrophy. Muscle tone defies gravity and can give our face a firm uplifted appearance. Furthermore, it is now known that the skin's nerves work together with the skin's immune system and you do not want to weaken your skin's immunity.

Nerve numbing injections may also age our brains! Recent studies reveal these toxins migrate to the brain and affect long-term memory and spatial navigation.

Fortunately, there is a way to reduce mimic wrinkles and this is by restoring the skin's natural elasticity with the help of SRCPs. The wonderful thing about this method is that you can get rid of your mimic wrinkles and still retain your ability to smile, laugh and even make faces if you wish.

Sagging and Loose Skin

There is one law that everybody has to obey—the law of gravity. Every living moment of our life, Earth's gravity pulls us down. That is why it is much easier to lie down then it is to stand up. Our skin feels this pull too. When we are young, our strong facial muscles and elastic resilient dermal proteins manage to defy gravity, keeping our skin from sagging. But as we age, muscle tension as well as collagen elasticity decrease, and this is where our skin's ability to stretch plays a bad trick on us, because we develop folds and flaps under our checks, eyes and chin.

Surgeons solve this problem by cutting off excessive skin and tightening up the remaining part. This is called a surgical facelift and it is a very efficient method of removing flaps and folds. With a facelift you can achieve tight skin that looks great from far away. However take a closer look, or if you get to touch this tightened up skin, there is a big disappointment—it is still the same old, floppy skin with the only difference being that it is now pulled tight! The reason is that a facelift does not change the structure of the skin. It does not remove old skin proteins nor does it facilitate the production of new ones.

Loss of Collagen Elasticity

The most difficult thing to deal with wrinkles are those that develop due to accumulating damage of the skin's collagen and elastin. This should be a very slow process, but it is greatly accelerated by excessive UV-radiation. When collagen and elastin are damaged, the skin's surface becomes uneven with dimpled, bumpy areas. A combination of collagen damage and mimic wrinkles along with the pull of gravity produces deep creases such as nasolabial folds.

Just as in the case of fine lines developed due to lack of moisture, if you swell skin with water, its surface will temporarily look smoother and firmer. However, under this seemingly younger skin there will still be vast areas of broken, damaged and inelastic collagen.

So as soon as you stop applying the "anti-aging" cream, the damage becomes visible again!

In contrast, the natural wrinkle-reduction methods described in this book restore skin thickness and elasticity, essentially transforming it to act more like biologically younger skin. The key goal here is to firm and moisturize, thereby bringing you back to the skin you were born with. The remodeling process tightens skin by replacing damaged proteins with new elastin and collagen, and it moisturizes by increasing the water-holding proteoglycans and glycosaminoglycans.

Remember, SRCPs were first discovered in the field of wound healing. Since the process of healing wounds works similarly to repairing skin, this makes SRCPs extremely effective. This repair process is just what the doctor ordered to naturally decrease the appearance of wrinkles. SRCPs in creams or serums, such as those made by Skin Biology, have been shown in many studies to firm, moisturize and reduce wrinkles. And as previously noted, many of Skin Biology's products work even better when combined with hydroxy acids which enhance the remodeling process.

FROM OUR CLIENTS:

"My nasolabial lines were largely reduced with 2-3 applications of Exfol and CP Serum (and BHO—Biological Healing Oils) daily." - J.W.

"I did something a little nutty to test the products. I took an eyebrow brush and brushed a deep line/wrinkle on my neck vigorously. It turned very red, but did not bleed. Then I treated it with Exfol Serum every morning and Super Cop every night. After only two weeks I noticed that it is 50% less visible. I am happy with that! Maybe I can get rid of it completely by repeating this procedure!" - U.A.

"I have seen a remarkable improvement in my skin elasticity. The improvement is most pronounced around my eyes. My large dark circles were beginning to turn into large bags that covered nearly half of my face... I have seen these wonderful results using the serum. Thank you." - L.E.

TYPES OF WRINKLES Not all wrinkles are created equal. We all have them and each and every one of us wants to get rid of our wretched wrinkles—yes, that includes you and me! Unfortunately, there is no one simple method for removing those time-telling lines. That is because we have two types of wrinkles and each have to be attacked differently. The first type includes lines on the forehead, around the mouth, on the cheeks, and at the edge of the eyes (known as crow's feet). The second sort forms lines around and under the eyes; these wrinkles require special care because thin skin surrounding the eye is prone to damage.

Treating Facial Wrinkles

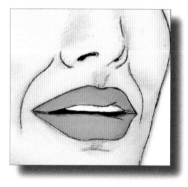

So how is that glass of wine doing? Are you feeling younger with each sip? Now bear with me. There is a wine analogy to the way we treat wrinkles. That fine glass of Merlot or Chardonney contains hydroxy acids which form part of our recipe for reducing wrinkles. In the days of Cleopatra, European ladies pampered their bodies with wine baths to have smooth silky skin. And guess what? We reduce the first type of wrinkle by alternating the application of hydroxy acids with SRCPs. As touched upon earlier in the book, hydroxy acids remove the skin in need of renewal, that is, the older skin on the upper layers, epidermis and upper dermis.

We use SRCPs, such as Protect & Restore and Super Cop, to help remodel and rebuild the skin. While stronger hydroxy acids work better in the short term, they have a tendency to irritate. Heavy duty hydroxy acids can lead to a rash or peeling when skin is removed by the strong acid concentrate. Over all, I recommend you take a slower approach to obtain the same result without irritation. Just apply lighter, less concentrated hydroxy acids for a longer period of time.

Nasolabial folds, those unflattering furrows that frame our sweet smiles, often concern clients more than any other wrinkles. These deep lines lie between the nose and corners of the mouth. They may run side to side, but most often appear vertical. They are associated with hanging skin. These furrows or folds tend to make a person seem sad or much older than their actual age.

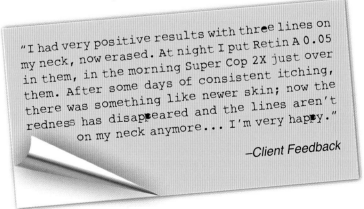

"I had very positive results with three lines on my neck, now erased. At night I put Retin A 0.05 in them, in the morning Super Cop 2X just over them. After some days of consistent itching, there was something like newer skin; now the redness has disappeared and the lines aren't on my neck anymore... I'm very happy."

–Client Feedback

TREATING WRINKLES AROUND THE EYES As the thinnest skin on our body, the delicate eye area presents us with one of the most difficult regions to repair, keep healthy and appear young.

This fragile skin tends to get irritated and may subsist in a condition of sub-clinical inflammation. Years of applying color cosmetics and other make-up, which contain a high concentration of dyes and metal salts, can produce extensive damage and sagging. In addition, the cleansers we use to remove make-up can cause further irritation by stripping away protective lipids from the skin. I have discovered that when Skin Biology clients use a progressively stronger remodeling system to treat their eyes, they obtain the best results.

Most clients start with Super GHK-Copper Cream or Super GHK-Copper Serum or CP Night Eyes Premier (a relatively weak cream), then progress to CP Night Eyes Regular. When the skin adjusts to the SRCPs and becomes somewhat thicker and more protective, many clients move on to stronger products like Super CP Serum, and then finally to Super Cop. I advise that you begin by using the last two products gradually at first and at low concentrations.

If a Skin Biology product should irritate your eye area, I suggest that you apply a biological healing oil to slow the uptake of the product as was mentioned earlier in the book. Applying either Emu Oil-S or Squalane before the SRCP product will result in a much milder response.

You will recall that if you apply a BHO after a SRCP product instead, the oil will push more of the SRCPs into the skin and intensify their effect. In this manner, it is possible to adjust the SRCP action to receive maximum results. In general, hydroxy acids, even at a very low concentration, should not be used around the eyes.

When you first begin to treat the delicate eye area, I suggest you follow these tips in order to help adjust to your new regimen:

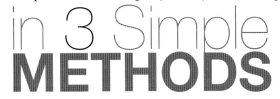

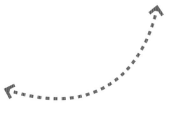Getting from here...

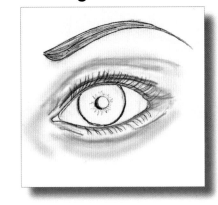

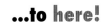...to here!

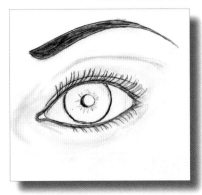

My Steps to **BEAUTIFUL EYES**

Start by cleaning around the eye area to remove make-up. Use a very mild make-up remover such as Emu Oil-S for Skin, Squalane, or Dr. Pickart Face & Body Cleanser. Rinse with clear water. Apply CP Night Eyes while the skin is still wet.

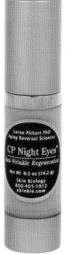

Because the skin may be badly damaged, start with a very light coating of Super GHK-Copper Cream/or Serum, or CP Night Eyes Premier, and then gradually increase the amount you apply over time. If you experience irritation, that means you have applied too much copper peptide through a very damaged skin barrier. In this case, you might try a gentler approach of alternating Emu Oil-S one night to replenish skin lipids and Super GHK-Copper every second night. Since everyone reacts differently to products, some people discover that Super GHK-Copper Serum feels milder than CP Night Eyes on damaged eyes.

As your skin barrier repairs itself, you will grow less sensitive to products. With time, the area around your eyes should tighten and firm and you can progress to more powerful products.

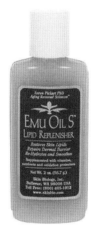

If you experience excessive dryness, use a little less of the SRCP product and cover it with a light amount of either Emu Oil-Skin or Squalane.

Super GHK-Copper Serum for Around the Eye Area:

"I love it! I've been using it morning and evening on my laser abrasions and around my eyes. There has been absolutely no puffiness; my eyes are tight and that is without using my usual DMAE... Bravo!"

–P.T., South Carolina

SKIN CARE GUIDE

How to Tighten the Delicate Area Around the Eyes

The key to remodeling this delicate area around the eyes is to go slow. By applying a thin layer of mild copper peptides underneath the eye, on the outside areas, or under the brow bone to affect a lift of the upper lid area.

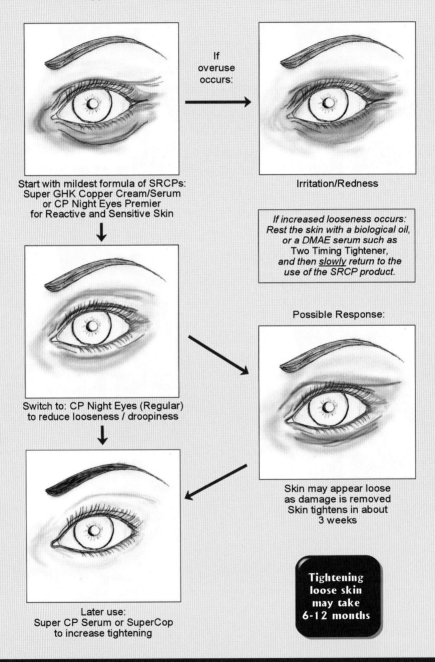

Start with mildest formula of SRCPs:
Super GHK Copper Cream/Serum
or CP Night Eyes Premier
for Reactive and Sensitive Skin

If
overuse
occurs:

Irritation/Redness

*If increased looseness occurs:
Rest the skin with a biological oil,
or a DMAE serum such as
Two Timing Tightener,
and then slowly return to the
use of the SRCP product.*

Possible Response:

Switch to: CP Night Eyes (Regular)
to reduce looseness / droopiness

Skin may appear loose
as damage is removed
Skin tightens in about
3 weeks

Later use:
Super CP Serum or SuperCop
to increase tightening

**Tightening
loose skin
may take
6-12 months**

SKIN CARE GUIDE

How to Remove Wrinkles with Hydroxy Acids and SRCPs (Natural Method)

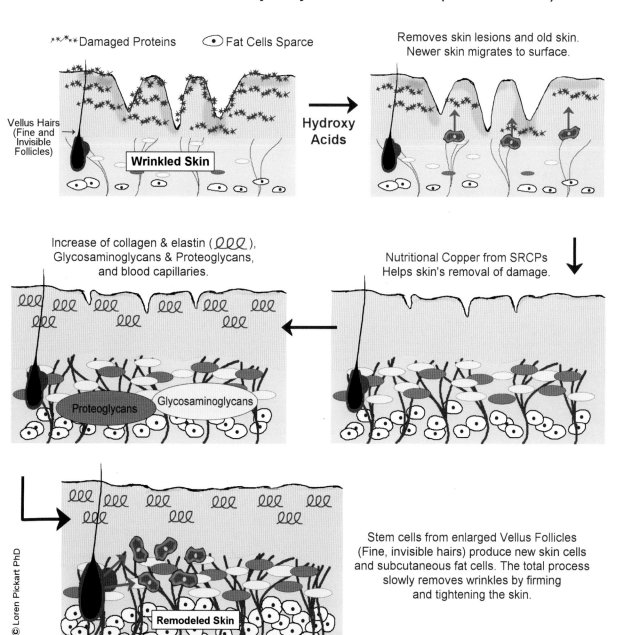

✶✶ Damaged Proteins

Fat Cells Sparce

Removes skin lesions and old skin. Newer skin migrates to surface.

Hydroxy Acids

Vellus Hairs (Fine and Invisible Follicles)

Wrinkled Skin

Increase of collagen & elastin (ℓℓℓ), Glycosaminoglycans & Proteoglycans, and blood capillaries.

Nutritional Copper from SRCPs Helps skin's removal of damage.

Proteoglycans

Glycosaminoglycans

Stem cells from enlarged Vellus Follicles (Fine, invisible hairs) produce new skin cells and subcutaneous fat cells. The total process slowly removes wrinkles by firming and tightening the skin.

Remodeled Skin

© Loren Pickart PhD

SKIN CARE GUIDE

How to Reduce the Appearance of Nasolabial Lines

"Laugh lines" are definitely nothing to "smile" about...

Super Cop 2X - Extra Strength should always be started slowly:

1. In the morning after cleansing, apply **Lactic Power 10** into the crease area.

2. At night, work in Super Cop 2X - Extra Strength very lightly directly into wrinkle.

3. REPEAT CONSISTENTLY...

Many clients report a significant reduction in fine lines after 3 to 4 months of applying this method. An eyebrow brush can be used to add a little abrasion while working products deep into the skin.

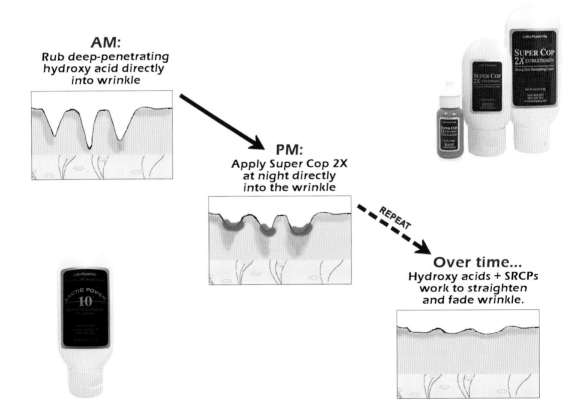

AM:
Rub deep-penetrating hydroxy acid directly into wrinkle

PM:
Apply Super Cop 2X at night directly into the wrinkle

REPEAT

Over time...
Hydroxy acids + SRCPs work to straighten and fade wrinkle.

BEFORE & AFTER EXPERIENCES Be patient when using SRCP products. Rebuilding the skin, particularly the delicate skin around the eyes, takes time, but eventually you will notice a difference. In some cases, your skin will appear worse before it begins to look better. But have no fear. You will look better as you continue to use the products. However, don't just take my word for it. Read on to discover what Skin Biology's clients have to say:

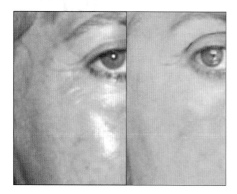

"I began working with Dr. Pickart's copper peptides consistently around November 2001...The changes in my skin within six months were just pretty unbelievable to me. I continued working with CP Serum, Exfol Serum and lots of oil. I began to introduce the Exfol cream to try to speed that sloughing off of the leathery old damaged cells that were migrating to the surface.

Quite evident [in the two pictures] is the reduction in wrinkles and crows feet. The discoloration during May 2002 was as a result of the copper peptides literally pushing or causing the damaged skin cells to migrate to the surface where they finally began to slough off. The sun-damaged spots are either gone or diminished greatly in size."
– *Courtesy of Diana Yvonne (www.dianayvonne.com)*

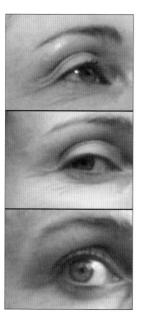

"Age 43: In November 2003, I introduced CP Night Eyes and I noticed two things: 1) the scales disappeared and 2) a little pin-prick-sized red mark that I'd had under my right eye for months and months was disappearing!

In comparing the progress pictures, the lid appears to have tightened up a lot. In the latest picture, looking down at the camera, the lines should be much more evident under the eye than when looking up as in the first photo.

The dynamic smile lines are smoothing out fast along with the long one that ran underneath my eye are almost gone!" Submitted by R.
– *Courtesy of Diana Yvonne (www.dianayvonne.com)*

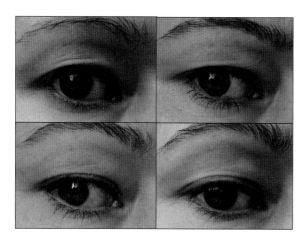

"I introduced CP Serum on May 26, 2004. I used it diluted the first night and felt no irritation. So I tried it full strength the second night (four drops for the entire face including around the eyes). As everything went fine, I've been using it undiluted since then. But I must say that my skin is really tough and that most people should really work their way up slowly. I currently only use CP Serum at night. In the last two months, the only new products I've included in my routine are: CP Serum, Exfol Cream and one 40 percent lactic peel weekly." Submitted by V.
– *Courtesy of Diana Yvonne (www.dianayvonne.com)*

First Message from Client:

I took a look at my eyes first thing this morning and man, I got to tell you, they looked awful! Big drooping, puffy half-moon ring underneath both of them. Much worse than the day before. At this time I look 100 percent worse than I did when I started CP Night Eyes two weeks ago. This is not good, but I haven't lost hope or faith in your products, I'm just concerned about what is happening and what I should do now. It would be nice to think that the puffiness is part of a reconstruction process going on under the outer skin. Is that possible? Are the effects of your products transdermal?

One Week Later:

My eyes are much better now! The puffiness is gone! I believe it was some deep rebuilding of the subdermal skin. The areas underneath my eyes are now filled out. I still have lots of small lines around the eyes, but I'm sure that the lines will vanish in time with continued use of your products. All and all a good experience using your product.

Thank You

-G.A., Washington

SKIN CARE GUIDE

Other Methods: Things to Keep in Mind
USING: Dermabrasion

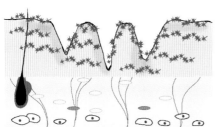

Dermabrasion
performed
on the skin

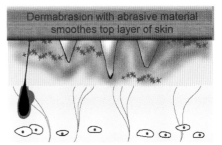

Dermabrasion with abrasive material smoothes top layer of skin

BETTER RESULT:
Follow with SRCPs and dermabrasion results in less redness and better healing.

SRCPs help activate the stem cells from enlarged vellus follicles to produce new skin cells and subcutaneous fat cells. Total process slowly firms and tightens skin after dermabrasion procedure.

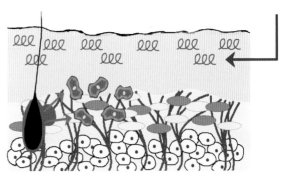

USING: Laser Resurfacing

Damaged proteins   ⊙ Few fat cells

Vellus hair follicles (fine, invisible hairs)

Laser burns off top layer of skin
Possible scarring may occur

Laser resurfacing performed

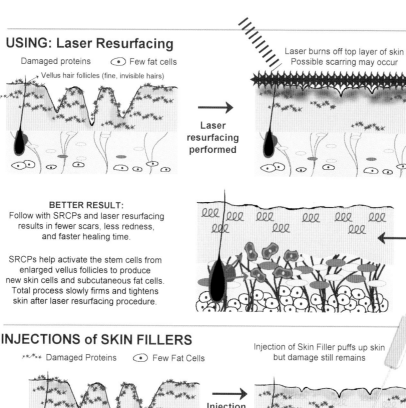

BETTER RESULT:
Follow with SRCPs and laser resurfacing
results in fewer scars, less redness,
and faster healing time.

SRCPs help activate the stem cells from
enlarged vellus follicles to produce
new skin cells and subcutaneous fat cells.
Total process slowly firms and tightens
skin after laser resurfacing procedure.

INJECTIONS of SKIN FILLERS

⚹⚹/⚹⚹ Damaged Proteins   ⊙ Few Fat Cells

Injection of Skin Filler puffs up skin
but damage still remains

Vellus Hairs
(Fine and
Invisible
Follicles)

Injection
of
Skin Filler

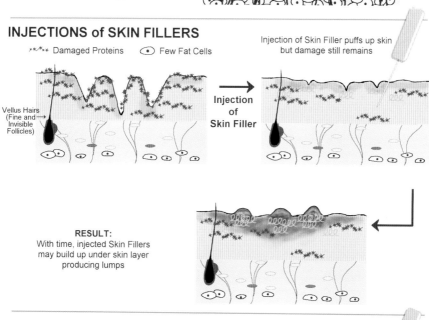

RESULT:
With time, injected Skin Fillers
may build up under skin layer
producing lumps

Botulinum Toxin Injections
or Skin Creams with Muscle Paralyzers

Injection of botulinum toxin relaxes muscles and loosens the skin
but damaged skin is still present plus paralyzed muscles

Injection of
Toxin

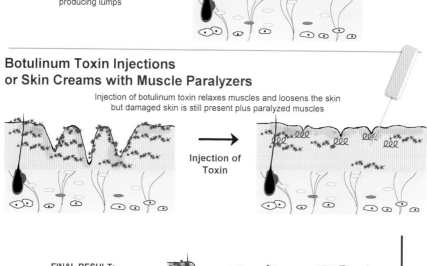

FINAL RESULT:
Toxin wears off and skin
may become worse with time.
Damaged skin now also has
paralyzed muscles as well.

Toxin also enters brain and
affects brain function.

c Loren Pickart PhD

wrinkle Busting Regimens

The best way to remove wrinkles and damage depends on your skin type. We recommend the following regimens:

Under Age 30

1. In the morning after cleansing, apply a light amount of CP Serum or Super GHK-Copper Serum. If acne is a problem, try Super CP Serum.

2. At night, apply Protect & Restore Classic Cream or Super GHK-Copper Cream over your face three nights weekly and Exfol Serum or LacSal Serum three alternate nights weekly.

3. If dry patches are a problem, use Emu Oil-S. This does not cause breakouts.

Over Age 30

1. In the morning after cleansing, apply a light amount of CP Serum or Super GHK-Copper Serum, and follow with a light coating of Emu Oil-S or Squalane.

2. At night, apply Protect & Restore with Retinol or Super GHK-Copper Cream over your face three nights weekly and Exfol Cream or LacSal Cream three alternate nights weekly.

3. After two months, you may progress to stronger hydroxy acids, such as a 30 percent lactic acid and Super Cop Cream. Be sure to use stronger products lightly at first.

Anti-Wrinkle/Rosacea

1. In the morning after cleansing, apply a light amount of CP Serum or Super GHK-Copper Serum followed by Emu Oil-S Lipid Replenisher.

2. At night, apply Protect & Restore Classic Cream or Super GHK-Copper Cream over your face three nights weekly.

3. Sometimes Exfol Serum or LacSal Serum also helps to reduce rosacea. Apply the product lightly at night when not using Protect & Restore Classic Cream.

4. Dr. Pickart's Face & Body Cleanser works exceptionally well on super-sensitive skin with rosacea.

TIGHTEN LOOSE & SAGGING SKIN
THE BENEFITS OF BIOLOGICAL SKIN TIGHTENING

Are you tired of those jiggly jaggly jowls that sag as they wiggle,
that sway on both sides and droop down the middle?
So go swoop it all up with skin so tight and taut by
using what nature gave you to remodel what you've got.

If those jiggles and jowls disturb you, please do not despair. One question I hear most often is: "How can I tighten my loose skin?" In this chapter I will present you with some natural techniques to tighten the sag that develops with age or as a result of weight loss. As many of my clients will attest, these painless methods can defer your need to go under the knife. Besides, skin-tightening surgery is not only painful, it costs a bundle. Not only that, but you can expect to wait at least a year before your rebuilt skin recovers. Who wants to wait that long? Here's a time saving tongue twister: Do not lose time while losing loose skin.

My customers tell me that they prefer to use their body's natural systems to tighten skin. They find this biological approach more appealing. My objective is to help you achieve your skin-tightening goals by working with the skin's natural remodeling system.

We can best demonstrate how the body tightens skin when we observe how wounds heal. Visualize it this way. You fall off a bike and scrape your knee. You put a bandage on the wound. After a very short time, perhaps a few days, the wound closes. As skin pulls together, new collagen forms to seal the wound. Often during the healing process, the skin-tightening action grows so intense that you can see stress lines on the skin as it pulls the sides of the wound together.

So I'll bet you wonder, "what pulls the skin together?" Well, it's certainly not spackle, cement or glue. You knew that? Bear with me. We're just having a little fun here as we learn how to appear sculpted. Wounds are closed by two mechanisms. First tissue rebuilds within the injured area; and secondly, the skin contracts around the wound. When we use SRCPs, we can enhance the process of healing wounds and thus tighten skin. In my work with SRCPs, one of my first discoveries was that they have a profound effect on tightening wounds. As one example, we treated the skin ulcers of many hospital patients with SRCPs. The results were truly astounding. We often observed strong wound contractions within 48 hours and the development of stress lines in the skin.

These lines result from the intense pulling on the skin by the tightening of collagen strands.

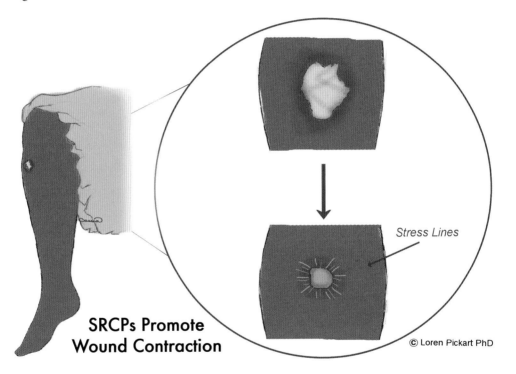

SRCPs Promote Wound Contraction

Stress Lines

© Loren Pickart PhD

The Natural Way to Tighten Skin

We can visualize young skin as the surface of a buoyant balloon; push it in or pull it out and it quickly returns to a smooth surface. Like a balloon, biological skin tightening arises as the skin's repair cells and the fibroblasts pull collagen strands together. The fibroblasts biochemically attach collagen strands to each other. This natural skin tightening process keeps the skin elastic and soft. The fibroblasts use an enzyme called lysyl oxidase to connect the collagen strands, which requires both copper (II) and vitamin C to work.

Biological Skin Tightening - How and Why It Works:

Youthful, healthy skin (much like the surface of a balloon) will be flexible and enjoy good elasticity. Copper-peptides help activate the skin's natural renewal systems to keep the skin that way!

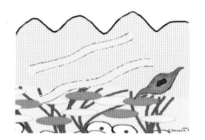

SRCPs Transfer Copper(II)

[Loose collagen + ascorbic acid strands (Vitamin C) $\longrightarrow$ Lysyl Oxidase + Copper (II) $\longrightarrow$ Attached tight collagen + dehydroascorbic strands acid]

We require adequate levels of copper (II) and vitamin C in order to tighten our skin. We can not attain a tightening effect without having a high level of each molecule in our skin. The best way to supply copper (II) is to apply SRCPs to the skin's surface. However, when we apply vitamin C products to our skin, they tend to produce far less collagen than topical SRCPs. Most vitamin C creams and serums contain forms of vitamin C and pH levels that prevent optimal absorption. We can most easily increase vitamin C levels in our skin by taking 0.5 grams daily as a supplement. For a more extensive discussion on this topic, see **Chapter 18: The Science Behind SRCPs**.

The use of hydroxy acids, such as salicylic acid and lactic acid, also helps tighten the skin. Hydroxy acids remove the older cells on the skin's surface by producing a very mild skin damage. This damage assists in the skin renewal process, most likely by increasing the number of fibroblasts.

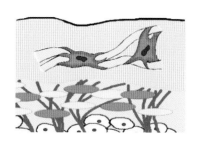

Collagen strands in loose skin:

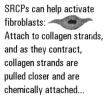

SRCPs can help activate fibroblasts: Attach to collagen strands, and as they contract, collagen strands are pulled closer and are chemically attached...

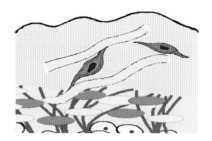

RESULT:
Tightened skin with elastic collagen that retains natural elasticity.

KIN CARE GUIDE

Recommended Regimen for Tighter Skin on Face and Body

The following regimen has helped many Skin Biology clients turn back the clock on their skin:

1. Use SRCP products, vitamin C supplements (0.5 grams daily), and hydroxy acids to tighten the skin. Be patient; this slow process may take several months and the hydroxy acids can produce a mild irritation. Many clients apply LacSal Cream or Lactic Power 10 in the morning and a strong SRCP cream such as TriReduction with Retinol or Super Cop at night. However, some sun lovers opt to reverse the regimen since hydroxy acids increase photosensitivity. In this case, they apply SRCP creams such as Protect & Restore Day Cover with Titanium Dioxide during the day and LacSal or Lactic Power 10 at night. After losing a large amount of weight, some clients have combined these products to effectively avoid surgical removal of excess skin.

2. For maximum effectiveness, some clients apply a SRCP cream and a hydroxy acid at approximately four to six-hour intervals. In this case, apply each product twice daily.

3. To speed things up, you might use a stronger hydroxy acid, such as a 10 percent to 30 percent lactic acid. Mild microdermabrasion can also help you see faster results.

4. Take a daily supplement of 1 gram methylsulfonylmethane (MSM), which supplies the nutritional sulfur needed to produce skin proteins.

Achieving a Slight Breast Lift You can also achieve a slight breast lift by following the preceding four-step regimen for tighter skin. I recommend trying Protect & Restore BND Cream and a 10 to 30 percent lactic acid as the best products to use for this purpose. Some women who were planning a surgical breast lift found this mild method gave enough improvement to satisfy them without surgery.

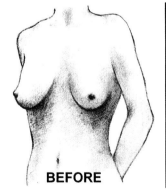

BEFORE

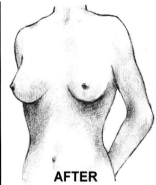

AFTER

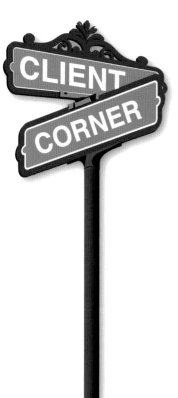

CLIENT CORNER

"The first pic is May 5, 2005, the second 6 weeks later, the third 6 months after...Look at my eyes, jowls, and most importantly my neck, which I believe is the foundation of everything! Touching it, it felt like tissue paper. I had creases, and below my adam's apple, I had those horrific vertical lines. Just check it out. By curiosity only, I took this pic myself. I was in shock when I looked at it! "That's Me???", I said! I have some opinions on facial exercises, and admit to doing them as part of my routine, but IT BEGINS WITH GETTING ON THE RIGHT REGIMEN TO REBUILD AND FIRM YOUR SKIN! I proved that with the recent pics I sent you, as I was curious as to if the exercises were helping or was it the skin products I was using (Skin Biology's of course!)...I credit the skin repair and firmness to the SRCPs, CASE CLOSED....No doubt about it, the SRCPs repaired and firmed my skin, plus greatly reduced the appearance of lines, etc..."

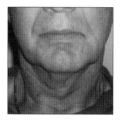 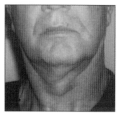 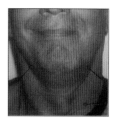

BEFORE PICTURE: Client's goal to improve neck, jowls, and overall skin tightening/condition.

6 WEEK MARK: Improvement in jowls, neck skin, overall tightening, texture, and color.

AFTER PICTURE: Notice blue arrows pointing out improvement on jowl area and neck area!

BEFORE PICTURE: Before using SRCPs.

AFTER PICTURE: Notice blue arrows pointing to skin tightened around orbital bone, lifting effect, and improvement of crows feet!

I have experimented with my face and skin so much, you wouldn't believe it! I've tried a lot of the "over-the-counter" products, but all ended up long on promises and short on results! I think I must have tried at least 20 products, LOL! Yes "Me", A GUY!...I wondered is it the skin products or the eye exercises. Thus, I took some pics after not doing any exercises or skin care for a few days. Then only applied the skin care products. Since then I hardly touch my eye exercises! Only Skin Biology products!...

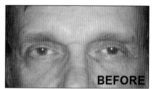

BEFORE

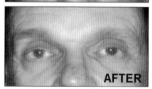

AFTER

SKIN CARE REGIMEN:
I started with three products! First of course, I used the Gentle Cleanser. Then Exfol Serum, which at the outset I found just a bit strong for my skin, so I diluted it with water 'til I used it all. Emu Oil-S - After exfoliating I would use Emu Oil-S next, and my face literally soaked it in like a sponge! I loved how my face felt after using it, as I actually massaged my entire face and neck with it twice a day! Next, I applied diluted CP Serum (2-3 drops of CP Serum mixed in the palm of my hand with a few drops water), as I had read to try it on top of an oil to avoid irritation and to give the skin time to adjust to the SRCPs. After first applying the SRCPs on top of the Emu Oil-S, I could feel a tightening effect. Plus my face and especially my neck began to have a nice glow to it! After a few months of reading on the Skin Biology site that the Retinol in Squalane was also suitable for my skin, I decided to try it and eventually I switched to Exfol Cream. On my eyes, at night only, I applied the Emu Oil-S first. Then, very diluted with water, CP Serum. Since I had gradually introduced my eyes to SRCPs by diluting it on top of the Emu Oil-S, I also ordered the CP Night Eyes as I thought they were now ready for direct application with an oil on top this time!

I now use Exfol Cream in the AM, followed by Retinol in Squalane, then only slightly diluted CP Serum...At night, after cleansing, I apply the diluted CP Serum first, then Retinol in Squalane on top, switching the order from the AM! On my eyes, I now apply the CP Night Eyes first on one night with the Squalane on top, and on the next night I reverse the order! P.S. About the scalp: Forgot to mention this! I added Folligen and first tried Folligen Cream, now Folligen Spray. I do feel a difference in thickness! Many thanks!

MY GOALS:
My goal is to apply CP Serum first, all of the time and CP Night Eyes too, followed by the Retinol in Squalane on top. But I'm just taking it slowly and enjoying it! I know how my skin felt and looked in May of 2005 (somewhat like tissue paper) and today over seven months later I see and feel a great difference! Thanks Skin Biology! I'm looking forward to trying other skin products from you!"

—C.K.

newfacenewbodynewmind@yahoo.com

Using Controlled Heating Methods to Tighten Skin

Have you ever spilled hot grease on yourself while cooking? Ouch! No one enjoys getting burned. However, you may have noticed that this heat burn caused your skin to contract. In serious burns, the resulting skin contraction can be so severe that it acts as a tourniquet to stop blood flow into the area. When this happens, a doctor may cut open the burned skin to relieve pressure and permit blood flow again.

So what if we could replicate wound healing in a controlled way? Well, that's where lasers, microwaves, and various types of lights enter the picture. These controlled heating methods produce a mild contraction and thereby tighten the skin. So it's out of the hot kitchen and into the weak not so hot fire. However, these methods are far from perfect; they do not produce collagen and may actually damage the vellus hair follicles that produce stem cells for rebuilding skin.

Those who use a controlled heating method must take care to treat the skin properly after the procedure. Their effectiveness depends on the skin's ability to regenerate after incurring damage caused by these treatments. To offset the potential harm, I recommend you apply CP Serum followed by Emu Oil-S, beginning one to two weeks after the procedure. By using these products, you will get the results you want. Your skin will rebuild collagen and elastin with less scarring and you will end up with softer skin.

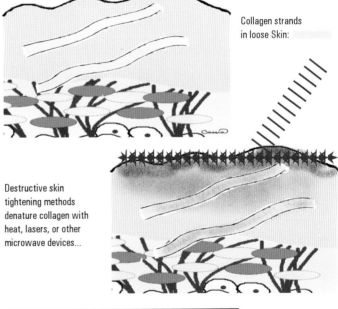

Collagen strands in loose Skin:

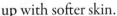

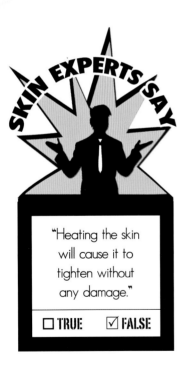

"Heating the skin will cause it to tighten without any damage."

☐ TRUE   ☑ FALSE

Destructive skin tightening methods denature collagen with heat, lasers, or other microwave devices...

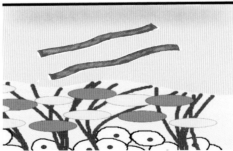

Collagen matrix shrinks like bacon in a pan, causing a general skin contraction.

RESULT:
Tighter skin with condensed damaged collagen

Just as weight training tightens the appearance of loose skin on the body, facial exercise firms the face. Similar to the body, facial skin sags over time. I recommend you add a regimen of facial resistance training. Facial resistance training does for the face what weight training does for the body. Facial exercise can provide a beneficial enhancement to the topical skincare regimen I recommend in this book.

When we exercise our facial muscles, we can help strengthen and lift, tone and tighten. Facial exercises create fullness and lift, especially in the cheeks, under the eyes, and around the chin and jaw. It fills in the hollows in the cheeks, flattens the areas under the eyes, and reduces sagging of the jowls, chin and neck area. The isometric, isotonic resistance training of FlexEffect can be successfully combined with SRCPs to achieve tighter, younger skin.

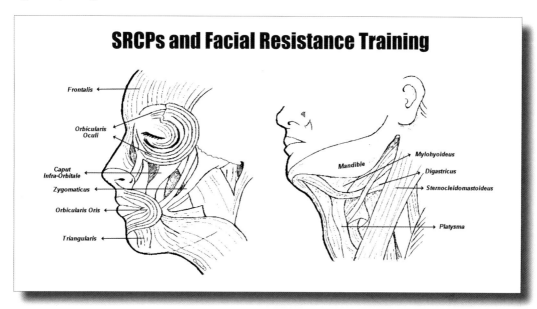

Information from FlexEffect (Facial Resistance Training: www.flexeffect.com)

Tightening Pores

Many of my clients complain about clogged and enlarged pores. SRCPs, hydroxy acids, pore cleaning strips and saunas can help to effectively reduce or tighten pores. Try the following suggestions:

1. In the morning, use a 2% salicylic acid pad (available at drugstores).

2. Apply a light amount of Exfol Serum or LacSal Serum and leave on the skin without washing off.

3. Apply a light amount of Super CP Serum (maximum of 4 drops daily when starting and then slightly increasing this amount if needed).

4. Apply pore cleansing strips every two weeks on problem areas as needed.

5. You might also enjoy occasional steam baths or saunas which help with pore size reduction.

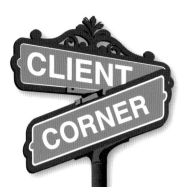

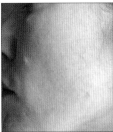

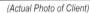
(Actual Photo of Client)

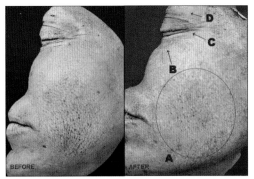
Before and After of facial replica mask)

A Section of Face: Shows marked improvement in overall texture, tightened pores, and very visible reduced appearance of fine lines and spots.

B Section of Face: Look closely to see improvement of under eye skin area and skin health.

C Section of Face: Fine lines around eyelids have decreased and tightened. Notice additional lines of the eyelid area shown in the Before picture that are reduced in the After.

D Section of Face: Above eyelid area has improved in texture and loose skin has remodeled.

(Replicas are produced using indicator tint that highlights pores and intricate details of your skin)

"I've been using Exfol, Protect & Restore, and Super Cop for over a year now, and have been meaning to write you for some time...Before I started using your products, I made a replica of my facial texture. Frankly, I was tired of wasting money on skin products that didn't perform as promised. I felt like my skin was softer and rosier right away. But then, over time, with good and bad days, I wasn't sure if I wanted to re-order. So, I made another facial texture replica and compared them side by side...I was so surprised at how much my skin texture had improved! Needless to say, I am using your products religiously, and I recommend them to friends...I am often complimented on my skin. I just wanted to let you know how nice it is to find an over the counter product that actually works, and can prove it!" – From Ohio, USA

How our Products Work for Tightening Pores:

"I have been using the Super Cop 2X on my enlarged pores on the nose (sparingly) and I have noticed in some of the areas they definitely appear to be smaller. I find it's great as my skin is oily and it doesn't make my nose any oilier either. Thank you so much!!!" -K.N.

"Salicylic acid is lipid soluble and can deep cleanse the pores... My nose pores "disappeared" after three days, and the facial pores diminished after 1.5 weeks. My skin texture and pores continue to refine even after two months of using Exfol Serum and SRCPs. You could also add steam facials (add favorite herbs and citrus peels for added aromatherapy) for deep cleansing and refinement of pores." -J.W.

"I have oily skin with large pores & have been using CP & Exfol Serums, Emu Oil or jojoba oil, & glycolic acid peels for about a year now. I've seen a definite difference in the size/appearance of my pores. They look smaller & are less noticeable - I don't know if it's because they are kept clear now or if they've actually tightened." -G.B.

"The combination of keeping the pores clear with salicylic and the rebuilding of skin makes the pores look smaller... Try using Exfol twice a day and be sure to wait 30 minutes after applying it, before applying any other products. This will work on pore exfoliation." -D.B.

"I have had great results using Exfol, Super CP Serum & Emu Oil, supplemented by 10% Lactic Acid and 5% BHA. The pores on my nose are improving everyday...I think the exfoliation is revealing pores that weren't noticeable because the skin had grown partially over them. And if skin had partially occluded the pore, that must be the reason why you could leave the house looking just fine and the next time you looked in a mirror there would be a pimple. I could never understand how it happened so fast, but when I think about it, it's almost like – how could you expect any other result. Those pores were ticking time bombs just waiting to mess up your world!" -A.M.

Diet and Exercise Helps Tighten Skin

Do not overlook diet and exercise to optimize your skin's natural tightening systems. When you eat a healthy diet, you enhance the body's ability to repair itself. Include plenty of vitamin C rich fruit and vegetables such as oranges and bell peppers to enhance the benefits of SRCPs.

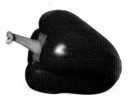

Get sulfur from tomatoes, kale, broccoli and brussel sprouts to produce skin protein. Vitamin A in dark greens, carrots and sweet potatoes are essential for a healthy complexion. When you enjoy almonds and other vitamin E rich foods, you encourage skin to heal and reduce scarring after injuries such as burns.

In other words, vitamin E can aid wound healing and thus assist the remodeling process. Add Omega 3 rich fish such as salmon and sardines. Essential fats add luster to your skin. Sardines also contain DMAE which increases tone in the skin. Minimize high glycemic processed foods such as white bread and sugar. Refined foods cross-link proteins, leading to aging skin and wrinkles.

Exercise enhances the skin's natural tightening systems. So build some muscle with weight training to reduce the appearance of saggy skin. If you are overweight, dieting will have a tightening effect on skin. Consider how people who have been starving for a long time never have areas of loose skin on the body; the body absorbs excess skin when it can't find enough energy producing calories in the diet.

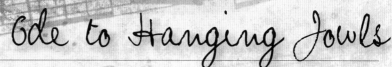

Ode to Hanging Jowls

Idelle Musiek

Sing to the tune of the children's song: "Do Your Ears Hang Low"

Do your jowls hang low as they wobble to and fro?
If they wiggle, squiggle, jiggle like a loose-skinned foe
Please do sing along but do not despair...
Are you tired of jiggly jaggly jowls
that sag as they wiggle,
to sway on both sides
and droop down in the middle?
So go swoop it all up
with skin so tight and taut
by using what nature gave you
to remodel what you've got.

However, when you lose too much too quickly, your fat cells will have retained their shape causing your skin to resemble an empty rubbish bag on the floor. Just as effective skin remodeling takes time, so does weight loss.

Never lose more than one to two pounds a week if you want to minimize loose skin. Follow up weight loss with weight training to rebuild muscle tone and minimize flab. Aerobic exercise also helps tighten the skin. Regular aerobic exercise tightens the internal muscles and enhances the rebuilding process.

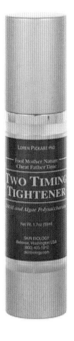

QUICK FIX TO TIGHTEN SKIN True skin tightening takes a few months of diligence. Many clients rave about their firm glowing complexions stating the journey is well worth it. However, at times, you may yearn for a quick fix to superficially tighten skin while waiting for copper peptides to do their magic. Thus, we created Two Timing Tightener which contains DMAE and algae polysaccharides. This quick fix elixir will two time mother nature with two times the skin tightener of any one product.

Our potent duo creates skin synergy unheard of in other products. Clinical studies show DMAE, first advanced by Dr. Nicholas Perricone, delves below the skin's surface where muscles contract to prevent facial sagging. In contrast, algae polysaccharides work on the skin's surface to immediately tighten the skin. The algae polysaccharides are carefully fermented to form Pepha-Tight® which has been proven to not only tighten the skin but also diminish fine lines.

So go ahead... fool Mother Nature and cheat Father Time with Two Timing Tightener!

8

THE BALANCING ACT
FOR REMOVING SCARS AND BLEMISHES
Help Skin Heal After Deep Peels, Laser Resurfacing, and Dermabrasion

We're all of us sentenced to solitary confinement inside our own skins, for life!
—Tennessee Williams

If you have been startled by those scary scars and blemishes that go bump in the night like a blotched house of horrors when you look in the mirror, you have come to the right chapter to salvage your flaws.

You may be tempted to remove these remnants of your blemished youth with resurfacing methods such as deep peels, laser resurfacing or dermabrasion. However, take heed of this warning. Laser treatments and other methods commonly used to reduce acne scars and other skin blemishes are far from ideal. Not only are they painful, expensive and only marginally effective, they often produce further scars, the very scourge you want to banish from your milky complexion.

So here's the good news: you can eliminate many blemishes and scars by using a combination of hydroxy acids and SRCPs. This painless low-cost approach utilizes your natural remodeling cycle and thus may take several months to achieve optimal results. Beware of methods that claim to work overnight. Instant miracles can also create instant disasters. As the saying goes, "Don't Fool with Mother Nature."

SRCPs provide a delicate balance to the process of removing blemishes. These miraculous molecules help calm and rebuild new skin, allowing skin lesions to be slowly dissolved and replaced by fresh, unblemished skin. They also help your skin heal properly without new scarring in case you were so eager to get rid of your flaws you preferred to burn down your old skin with strong acid or lasers.

Caution: These methods are not intended to replace regular skin care by a physician. Lesions that are dark and irregular, those that bleed, or are infected should be promptly checked by a physician.

WHAT CAN I USE TO GET RID OF SKIN DAMAGE?

Unsightly acne and scars crop up when cellular damage prompts our skin cells to grow in an abnormal manner. Many triggers can disfigure our skin including viruses, bacteria, heat, UV or X-ray radiation, and scar tissue that results from incomplete wound healing. This abnormal skin must be removed so that normal healthy skin can re-fill the area and create a smooth, unblemished complexion.

However, many modern methods that allow quick removal of such abnormal tissue can damage the skin too much, causing inflammation and incomplete healing resulting in... new scars! So the question is how can we break this vicious circle and achieve flawless healing and radiant beautiful skin?

First let's ask ourselves, what causes the skin to heal abnormally in the first place? Today we know that healing requires a certain kind of environment, meaning that a number of molecular factors should be present in right concentrations to orchestrate and guide the extremely complex healing process, preventing it from going awry.

The deficit or excess of such factors can turn healing into pretty messy business, resulting in prolonged inflammation, delayed healing, and hypo- or hyper-pigmentation. So here is the key to reversing damage: We selectively remove the blemish as gently as possible while creating an environment that fosters the creation of new healthy skin.

1. Blemish develops after skin damage followed by inadequate healing. Healing process can be further assisted by the following methods...

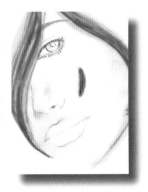

3. Skin Remodeling Copper-Peptides help the skin repair itself.

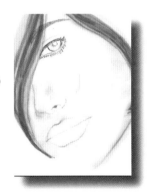

2. Exfoliation with salicylic acid helps to remove damaged skin proteins. Blemish decreases in size and edges may "dry" up and flake off.

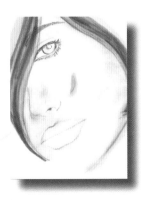

4. Process is repeated over and over again, leaving the skin healthy and unblemished!

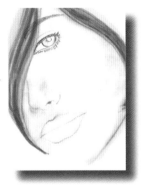

What is "The Gold Reserve" of Your Skin and How to Preserve It

Most "old school" dermatologists know that they can remove almost any skin lesion by applying hydroxy acids and/or retinoic acid or liquid nitrogen over a sustained period of time. However, these approaches can inflame the skin. The lesion may be removed, but it takes time and can be very irritating. When irritation and pain outweighs any gain, are you willing to pay the price?

Today more and more dermatologists resort to a "quick fix" approach. They use either laser beams that evaporate the upper layer of the skin, taking with it damaged tissue, or they abrade it with rotating brushes, or burn it away using medium (TCA) or deep (phenol) peels.

Instead of a series of liquid nitrogen or salicylic acid applications, they deal with damage in one mighty sweep: burning old skin away. But after scar tissue is removed, it is up to the skin to rebuild itself. Have you ever wondered how your skin does this? Why it is possible for it to rebirth just like a legendary Phoenix that burns itself and then rises from the ashes again?

Today we know the answer. The source of the skin's renovating power, or "gold reserve", is hidden in the lowest part of the epidermis. They are called the stem cells— wonder cells that alone are endowed with an amazing capacity to transform into any cell that your skin needs to rebuild itself. Whenever there is considerable damage to the skin, which cannot be filled by existing skin cells, the stem cells start to grow and transform into cells needed for repair.

The problem is that as we grow older, stem cells seem to gradually lose their ability to grow and produce repair cells when needed. That explains why the older we get, the longer it takes for our skin to heal after wounding or skin resurfacing.

The good news is that SRCPs have been scientifically proven to re-charge the regenerative power of aged skin's stem cells by restoring their production of p63—the stem cells' anti-senescence protein. The renewed power of skin's stem cells allows the skin to recover after resurfacing procedures faster and without side-effects.

Another way SRCPs help your skin's stem cells is by regulating copper level. Low tissue copper causes skin's stem cell to proliferate, while high tissue copper cause them to differentiate into cells needed for repair.

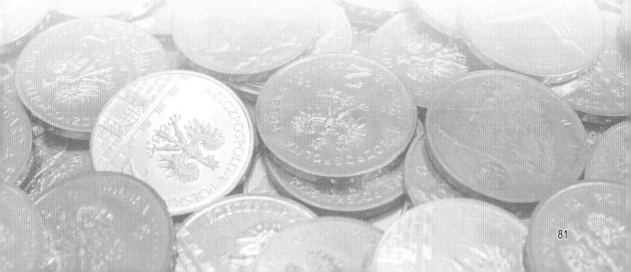

Decorin—Your Collagen Building Anti-Scar Protein!

Scar tissue is formed from coarsely organized loose collagen, while proper skin structure requires well-organized, uniform collagen fibers that are woven into a tight and resilient network. The protein that oversees collagen formation is **decorin**—a small proteoglycan produced by skin fibroblasts. When there is not enough decorin, scars are formed. An addition of decorin to wounds prevents scar formation.

SRCPs have also been scientifically proven to increase decorin production in fibroblasts thus creating a proper wound healing environment. Not only do they ensure that the skin puts collagen to its proper use rather than re-creating the scar tissue again, but they also help tighten the skin making it more resilient and elastic after healing. No scars and fewer wrinkles—now isn't that a dream come true!

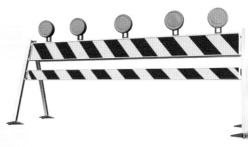

· · · · · · · · · · · When Too Much Really Is Too Much
Every healing process goes through some inflammation stage that helps the skin to get rid of bacteria. This inflammation process is regulated by certain molecular factors such as TGF-beta, TNF-alpha and prostaglandins. However, if those factors are produced in excess, both chronic inflammatory conditions and scarring can occur. Fortunately, SRCPs work beautifully controlling inflammatory chemicals and curbing inflammation.

First Restore Health, Then Remove Blemishes

No matter which method of scar removal you may choose, whether it is gentle methods that I recommend such as hydroxy acids and retinoic acid or harsh skin resurfacing methods, the first step for removing blemishes is to baby your skin back to health.

Before you can remove lesions, you need to heal your skin and strengthen it. My recommendation is to use a combination of SRCPs and biological healing oil, such as Emu Oil-S or Squalane, for two weeks to a month to help nurse your skin and revitalize it. SRCPs used several weeks before scar removal ensure high activity of skin's stem cells and prompt regeneration. When your skin is in better shape, you can then add the use of hydroxy acid and/or retinoic acid to speed skin-lesion removal. I recommend that you wait before using more aggressive methods and give gentler approaches a fair trial first.

THE BALANCING ACT FOR REMOVING SCARS AND BLEMISHES

Rather than pain outweighing gain, I have found ways to remove blemishes while reducing irritation. It's a balancing act that performs slower than some methods. However, it works gently and you will emerge with a clear radiant complexion. Over years of observations, I discovered a number of routines that help remove many types of blemishes (scars and pitted scars, skin tags, moles, sun damage, stretch marks, warts, hyperpigmentation, discoloration, and so on).

If you use both hydroxy acids and SRCPs, they work together in a balanced way to lessen irritation and eliminate blemishes. I recommend you alternate applications of moderate-strength hydroxy acids and SRCPs. The hydroxy acids gradually loosen and dissolve the blemished tissue, while the SRCPs help rebuild new skin. This method is slow, but effective and does not cause excessive skin irritation.

To remove blemishes, I suggest applying an SRCP product in the morning. In the evening you can rub hydroxy acids into the trouble spots. The most potent hydroxy acids (those higher than 5%) and Skin Biology products work fastest, but they can irritate the skin so use them with caution. Many of my clients also find that retinoic acid and/or abrasion, such as dermabrasion, pumice stones, and needling (subcision), can also help speed the removal of blemishes.

Perfecting The Balancing Act

The hydroxy acids and SRCPs work best when used daily. Some clients with severe scars have experienced radiant results by applying the products up to four times daily (for example, a hydroxy acid at 8 a.m., a SRCP product at noon, a hydroxy acid at 5 p.m., and a SRCP product before bedtime). You should see an improvement in about a month, but some old scars, such as stretch marks and keloid scars, may take six to eight months to slowly fade. Skin usually reverts to its pre-damage color.

Strong hydroxy acids can make your skin more sensitive to sunlight. So use a sun protectant that contains a physical sunblocker such as pure titanium dioxide if you decide to apply hydroxy acids during the day. Or as mentioned earlier, apply hydroxy acids and/or retinoic acids at night and SRCPs in the daytime.

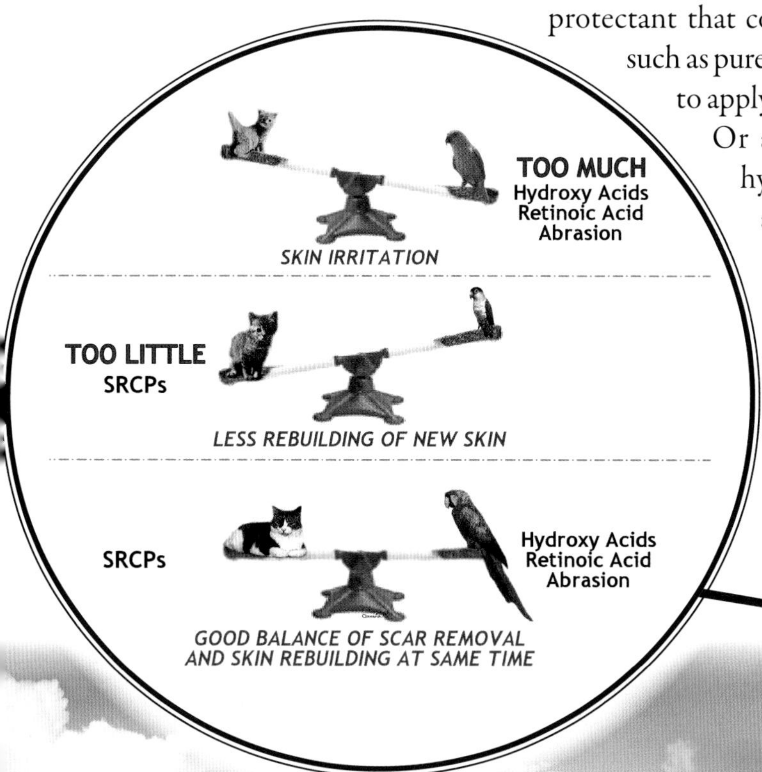

TOO MUCH
Hydroxy Acids
Retinoic Acid
Abrasion

SKIN IRRITATION

TOO LITTLE
SRCPs

LESS REBUILDING OF NEW SKIN

SRCPs

Hydroxy Acids
Retinoic Acid
Abrasion

*GOOD BALANCE OF SCAR REMOVAL
AND SKIN REBUILDING AT SAME TIME*

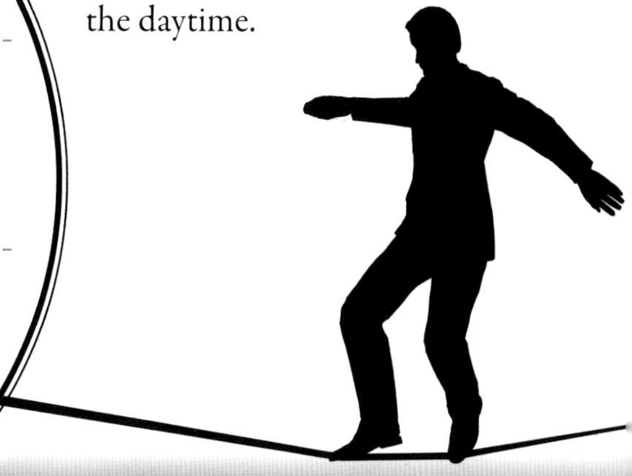

Remember, blemish removal is a balancing act. If you remove too much blemished skin with hydroxy acids, you may end up with a gaping hole marring your beautiful complexion; if you use too few SRCPs, you may not rebuild your skin enough to see results. Depending on your skin type and condition, you may have to use more or less of the blemish-reduction products. In general, it is best to go slowly. Your skin can only change and improve so fast. When it comes to glowing skin, patience is a virtue.

How Hydroxy Acids and SRCPs Work

In a sense, hydroxy acids do their magic by inflicting damage in order to remove scars and blemishes, which are also forms of skin damage. Hydroxy acids, such as salicylic acid and lactic acid, are widely used as exfoliating agents and for skin peels. They remove dead skin cells and can also loosen and slowly dissolve skin lesions such as acne scars, skin tags, stretch marks, sun-damage marks, and moles.

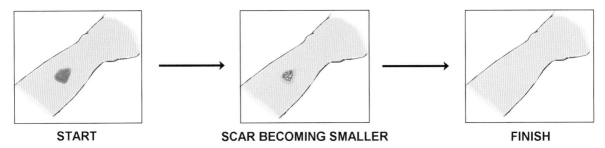

START   SCAR BECOMING SMALLER   FINISH

It may appear ironic that hydroxy acids need to cause damage in order to remove damage. Aaah, life and skin can be an enigma as we balance cosmetic contradictions! So here is the nitty gritty secret behind the action of hydroxy acids. Normal healthy skin can resist the damage inflicted by hydroxy acids where as unhealthy lesions cannot survive this acidic assault. When healthy skin is treated with hydroxy acids, it quickly repairs with the aid of the SRCPs. The only difference is that this time it heals properly without bothering to restore skin lesions and imperfections. This means that your newly restored skin will be healthy, smooth and blemish-free, provided that this repair process goes through without a hitch. And that's what SRCPs are there for—to ensure correct and flawless regeneration.

The acidic environment created by the hydroxy acids also activates some enzymes and immune cells that help remove damaged skin and lesions. As a result, hydroxy acids will dissolve most skin lesions when used over a period of a month or longer allowing new unblemished skin to rise to the surface. This approach offers a gentle alternative to normal skin-peel techniques that employ a very strong hydroxy acid (or other peeling agent such as TCA or phenol).

Skin peels work well under perfect circumstances. However, they can severely irritate skin when it is unable to fully regenerate and heal as a result of strong acid treatments. In other words, if too little skin rebuilding takes place, the peeling agent may cause further scarring or inflammation. However, by using an SRCP product after the hydroxy acids, you create an environment that prompts the regeneration of normal, healthy skin. Hydroxy acids and SRCPs complement one another; while the repeated application of hydroxy acids slowly dissolves skin blemishes, SRCPs aid in the rebuilding of healthy, smooth skin. As the skin is rebuilt and scars are removed, the elastic properties of the skin pull it into a smooth surface.

REDUCTION OF ACNE SCARS AND PITTED SCARS

Now this may sound obvious. But if you want to reduce acne scars, you need to avoid new breakouts.

The following regimen has been found effective by many of Skin Biology's clients, both for preventing and reducing acne scars and other pitted blemishes. As with all scars and blemishes, the key is to be patient and keep working on the scar.

1. In the morning, wipe your face with a 2 percent salicylic acid pad (available at drugstores).

2. After the salicylic acid pad, apply Super CP Serum (a SRCP cream which contains a small amount of salicylic acid) and leave it on. Start with a maximum of four drops daily, and then slowly increase the amount. If you have sensitive skin, start with Super GHK-Copper products which provide gentle healing.

3. In the evening, apply a light amount of LacSal Serum (8.5% lactic acid + 1.5% salicylic acid in a supportive liquid) and leave it on.

4. For pitted scars, some people use stronger hydroxy acids and/or retinoic acid at night.

5. About every two weeks, use pore-cleansing strips (available at drugstores) on acne-prone areas. Be careful not to overuse the strips to the point of irritation.

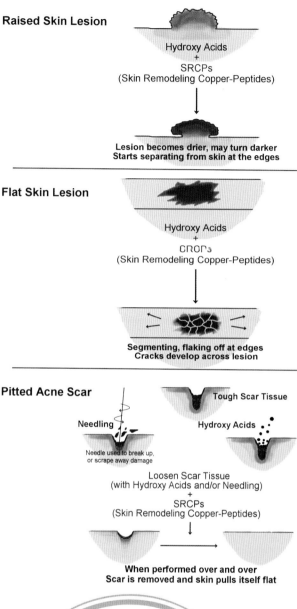

Raised Skin Lesion

Hydroxy Acids
+
SRCPs
(Skin Remodeling Copper-Peptides)

Lesion becomes drier, may turn darker
Starts separating from skin at the edges

Flat Skin Lesion

Hydroxy Acids
+
SRCPs
(Skin Remodeling Copper-Peptides)

Segmenting, flaking off at edges
Cracks develop across lesion

Pitted Acne Scar

Tough Scar Tissue

Needling

Hydroxy Acids

Needle used to break up, or scrape away damage

Loosen Scar Tissue
(with Hydroxy Acids and/or Needling)
+
SRCPs
(Skin Remodeling Copper-Peptides)

When performed over and over
Scar is removed and skin pulls itself flat

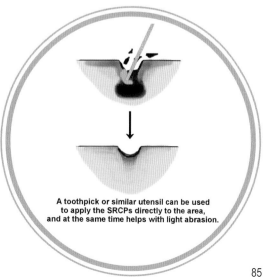

A toothpick or similar utensil can be used
to apply the SRCPs directly to the area,
and at the same time helps with light abrasion.

6. Some people use this method one day and anti-acne products on alternate days.

7. Anti-acne products and Super CP Serum can be somewhat drying to the skin. Emu Oil-S works well as a moisturizer and rarely increases breakouts.

REDUCTION OF SKIN TAGS
How would you like to reduce your skin tags? What?... You've never heard of a skin tag? Well then tag, you're it! Skin tags are small, generally benign skin growths. They often fall off naturally, and hydroxy acids are known to speed up their removal. Applying SRCPs also seems to help by aiding the recovery of normal skin around the skin tag.

The following regimen has been found effective by many of Skin Biology's clients. Some skin tags are more resistant than others, but you should see significant results in about a month.

1. In the morning, apply Super CP Serum very lightly on the skin tag.

2. In the evening, apply LacSal Serum or LacSal Cream (a 10% hydroxy acid product) to the tag.

3. On alternative evenings, you can apply stronger SRCPs such as TriReduction Cream with Retinol or Super Cop 2X - Extra Strength.

Sometimes LacSal Cream's salicylic acid irritates the skin tag and it becomes reddened. If this happens, you may want to reduce the frequency of application, but try to find a schedule that allows you to keep applying the cream on a regular basis.

REDUCTION OF STRETCH MARKS
Stretch marks arise when your skin needs to stretch rapidly and ends up getting over extended as a result of pregnancy, body building and weight gain.

The following regimen has been found effective by many of Skin Biology's clients. It will take about a month before you notice an improvement, and the

DEPRESSED SCARS
Why Things May Appear to Look Worse Before They Look Better

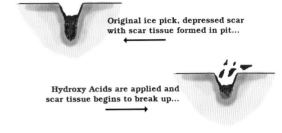

Original ice pick, depressed scar with scar tissue formed in pit...

Hydroxy Acids are applied and scar tissue begins to break up...

As scar tissue is removed, scar may become deeper for a time...

But this does not last, SRCPs help rebuild healthy skin and slowly the depressed area fills in!

LAYERS OF DAMAGE
What Truly Lies Beneath Your Skin

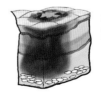

Damage from acne infection appears on top of skin layer, but reaches deep into skin...

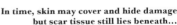

In time, skin may cover and hide damage but scar tissue still lies beneath...

As hydroxy acids + abrasion + SRCPs work on the skin, the damage that was below may be revealed...

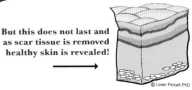

But this does not last and as scar tissue is removed healthy skin is revealed!

© Loren Pickart PhD

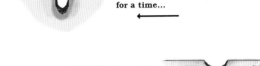

best results may take several months. Be patient; we have had reports from women saying they were able to remove stretch marks from pregnancy that were up to 30 years old!

1. In the morning, apply TriReduction Cream, Super CP Serum, or Super Cop Cream 2X - Extra Strength to the stretch mark.

2. In the evening, apply LacSal Cream or Lactic Power 10 to the stretch mark.

3. On alternative evenings, apply another application of the SRCP Cream of your choice (TriReduction Cream or Super Cop 2X - Extra Strength).

REDUCTION OF SUN DAMAGE Sun worshipers beware: many years of ultraviolet light can darken the skin and cause precancerous lesions such as actinic keratoses. This type of sun damage can be markedly reduced or removed by using a combination of SRCPs and beta hydroxy products and/or retinol. After about a month of treatment, the lesions should appear less noticeable as they diminish in size and thickness. After a week, you may notice a slight flaking of the skin around the periphery of the damage. This is usually followed by a shrinking and thinning of the lesion.

The following regimen has been found effective by many of Skin Biology's clients:

1. In the morning, apply a light amount of Super CP Serum to the sun-damage mark. If you have sensitive skin, start with Super GHK-Copper products which are gentle to sun-damaged skin.

2. In the evening, apply LacSal Cream lightly on the sun-damaged area.

3. On alternative evenings, you may want to apply TriReduction or Super Cop Cream to treat sun damage. Start with a light application. For the sensitive breast and décolletage area, use Protect & Restore for Breasts, Nipples, and Décolletage.

HYDROXY ACIDS
How They Work to Reveal HIdden Buried Damage

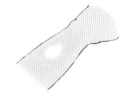

1. Damaged skin with blotchy tone

2. Damage starts to heal and is covered with new skin

3. Years later: Damage seems to fade

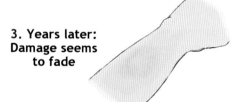

4. Exfoliation with hydroxy acids may uncover scar lines

REDUCTION OF MOLES You can slowly reduce and remove moles. No, I'm not talking about the burrowing mammals with small eyes staring at you. I'm talking about that dark pigmented growth on your skin. What did you think? You remove these unpleasant growths with mild hydroxy acids and copper peptides. However you can achieve faster results with stronger products. Some skin clinics apply 70 percent glycolic acid to moles with a cotton-tipped swab for six minutes. This must be done by a skin-care expert. When the acid is washed off, you can apply a copper peptide product such as CP Serum. Continue to apply CP Serum at bedtime for a few more days. After this procedure, many moles drop off in two to three days' time.

If You Want Faster Results

If you want to see quick results, you may use stronger hydroxy acids with most of the skin-care regimens in this chapter. However, these potent hydroxy acids also increase the chances of irritation or chemical burns. The strongest Skin Biology product is LacSal, a 10% hydroxy acid solution (8.5% lactic acid and 1.5% salicylic acid) at pH 3.2 and Lactic Power 10 (10% pure lactic acid). Some estheticians and clinics use 20 percent salicylic acid or 30 to 70 percent alpha hydroxy acids to loosen scar tissue followed by the copper peptide product. You can obtain these potent hydroxy acids from estheticians and dermatologists or from the resellers in the Resources Chapter.

A number of our clients use the pads (17% to 40% salicylic acid) and salicylic acid (12% to 17%) solutions that are used to remove calluses and warts. These work well on many types of skin lesions, but again be cautious to not over use such products. Apply the pads or solutions at one time of the day, or on alternative days, and use SRCPs at different times.

Skin Abrasion and Scar Reduction

Methods that mildly abrade skin can also hasten the removal of scars, especially when you combine them with hydroxy acids and SRCPs. These abrasive techniques include microdermabrasion, microdermabrasion sponges or cloths, and needling (subcision). Some old scars get especially tough, fibrous and difficult to decompose. Physically abrasive techniques break down scars and thereby allow the hydroxy acids to start dissolving them.

Microdermabrasion works well for elevated or flat scars. Microdermabrasion sponges or cloths work especially well for small skin lesions since you can focus on abrading a small area. The cloths cost about $10 each. But be careful, they are deceptively potent and you can easily overuse the product.

Subcision, performed by an esthetician, can break up depressed scars such as pitted acne tissue. In this procedure, a needle (similar to a tattoo needle) disrupts the scar collagen and stimulates its replacement by newly formed collagen. The best results are achieved with several sessions.

Some estheticians tell us that they use CP Serum or TriReduction after the needling and see a much improved and faster clearing of the scar.

However, do not apply the copper peptides until the wound has scabbed over and is no longer open or oozing liquid.

POST-PROCEDURE HEALING
After Peels, Laser Resurfacing, and Dermabrasion

In addition to reducing many types of scars, hydroxy acids and SRCPs can enhance healing after skin peels, laser resurfacing, and dermabrasion. The rest of this chapter will describe how to use hydroxy acids and SRCPs effectively during post-procedure recovery.

After a Chemical Peel

While medium and deep chemical peels may improve damaged skin and promote a rosy glow, they also can produce severe irritation that leads to scars and prolonged redness. Oh no! I can read your mind now. How can a treatment that improves skin also damage it? Well, as we discussed, proper skin care requires a balanced approach. Although medium or deep peels may remove abnormal tissue faster, to ensure that the skin heals properly this time you need to create the right environment.

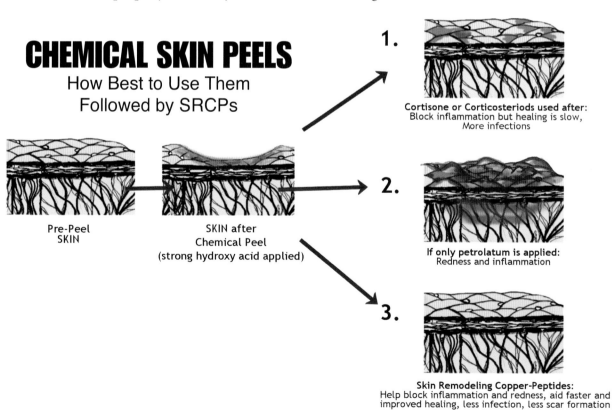

CHEMICAL SKIN PEELS
How Best to Use Them
Followed by SRCPs

Pre-Peel
SKIN

SKIN after
Chemical Peel
(strong hydroxy acid applied)

1.
Cortisone or Corticosteriods used after:
Block inflammation but healing is slow,
More infections

2.
If only petrolatum is applied:
Redness and inflammation

3.
Skin Remodeling Copper-Peptides:
Help block inflammation and redness, aid faster and
improved healing, less infection, less scar formation

After a peel, you will probably want to apply some type of moisturizer and/or anti-inflammatory to reduce irritation. However, I do not recommend petroleum jelly or other simple coverings since they do not prevent redness and inflammation. I must also discourage you from applying cortisone, often used as an anti-inflammatory. Cortisone can defeat the healing process since it inhibits skin repair.

Then what do you end up with? Thin skin! Now you may wish to appear slim and trim in your designer jeans, however thin skin loses elasticity... not a pretty sight to behold.

Fortunately, SRCPs can rebuild our skin and reduce irritation. So it's good-bye thin skin and hello to a beautiful complexion. Unlike cortisone, which inhibits skin repair, SRCPs are anti-inflammatory and enhance repair; they inhibit the action of interleukin-1, a cytokine that increases skin damage after injury, and TGF-ß-1, the scar-forming protein.

After a chemical peel, some of our clients have experienced dramatic results by following these steps:

1. In hot climates, apply TriReduction after the peel. This product contains SRCPs and high levels of squalane and octyl palmitate as skin protectants.

2. In cool climates, apply CP Serum followed by Emu Oil-S after the peel.

3. The first use of SRCP products should be within two hours of the peel, then on a twice-daily basis. Use the products lightly.

After Laser Resurfacing and Dermabrasion

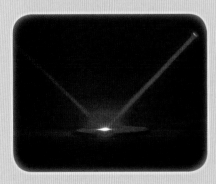

Again, some of our clients have experienced dramatic results by following these steps.

1. Apply CP Serum to the skin within two hours of the procedure.

2. Apply a thin coating of CP Serum daily to the healing skin. Be careful to use only a light coating. Too often, people think more is better.

SKIN THAT IS IRRITATED, REDDENED, OR HAS NEW SCARS

As we discussed, chemical peels can irritate the skin and make it sore. This may sometimes lead to visible burns and hyperpigmentation. Unfortunately, this unpleasant phase can last for a year or longer after the procedure. The following regimen should assist in the recovery and hasten the healing time.

1. Apply Emu Oil-S until all of the soreness is alleviated.

2. When the soreness is gone, apply CP Serum followed by Emu Oil-S on a daily basis. Be careful to use only a light coating of CP Serum. A small amount of CP Serum is quite effective.

This road to recovery may take time. However, you should notice a significant improvement in a month. If you suffer from severely burned or irritated skin, it may take several months for a full recovery.

ROSACEA

Often rosacea (The Curse of the Celts) can be controlled by the use of mild skin cleansers, such as Skin Biology's Dr. Pickart's Cleanser, followed by CP Serum and Emu Oil-S.

HELP FOR HYPERPIGMENTATION AND HYPOPIGMENTATION

When sun, chemicals, and other elements discolor and damage the skin we end up with either too much melanin (hyperpigmentation) or too little (hypopigmentation) which can create the illusion of a blotchy pincushion. Now that's no fun! Hyperpigmentation often contributes to brown and red spots and highly pigmented lesions. In cases of hypopigmentation, the loss of pigment can appear as a white rash as seen in cases of vitiligo and albinism.

We recommend that you treat hyper/hypopigmented areas in the same manner as you would treat blemishes and scars. You can remove almost any skin blemish (this includes hyperpigmentation or hypopigmentation) with a combination of hydroxy acids, skin abrasion, and Skin Remodeling Copper Peptides (SRCPs). The hydroxy acids and abrasive methods slowly loosen and dissolve the blemished tissue while the SRCPs help to rebuild new skin.

Many of our clients have shared their success stories as they successfully reduced scars and hyperpigmentation. It may take a while...but it has worked for many.

1. If you have oily-to-combination skin, apply Super CP Serum in the morning and LacSal Serum at night. Start the products lightly and then slowly increase the amount over time.

2. If you have dry-to-normal skin, use TriReduction P&R with Retinol in the morning and LacSal Cream at night.

3. If you are not getting enough effect, try Super Cop or Super Cop 2X Extra Strength.

4. If you still are not getting enough of an effect, then slowly work up to a stronger percentage hydroxy acid product.

5. Microdermabrasion sponges or cloths often work well on reducing scar tissue.

6. Daily supplements of 0.5 gram Vitamin C, 1 gram MSM, 1 gram of Flaxseed Oil and 500 mg of Borage Oil also help skin rebuilding.

7. Stress inhibits skin repair and the rate of scar reduction as it increases blood cortisol. DHEA (75 to 100 mgs daily) may help block the cortisol effect and stimulate skin repair. But only take DHEA for short periods of time, such as one month, if you are experiencing great stress.

8. Regular aerobic exercise increases blood flow into the skin and speeds skin repair and scar reduction. According to recent studies, it also causes the DNA to produce more proteins that are characteristic of young skin, so you get a double benefit—faster healing and younger looking skin.

Skin color will usually revert to its pre-damage color.

SKIN NEEDLING AND ROLLERS FOR SCAR REDUCTION
The following article, written by **Dr. Phillipa McCafferey** of **Clear Skin Care** in Australia (clearskincare.com.au), is designed to make clients aware of a technique for scar reduction utilizing skin rollers or needles. Many clients have used this method successfully along while using copper peptide products.

"Skin Needling has been performed for many years, using a variety of instruments, to soften depressed scars and deep lines. Dr Philippe Simonin, a Swissfrench Dermatologist, published his results in Baran's Cosmetic Dermatology 1994, but his ground breaking technique, which he named Electroridopuncture (ERP), remained largely unknown to the wider medical community. In his study of 600 patients, he examined results for 2 patient groups—one with Skin Ageing and the other with old Scars. He performed 10 treatments on all patients.

In the patient group with Skin Ageing, 40% showed significant improvement, 22% moderate improvement and 13% some improvement—as measured by comparative skin imprints. In the patient group with old scars, 60% improved with 5-6 treatments. Best results were obtained for old fibrous and depressed scars.

Another pioneer of Skin Needling was Dr Andre Camirand, a Canadian Plastic Surgeon who made a chance observation of improvement in the texture and depression of the scars of some of his facelift patients, who had undergone tattooing for scar camouflage. He experimented with tattooing facelift scars without pigment, and noted improvement in texture and colour. He published an article on his results in JACPS in 1992. Dr Camirand postulated that hypochromic (depigmented) skin repigmented through the transplantation of melanocytes (pigment producing cells) from normal skin into the hypochromic (depigmented) skin during the needling procedure. He also reported flattening of hypertrophic (overgrown) scars. He performed his needling procedures using a high speed tattoo gun, under local anaesthesia and treated each scar to pinpoint bleeding. He repeated the procedure every 2 to 8 weeks and no side effects or complications were reported.

Skin Needling can be safely performed on all skin colours and types. There is no risk of post-inflammatory hyperpigmentation (pigmentation of the skin as a result of skin trauma) as the melanocytes remain, like the dermis, intact during Skin Needling. This is the major distinguishing safety feature when comparing Skin Needling and other invasive procedures that are used to treat deep lines and depressed scars, ie laser resurfacing, deep chemical peels and dermabrasion. Skin needling with a skin roller produces hundreds of tiny dermal injuries. Each dermal injury triggers the body's natural wound healing response within the skin, producing and depositing new collagen in the treatment area. Each successive treatment triggers the production and deposition of new collagen that progressively fills in depressed scars and deep lines. This infilling process can continue for up to 12 months after a treatment has been performed.

Distinguishing safety features of skin needling include:

- Reduced risk of infection
- Significantly reduced downtime period for healing
- Significantly reduced comparative cost

Results vary between patients, with some achieving 90%+ improvement in scarring and others less than 50%. However, all patients achieve some improvements. There are now a number of skin rollers available for home use and they come in many different needle lengths, needle diameters and needle numbers, which can make it very confusing for their users. In my own practice, I have tried many different needle lengths and needle diameters, in an attempt to determine the best combination for treating scars and rejuvenating the skin. The number of needles on a roller is the least important feature, as repeated rolling causes numerous dermal injuries. Needle diameter is very important as we are seeking to maximise the dermal injury without creating a new scar. In my experience, 0.25mm needle diameter is the maximum that can be used without causing a new scar in the skin. Smaller diameter needle skin rollers can be used but do not maximise the dermal injury and therefore will be slower to produce results.

Needle length is also a critical issue. The target when we needle the dermis is a layer in the upper dermis called the intermediate reticular dermis. This dermal layer contains the highest number of stem cells which are able to produce new collagen.

The epidermis (the outer layer of the skin) varies in depth from .05mm on the eyelids to 1.5mm on the soles of the feet. The epidermis of the face (other than the eyelids) varies from 0.3mm to 1mm in depth and therefore a 0.75mm to 2mm needle length is more than adequate to reach the intermediate reticular dermis. In my experience, needles more than 2mm in length have a tendency to catch and tear the skin.

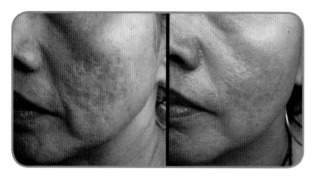

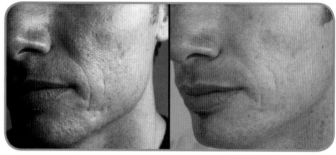

Skin needling is now well established as a treatment option for depressed acne scarring. It is a far more cost effective option than fractional laser therapy and delivers very similar results with repeated treatments. As the skin has a memory and will seek to return to its previous state, I recommend repeated Skin Needling treatments over a period of 1 to 2 years. I also recommend that my patients continue home needling to ensure the longevity of their scar improvement. And home needling can be safely combined with the use of CP Serum and /or tretinoin to maximise improvements in depressed scarring."

Skin Needling plus Copper Peptides
Skin Biology clients are using the following techniques to gain great results in diminishing scars and deep wrinkles.

Note: Use all skin needling rollers as directed by the manufacturer. Do not misuse by performing skin needling more often than the instructions indicate. In the following graphic it mentions that one could use the device "later" after an application of hydroxy acids. "Later" means the next time you use the device. It does not mean these devices should be used twice a day.

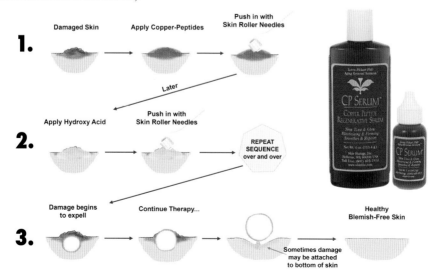

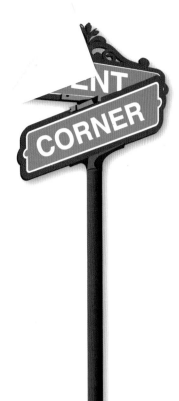

CAN COPPER PEPTIDES + HYDROXY ACIDS WORK FOR STRETCH MARK REDUCTION? YES!

"I just ordered the products and I'm going to begin treating my stretch marks just as soon as the products arrive. Here is a picture of my 9-year-old stretch marks…I'm in this for the long haul so I think I'll take pictures once a month. I'll post them no matter what the results are.

I'm also using glycolic acid that I bought from Platinum Skin Care. I bought the 70% which can be diluted to whatever percent you want. The glycolic acid breaks down the scar tissue, the copper peptides restore the collagen and elastin to your skin and the Emu Oil helps it penetrate into the skin. My goal is to be back in my bikini and hip hugger jeans by next summer so I'm going to be aggressive and consistent.

These are the products I'll be using:
Exfol Cream or LacSal Cream
TriReduction Cream
Emu Oil-S Lipid Replenisher
Glycolic Acid

I'll be exercising and drinking lots of water too."

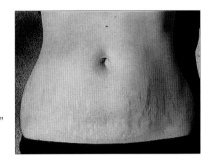

THREE MONTH UPDATE:

"Three months into treatment. I love the results so far!!! I'm working the area very hard right now. I use 40% glycolic acid in the morning (I leave it on for 5-10 minutes). I then use Super CP Serum and a thin layer of Emu Oil. In the afternoon I repeat this. At night when I'm in the shower I use a micodermabrasion cloth and scrub like crazy. After I'm out of the shower I put Super Cop and Emu Oil on right before bed. I'm also taking MSM, Vitamin C, Multi-Vitamins, and Vitamin B.

Some of the small marks are definitely fading. The bigger ones are not as deep and are very smooth. When I would lie down and rub my hand across my stomach I could feel the stretch marks – I CANNOT feel them anymore (except for one on my right side by my hip bone – but that one is much smaller....I can't wait to see how much things improve in the next several months. I'm hoping I can be in my bikini next summer. Thanks Skin Bio!…

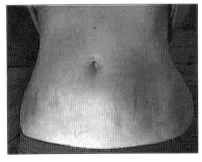

The [Skin Biology Chat] forum has really helped me with and during this treatment…This treatment has truly worked and is still working. My stretchmarks are not completely gone—but they are hardly noticeable now (some of the smaller and not so deep ones are GONE). I honestly believe if I keep at it they will disappear.

Now, I don't mind it when my shirt rides up and my stomach shows because you can't see my stretch marks unless you're right up on them. Before you could see them across the room because they were bright white/ silver. As you can imagine I'm very happy with this!! Yippee!!

I'd like to add that I also use TriReduction several times a day too (sometimes 3 or 4 times). I have a tendency to use it like a lotion. I use Exfol Cream (very rarely) only when I don't have time to wash off the glycolic acid. I bought the microdermabrasion cloth off of Ebay and use that every day…Everyone is different[,] so find what works for you (some people might not have to be as aggressive as I have been, others might need to take it to the next level).

I told myself (and my hubby) that I'll give this a year and then I'm getting a tummy tuck...my husband didn't want me to go that route. So, this has literally saved me from surgery. I can't thank Dr. Pickart enough! What he has created gives people hope and can really change their lives—just amazing!" -B.W.

PLEASE HELP MY SKIN THAT HAS HYPO-PIGMENTED!

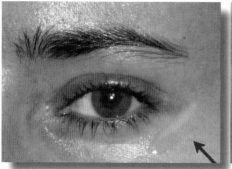 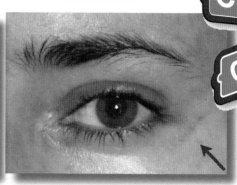

"Hi, I had a light Erbium laser on my face and have been experimenting a little with regular CP Serum and Emu Oil....I will try a drop today mixed with some emu and check for reaction....(After a couple of weeks pass:)...Thankfully, it is most definitely improving but I was getting a little itchy with a slightly darker rim around...I've been using the drop gently applied on and around the area topped with emu twice a day...I have never had hypopigmentation before but am hoping it will continue improving like this. Still there but definitely not so obvious!"

Latest Update (about a month thereafter):
"Although it suddenly turned a bit hyper pigmented early into using the CP's I was still relieved, very much preferring that to hypo and I consider it something of a triumph because at least I can do something about that...The white patch in the before picture wasn't a blister any longer at that point, as it seemed to heal pretty quickly into a flat white patch. I used a drop of CP on it morning and night at that point which was overdoing it because of my haste and it was getting a bit itchy. A diluted drop perhaps once a day would probably have lessened the pigment that developed but I can easily work on that later."

OTHER SCAR REDUCTION TESTIMONIALS

"I've been using the Copper-Peptide Serum for approximately two months....Within the past couple of weeks, I've seen incredible results – both visible and tangible! I've tried countless products in an attempt to address my post-acne problems, but SRCPs have proven that I can remedy them using the 'remodeling power of my own skin!'...

This is just one example I cannot help but share: I had tried to heal hypertrophic scarring I had along my jaw line. SRCPs had removed them entirely. Not only do I feel more confident about their removal, but I no longer experience the intense itching associated with their presence. I used to go to the doctors to get injections directly into the lesions – very painful and expensive AND they still persisted!! They even persisted AFTER I visited another doctor to get pulsed-dye laser treatments done!! I would avoid touching my jaw area because they were so discomforting... now I must get used to touching the smooth, healthy skin!! It's such a relief. I couldn't have imagined that my skin itself could be encouraged to remove the damage.

I have so many positive things to state about SRCPs – so many more things that it's probably not a good idea to keep rambling on! It has given me a renewed hope about gaining control of my skin...of returning it to the state before I had my unfortunate bouts of acne. I was once considering getting more laser treatments for my scarring. I don't think so any more. I don't have to spend millions on questionable procedures or risk further damage to my skin. I cannot wait to see the improvements a month, two months, three months from now. This is truly the greatest investment I could have made, and I thank Dr. Pickart for bringing us such a marvelous product. SRCPs are nothing short of miraculous. Not only have they improved my skin quality, but they have given me a significant boost in self-esteem – that is golden." -R.O.

"I had a biopsy scar on my neck...It was about as large as a dime. Without using the SCRPs on it, it had stabilized in about 3 months. It was red (I have scars that are still red after years), the walls on the side were vertical, it was much lower than the rest of the skin, and it was very noticable.

I started using Exfol Serum on it, then immediately plopping Super CP Serum on it (one full drop from the bottle originally filled the scar indentation - it was pretty large). Well the edges are sloped now, the bottom of the scar is rising, and it's pink, not red. The skin in the middle of the scar is even with the non-scarred surrounding skin. A nice bonus - since I'm not terribly careful about where I plop the stuff, there's a surrounding area of skin that is FANTASTIC, and the freckles that were there have faded, some have even disappeared (I did not like my freckles)!!!! I use it twice a day when I remember, which isn't as often as I should. When I put it on, I'll also pinch the skin between my thumb and pointer finger and gently rub - one of my friends who is a massage therapist and works with people who've had car accidents says that helps break up scar tissue a little, but very gently.

I wish I'd taken before pictures now, but I didn't terribly want a reminder of the scary skin cancer biopsy stuff. If the scar is completely gone by the time I'm done, I will actually be glad to have no reminders of that horrible time. Yay!" -MBP

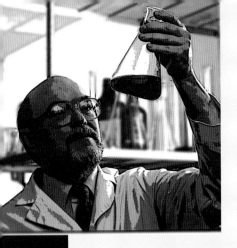

PIGMENTATION PROBLEMS There are at least three mechanisms of skin darkening. The first, includes an increase of melanin production in response to skin injury. The second results from local accumulation of dead skin cells (keratosis) which leads to a darkening of the skin color. Finally, abnormal proliferation of melanocytes in response to a chronic damage can result in lentigo (or what is commonly referred to as age spots).

Hyperpigmentation that occurs after aggressive cosmetic procedures such as lasers, deep chemical peels etc., or after acute skin traumas, is usually because of melanin. Stressed keratinocytes (skin cells) produce signal molecules that command pigment cells (melanocytes) to increase melanin production. In the case of very acute or repetitive stress injury, skin cells may become permanently hyper-activated (or "reprogrammed") and the darker spot will persist.

Keratosis also results in skin discoloration, since areas with thick horny layers look darker. This can be corrected by consistent alpha hydroxy acid application. Dark spots on the skin of elderly people (lentigo) may be the result of decades of sun damage and possibly from other damaging factors as well. In case of lentigo, there is an increased number of melanocytes in the darker area. Lentigo may be more difficult to remove than normal hyperpigmentation.

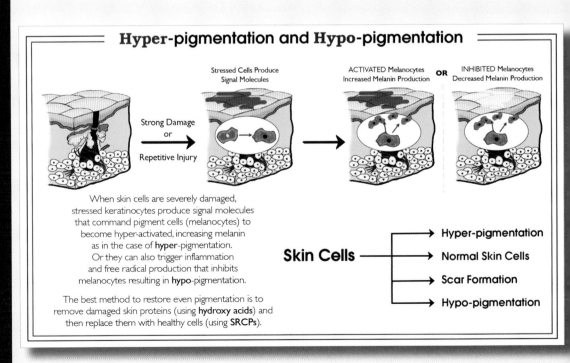

Hyper-pigmentation and Hypo-pigmentation

Stressed Cells Produce Signal Molecules

Strong Damage or Repetitive Injury

ACTIVATED Melanocytes Increased Melanin Production **OR** INHIBITED Melanocytes Decreased Melanin Production

When skin cells are severely damaged, stressed keratinocytes produce signal molecules that command pigment cells (melanocytes) to become hyper-activated, increasing melanin as in the case of **hyper**-pigmentation. Or they can also trigger inflammation and free radical production that inhibits melanocytes resulting in **hypo**-pigmentation.

The best method to restore even pigmentation is to remove damaged skin proteins (using **hydroxy acids**) and then replace them with healthy cells (using **SRCPs**).

Skin Cells →
→ Hyper-pigmentation
→ Normal Skin Cells
→ Scar Formation
→ Hypo-pigmentation

WHAT IS "BURIED SKIN DAMAGE"?
At times removing damaged skin can cause deeply buried scar tissue to become more visible. It is this buried skin damage that is often covered over with normal skin. As such deep damage becomes visible, it is important to focus on the use of SRCPs (to trigger faster production of healthy skin cells) and hydroxy acids (to break down and remove damaged tissue).

Can you see buried skin damage?
Dr. Austin Richards (of Oculus Photonics LLP) is a consultant in the field of infrared and ultraviolet imaging. He has years of industrial experience developing invisible-light imaging systems and applications. Dr. Richards developed the UVCorder™ out of the necessity for a digital imaging solution in the near-ultraviolet band. He is the author of the book *Alien Vision: Exploring the Electromagnetic Spectrum with Imaging Technology*, as well as numerous articles and papers on the subject of invisible-light imaging. For more information see: www.UVCorder.com

What can the UVCorder™ reveal?

UVCorder™ is a hand-held digital ultraviolet imaging solution that serves a very practical purpose. In the case of revealing buried skin damage, excess melanin production is much easier to show in the UV light band than in the visible band. Scars and blemishes can be seen in the UV months after they have faded to the naked eye.

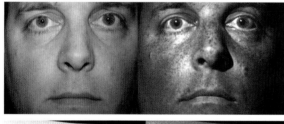

Facial skin with mild sun damage.
Left-Visible, Right-UV

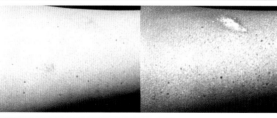

Burn mark on skin.
Left-Visible, Right-UV

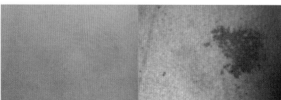

Injection mark on skin.
Left-Visible, Right-UV

The only method to remodel the skin is the removal of buried skin damage and subsequent stimulation of healthy skin cell production. This formula of using copper peptides plus abrasion to repair damage is not a cosmetic cover up or "quick-fix". It takes time, patience, and consistency. But many clients have found it effective in helping remove damage from the inside out—in time revealing younger, healthier, tighter skin.

"Dear Skin Biology, I just wished to thank you for your excellent products. I have been using copper-peptides for about 7 weeks now, for the last few weeks I have been using Super Cop 2X, putting it on my acne scars with a small metal spatula...For exfoliation I have been using Exfol Cream and a dermabrasion cloth. For the last week I have been using the dermaroller. The effect on my skin and in particular upon my scars is amazing. My scars have improved so much I no longer need to wear make up. And from being quite noticeable on both cheeks you now have to peer hard to see them. Thank you so much. I shall be building my collection of Skin Biology products as and when I can." -N.A., Scotland

"I've been using a soft-bristled toothbrush to apply copper-peptides. I dipped the toothbrush into the CPs, sometimes diluting the CPs with a bit of water to adjust the strength; then, I gently rubbed and abraded the areas of pitted scarring with the CP-soaked bristles. This is just a modification of the 'toothpick' method Dr. Pickart recommended for more expedient scar reduction, but I had difficulty utilizing that technique. I think that the 'toothbrush' technique helps breakdown the scar tissue, and allows the CPs to penetrate into the depression more effectively. I found it very easy to overdo the toothbrush abrasion, and I had a bit of slight pinkness and tenderness of the skin when I became too overzealous in the scar removal. I have noted quicker improvements in the appearance and feel of my scars since I have been applying the CPs in this manner as compared to when I just rubbed the CPs in with my fingers... My experience so far leads me to believe that I may have found a quicker way to reduce the appearance of pitted scarring for my skin." - Client Submission

"I woke up today with massive improvements over yesterday. I can't believe this stuff actually works. Dr. Pickart is truly onto something here." - Client Submission

"I have been using a flat foot file on my scars, pulling my skin tight I abrade my skin...It sounds awful but since my skin has peeled I can see a huge difference. It must be done carefully, but it's definitely working on my stubborn scars that strong TCA peels cannot fix." - Client Submission

"I've been using SRCPs for almost a year now off and on. After making the mistake of being too aggressive initially, I've finally reached the point where I can apply Super Cop 2X all over my face with no irritation...I just wanted to pass on a trick that really helped me with irritation, dry skin and blemishes. One of the products I use (Royal Jelly) came with instructions to 'compress' it on the skin. To do this you just run the washcloth under warm water, squeeze out the excess then apply your product in a layer over the cloth and press it on your face for 5 minutes. (I do it in 5 sections - each cheek, nose, chin and forehead). I was curious to see if this worked with other products so I tried it with Emu Oil and also with CP Serum after using a dermaroller. And wow....it does. The Emu Oil seemed to just melt into my skin and there was less of a residue after I removed the cloth. I just rubbed the excess in. The next morning my face felt great. I try to do this at least 2-3 times a week with various products and have noticed a great improvement in my skin. Less blemishes, redness and flakes. I highly recommend it!" - W.N.

"I've had great improvement to a very old and tough scar with regular application of lactic acid, some needling, and Super Cop 2X. The scar is still visible and I've still got some ways to go, but the change is quite remarkable. I've got hair regrowth to the scar, and its much flatter and softer. Its also regained its sensitivity like normal skin has. Before, I would feel no pain at all if I pricked the scar with a needle." - M.Y.

"I'm really surprised to see results already on my facial skin just using your new Super GHK-Copper Serum around my mouth, and it's not been a full month. It takes months to rebuild serious collagen, I know. However, last November I did a TCA peel (18%) around my upper lip area. It "took away" what vertical lip lines I had but left superficial, thin "line-like" red marks in certain areas that had not yet faded. I was covering these with makeup. Well, those reddish marks are no longer visible...They were there before I started, but after 24 or so days of use, I can't see these red marks left from the TCA peel. It's gotta be the copper." - V.C.

"I just wanted to report that another mole disappeared from my face. This one was the biggest of the entire face and was slight raised. Was about 1.5 millimiter diameter. Overall, it took about 6 months of strong CPs and 3 months of strong acids....I cannot see any brown spot under it, so I am fairly sure it wont come back... What has been more effective for me, for the last mole, has been pressing the 70% glycolic (pH 0.6) hard into the skin. I use a sort of Q-tip, which was originally designed for lip gloss. Its harder than Q-tips and sharper so it's perfect for small moles. Lately, I have been applying the glycolic acid for about 7-8 minutes, re-applying 3 times in those 7-8 minutes, and each time pressing the Q-tip hard into the skin. Super Cop 2X to follow and once a day every day.... I am really happy the big [mole] is gone. I have had it since the very first years of my life. Thanks everyone for the advice, and thanks Dr Pickart for your fantastic products!!" - R.

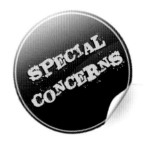

9

WHEN MAKEUP RAVAGES THE SKIN
FOR MODELS, ACTORS, AND MAKEUP LOVERS

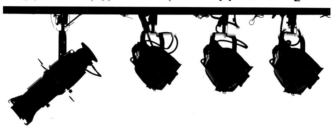

"**A**ll right, Mr. DeMille, I'm ready for my close-up." Most of us have that famous quote imprinted in our memories. Gloria Swanson, an aging starlet, walks into a scene of flashing cameras believing she still radiates the glow of her youth. Instead, we see decades of wrinkles earned from acting under hot lights. Yet, age is not the only factor that hampers an actor's skin. Even young actresses develop flaws that result from hot lights and harsh make up. From afar, we see a young star's silky skin sweep the screen. However in the close-ups and high definition we notice that she actually has skin riddled with moles, spots, or other skin damage. How can this be?

Many actors who make it in show business start out as stunning beauties with flawless skin. They often begin their careers as models before ending up on the big screen, and no doubt are successful in part due to their healthy, glowing complexions. However the celebrity life style can also damage an actor's beautiful claim to fame, a sad irony that is preventable.

"SPOTTED-FACED" BEAUTIES Actors and models lead unique lives. They face the spot light of fans and paparazzi who scrutinize their every move on screen and in magazines. No other profession requires the same dedication to appearance. Sadly, the celebrity lifestyle, which includes the constant application and removal of makeup, the harsh effects of stage lighting and a high level of stress, can take its toll on skin. This especially holds true for actresses and female models. However, makeup and stress plays havoc on all who love cosmetics.

Most damaging of all is the constant application and removal of foundation, eye shadow, blusher, and a whole bucket load of cosmetics. Both makeup (with its colored salts and chemical dyes) and make-up removers (which remove the protective acid mantle) are harsh on the skin. Actors and models need to quickly change makeup between photos and scenes. And many who don't live under the spotlights still like to change their makeup after work, before going out for an evening of festivities. This requires that they apply, remove and re-apply many coats in quick succession *(See dramatization)*. Other times, actresses wear heavy foundation for hours at a stretch before they strip away the pasty gook with a make-up remover at the end of the day.

Whatever the circumstances, the frequent application and removal of make-up makes the skin more susceptible to the development of skin damage, warts, moles, sun damage, and skin lesions. Therefore, it is essential for actresses, models, and all who adore makeup to learn how to properly protect and care for their skin.

SKINCARE TIPS FOR ACTORS, MODELS, AND MAKEUP LOVERS

Here are some easy steps to follow that are designed to address the specific concerns you may face...for your beautiful face.

General Guidelines

1. Before putting on makeup, apply a mild Skin Biology serum such as Super GHK-Copper Serum as a base to protect the skin. Super GHK-Copper creates an invisible shield to gently cushion your complexion against environmental havoc.

2. Hydroxy acids work well to remove dead skin cells and damaged skin proteins, dissolving flaws that impair a beautiful complexion. Use them if you will not be wearing heavy makeup under hot lights. Avoid using hydroxy acids in sunlight since they make skin photosensitive. You may want to use hydroxy acid products in the evening and SRCP products during the day.

3. Morning application of hydroxy acids or Super GHK-Copper products: When using hydroxy acids, exfoliate with a product such as LacSal Cream or LacSal Serum (which contain 10% hydroxy acids: salicylic and lactic acid). Apply lightly. When using Super GHK-Copper products to counter environmental damage, wash skin with a gentle cleanser such as Dr. Pickart's Face and Body Cleanser and follow with a light application of Super GHK-Copper Serum.

4. Evening use of SRCPs or hydroxy acids: SRCPs repair skin. Spot treat damaged areas with TriReduction Cream, Super CP Serum, or Super Cop Cream. Serums work best for combination or oily skin and creams work well, for drier skin. Apply hydroxy acids during the evening if you have used Super GHK-Copper Serum or CP Serum during the day. Some of our clients alternate their evening application between SRCPs and hydroxy acids.

To Protect the Skin After Makeup Sessions
1. Use only biological healing oils (BHOs) to remove make-up. BHOs are much healthier for the skin than harsh chemical removers, which have a drying effect. Oils such as Emu Oil-S, CELES Therapeutic Oil or Squalane work well.

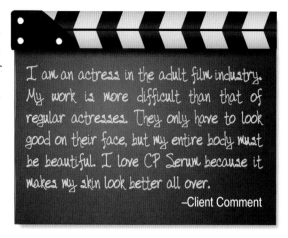

I am an actress in the adult film industry. My work is more difficult than that of regular actresses. They only have to look good on their face, but my entire body must be beautiful. I love CP Serum because it makes my skin look better all over.

–Client Comment

2. To remove makeup, first apply a BHO lightly to the face, and then rub gently to remove the makeup. Finally, rinse thoroughly with warm water. Any remaining oil helps replenish the skin's natural oils.

3. After you remove makeup, follow with a mild cleanser. Dr. Pickart's Face and Body Cleanser, with a pH of 7.5, is a good choice. Many soaps and cleansers not only remove surface dirt and oils, but actually damage the skin. Soaps that are alkaline, with a pH of around 10, destroy the skin's acid mantle. These harsh cleansers interfere with the natural protection imparted by the skin's protein/lipid barrier. A gentle yet effective cleanser keeps skin looking its best. Never over cleanse your skin.

4. Next lightly apply CP Serum to the face to help repair the skin's protective barrier and antioxidant defenses. In clinical studies at the University of California, SRCPs were able to stimulate skin-barrier repair within 24 to 48 hours. You may also want to alternate with applications of hydroxy acids especially if you use SRCPs during the day.

5. When applying CP Serum at night, finish with a light application of Emu Oil-S to help the skin retain a healthy glow.

FOR ANYONE WHO LOVES MAKEUP Although not everyone reading this chapter is a model or actor, many love to wear makeup. They enjoy dabbling at the cosmetic counter and find their vanity tables pouring over with colorful potions. They also may be aware that many products can harm skin. Yet the temptation to enhance lures them back to makeup bags brimming over with goodies and gook. Therefore, anyone with a passion for makeup can benefit from these skin-care tips.

Besides, if after adorning your face, you feel like a movie star... well what's the harm with that? Just take care of your skin and it will take care of you. In fact, if you use Skin Biology products, you may just find you look beautiful without makeup.

SKIN CARE GUIDE

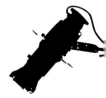

Special Concerns of Models & Actors

Consistent applications and removal of makeup (with its colored salts and chemical dyes) along with makeup removers (which damage both the protective acid mantle and the skin's protein/lipid barrier) are harsh on skin. Long hours of heavy makeup on the skin, scene changes, and touch ups, lights used in the industry and the stress to keep skin looking blemish-free can take its toll.

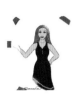

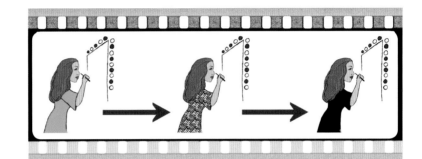

1. Before applying makeup, use a light protective layer of CP Serum on the skin.

2. Remove makeup with Emu Oil-S or Squalane, instead of harsh makeup removers.

3. Cleanse the skin with Dr. Pickart's Face and Body Cleanser.

4. Repair your skin with CP Serum or Skin Signals Solution and Emu Oil-S.

5. Remove damage marks with LacSal Cream, LacSal Serum, or Lactic Power 10.

6. Repair deeper damage with TriReduction, Super CP Serum, or Super Cop Cream.

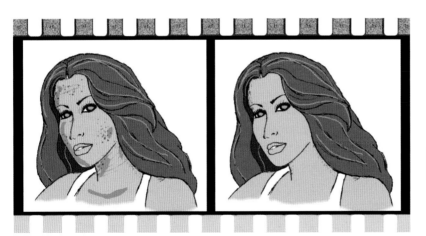

A SKIN BIOLOGY HOW TO GUIDE - DESIGNED FOR MY SKIN

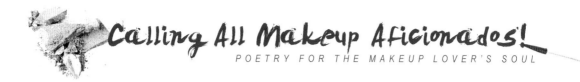
COSMETIC COUNTER ENCOUNTER

Today at the cosmetic counter

I cringed in a caustic encounter

with baby faced Jane,

age 18 and inane,

pushing products she can't even ponder.

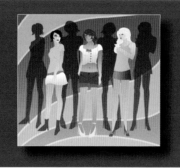

Modeling her wrinkle-free skin,

Jane claimed I could begin

to erase years from my face

and tighten my chin.

Clueless, her pitch made me flounder.

A wee babe in the woods has a hunch

That even pork rinds will make young skin glow.

The only miracle a sales clerk knows

is to sell enough junk to make money for lunch,

pushing potions in a corrosive road show.

Idelle Musiek

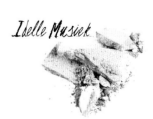

CARING FOR SENSITIVE AND EXTRA DRY SKIN
BioHeal, CP Serum, and Super GHK-Copper for "At-Risk Skin"

> "When they check for skin sores in the nursing home, the nurses, physicians, and technicians for blood-drawing come in and everyone is nervous. If you have a skin sore, they just slap an expensive bandage on it, which does nothing."
>
> –Comment from a client in California

The above quote, that came to me from an elderly client, demonstrates a sad reality regarding American health care. Although an "ounce of prevention" is worth a "pound of skin cure," it is difficult to convince the medical establishment to invest in the largest organ of our body. Hospitals and nursing homes often fail to maintain a patient's basic skin health. While Medicare will pay for complex bandages, they focus on selling expensive dressings to cover sores and offer little incentive to try low-cost measures to prevent complications (aka, Looting the U.S. Treasury). Just slap on a bandage to hide the symptoms: out of sight is out of mind when extra dollars can be made at the cost of health.

COMMON SKIN DAMAGING CONDITIONS

CONDITION PRODUCING SKIN DAMAGE	DEFECT INVOLVED
Diabetes	Inadequate protein synthesis
HIV/AIDS Condition	Insufficient immune cells for skin repair
Eczema / Dry Skin / Sjogren's Syndrome	Damaged skin barrier causes excessive water loss
Contact Dermatitis	Damaged skin barrier allows entry of irritants
Thermal & Radiation Burns	"Zone-of-stasis" around injury blocks blood vessel growth and wound repair
Post-Chemotherapy	Lack of sufficient immune cells for skin repair
Skin Allergies	Antigens cause free radicals that produce an inflamed state
Psoriasis	Abnormal production of skin cells that lead to skin barrier damage

Complications Caused by Damage to Skin Barrier

Skin barrier damage can be rapidly healed at an early stage of breakdown

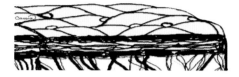

- -

IF NOT

Damage to the skin barrier may cause the following:

Irritants may enter causing eczema, skin allergies, and dermatitis

Viruses, fungi, and bacteria may enter causing infection

May start skin ulcers (diabetic, bedsores, venous stasis)

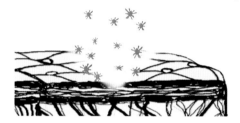

Symptoms of a compromised skin barrier include:

- *Irritation*
- *Skin Allergies*
- *Dermatitis*
- *Extreme dryness*
- *Inflammation*

In addition to helping the elderly, we can prevent skin problems for all who suffer from extra-sensitive skin conditions such as:

- Eczema
- Psoriasis
- Very dry skin
- Sjogren's Syndrome, an autoimmune disease with symptoms of dry/cracking skin
- Thermal or radiation burns
- After chemotherapy treatments
- Skin allergies to materials such as nickel, poison ivy, and poison oak
- Contact dermatitis
- An immune-compromised status (such as HIV or AIDS)

BIOHEAL AND CP SERUM CAN HELP If you suffer from extra-sensitive skin, you know that the pound of prevention analogy I mentioned is worth far more than the pound of pain you feel from developing open sores or cracks. The key is to prevent such unpleasant consequences with the aid of SRCPs. These products maintain skin health while preventing problems.

Besides not having to suffer from a painful wound, SRCPs offer important health benefits that can prevent serious damage from ever occurring in the first place.

Healthy skin possesses a strong resistance to irritants and microorganisms, but once damaged, it is prone to infections, inflammation, and allergic reactions. The result is direct damage to the skin itself, an inhibition of the normal repair process, the chronic generation of free radicals in the damaged area, or a combination of the three.

For individuals with limited mobility (such as people in wheelchairs), the attempt to maintain skin health poses a constant quandary. Chronic rubbing and pressure can cause irritation, bedsores and skin ulcers. It is vital that we heal these conditions rapidly in order to avoid serious complications.

I recommend three Skin Biology products particularly effective for those with extra-sensitive skin: BioHeal, Super GHK-Copper Serum or Cream, and CP Serum. BioHeal, a gentle, safe mineral cream, contains protective lipids that help the body heal damaged skin. I find BioHeal offers a safer alternative to cortisone and corticosteroids. Super GHK-Copper, milder than our second generation products, gently pampers the complexion. Super GHK-Copper provides a sensuous treatment that can help revitalize sensitive skin. CP Serum is a mild water-based liquid SRCP that easily spreads on the skin. I also recommend Dr. Pickart's Face & Body Cleanser (bar or liquid) to mildly cleanse the skin and Emu Oil-S to replenish natural lipids. In this chapter, I will also show you how these products can help improve the health of extra-sensitive skin while repairing damage.

PHOTOGRAPHS AT RIGHT – Example of healing "at-risk" skin: In the top photo, the patient has two open skin ulcers visible in the left, top and bottom of the photo. On the right side of the top photo, there are reddish fissures developing into skin ulcers. In the bottom photo, the application of SRCPs to the periphery of the skin ulcers has healed the fissured skin while the open ulcers still remain. It is in the early stages of skin breakdown that skin can be quickly healed.

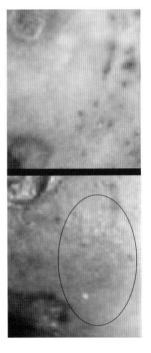

BioHeal helps rebuild the protective skin barrier formed by the acid mantle and underlying epidermal lipids. This barrier prevents the entrance of bacteria, viruses and irritants into the skin, limits water loss and keeps our skin healthy, smooth and well-moisturized. The acid mantle is the combination of sebum (oils) and perspiration that forms a protective emulsion on the skin rendering it less vulnerable to damage and attack by environmental factors, such as sun and wind, while leaving it less prone to dehydration. A healthy acid mantle maintains moisture and provides a soft appearance.

Caution: BioHeal, CP Serum, and other Skin Biology products are designed to improve skin condition, but are not substitutes for regular medical care by a qualified health-care professional. They should not be used on broken skin or large, deep wounds. If skin problems persist or worsen, consult a physician.

It Worked for Her!

To understand the dramatic benefits SRCPs have on extra-sensitive and damaged skin, consider the story of Joy Dawson (adapted from the Witchita Eagle newspaper). This 75-year-old middle-school substitute teacher suffered from eczema, a painful skin inflammation, on her index fingers and thumbs. After reading an article in the Witchita Eagle about non-surgical ways to reduce wrinkles, Joy tried CP Serum on her hands. She had previously tried lotions and salves from her dermatologist, as well as alternative medicine, without success. She even wore gloves to bed at night at the suggestion of her son, who is a doctor.

Joy commented that her hands had been so inflamed that "there would be cracks and splits, and they'd be bleeding." So she was intrigued by the newspaper article's reference to studies that reported how copper peptides reduce pigmentation, wrinkles, and retain moisture. The article went on to describe how copper peptide creams were originally developed for burn victims and diabetics whose wounds don't heal properly. Since Joy also suffers from type 2 diabetes, she didn't have to think long about trying CP Serum, which she ordered over the internet. Within a few weeks, her eczema and cracked skin vanished. Joy was full of joy as she reemerged with new healthy hands.

The mantle also has strong antioxidant properties since it contains lipo-soluble antioxidant vitamins such as retinol and vitamin E. Normal skin is somewhat acidic, falling into the pH range of 4.2 to 5.6. This acidity inhibits the growth of foreign bacteria and fungi and the skin remains healthier. Many cleansers and other skin-care products are alkaline (often having a pH of 9 to 10), which can strip off protective oils and exacerbate acne, allergies, and other problems.

The epidermal barrier is the next line of skin defense and it is formed by dead skin cells filled with hard proteins called keratin and glued together with a special kind of oil. It is like a fortress wall that keeps away allergens, irritants, and microorganisms. Strong detergents and solvents such as acetone can dissolve barrier oils and weaken skin barrier.

BioHeal is designed to adjust the skin's pH level into the acidic range. The product contains high levels of lipids such as squalane, cetyl alcohol, glyceryl stearate and stearic acid that resemble the fats of the acid mantle. Squalane/squalene are the skin's most important protective lipids, but they decline as we age (from levels of up to 15 percent in teenagers' skin to less than 5 percent in adults over age 60), resulting in dryer skin. BioHeal also contains allantoin, aloe, vitamin E, and retinol to aid the mantle's protective antioxidant properties.

Extra-sensitive skin is usually skin with a disrupted barrier and it carries a special danger in that it is prone to infection. Immune cells in the skin naturally produce hydrogen peroxide to fight bacteria. Many Skin Biology clients report good results by pre-washing the skin with 3 percent hydrogen peroxide for sterilization and blotting

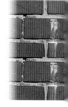

it reasonably dry before applying BioHeal. Some clinicians do not recommend the use of hydrogen peroxide because they say it increases skin damage. In contrast, my review of medical literature has found many reports of improved healing after washes of hydrogen peroxide at low concentrations (1 to 10 percent). However, skin damage is occasionally observed when applying higher concentrations. So any use of hydrogen peroxide on injured skin should be with strengths of 1 to 3 percent and no higher.

Treating Eczema

As Joy discovered, eczema responds well to SRCPs. This common disorder is caused by a combination of factors including slow skin-repair, exposure to irritants and an alkaline shift in the skin's pH. The mechanism of eczema is complex, but the trigger point is usually continuous damage to the skin barrier that allows the entrance of irritants. Therefore, the first and foremost step in preventing eczema complications is skin barrier restoration. Many clients have found relief from eczema by applying a light coating of BioHeal or CP Serum to the affected area daily, as the following letter shows.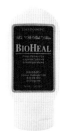

"Dear Sirs:

    Thanks for letting me try your BioHeal skin cream on my hand...The area of eczema on my right hand was about 2" long and 1.5" wide, very inflamed, sore, and continuing to spread. The problem started in October 1992 and I had given up hoping for a recovery—all the ointments I had been using allowed, at best, a temporary relief of the itching and burning. These ointments included a 1 percent and a 0.5 percent cortisone cream, a steroid cream prescribed by a doctor, and a coal tar from a health shop. Every time the hand started to look or feel a little better, the eczema would flare up again and I would be back to square one. Conditions that aggravated the eczema included chlorine in our swimming pool, bleach, and perfumed hand creams. I do not know how or why it started in the first place...

    Within the first few days of using your cream, I noticed the inflammation was reduced and the eczema had stopped spreading. About two weeks later, the cracks were healing well and the area was no longer tender. Now, three weeks later, there are just a few little scars that are quickly disappearing.

    I wish you the best success with the cream. I really thought my problem was here to stay, so thanks again." -Z.S., London, U.K.

Treating Very Dry Skin

As we age we tend to develop drier, less oily skin, prone to cracks and fissures, causing it to grow irritated, inflamed, and itchy. The condition worsens in areas with relatively few oil glands, such as the arms, legs, and trunk. We develop dry skin more often during the fall and winter due to a combination of low humidity and frequent bathing. Some dermatologists believe that dry skin has worsened in recent decades because we take more showers and baths today than in the past. People used to bathe only once or twice a year allowing their skin a chance to replace its natural oils between cleansings.

Conventional oil/water moisturizers can temporarily relieve parched skin, but they do not address the fundamental problem and can worsen the condition over time by weakening the outer protective proteins. Biological healing oils, such as Emu Oil-S and Squalane, are the best moisturizers for extremely dry skin.

Sjorgren's Syndrome

Clients with Sjorgren's Syndrome often prefer TriReduction with Retinol. This product alleviates dry skin while also helping to heal old scars that result from the syndrome. I received the following letter from a satisfied client who loved the product:

"I have Sjorgren's Syndrome and Lupus causing severe problems with very dry skin. I am prone to 'cracks' in my fingers due to Raynaud's, and 'burns' in other areas of my skin, including my face. I have used many expensive products trying to help the situation, with minimal results…I have never written about a product before, but the improvement has been so significant…I have been using Protect & Restore and BioHeal for about one month. Since using these creams, my skin is greatly improved with better texture and is significantly less dry. I was afraid to try anything on the burned areas of my face, but went ahead when I saw the improvement in other areas. The burns healed within days. More impressive, the unsightly scars from the steroids have been replaced with healthy skin. I have not had further problems of that type. In the past two weeks, I have received numerous compliments on my skin." –L.A., California

Treating Diabetic Skin Problems

Diabetes causes many skin-related problems. The most visible signs include slow wound healing, dry and cracked skin with loss of elasticity and tone. It is vitally important to rapidly repair broken and cracked

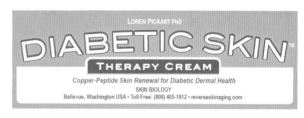

skin before an infection sets in. Leg and foot sores are the leading cause of amputations associated with broken skin that becomes infected.

Many diabetic clients who apply BioHeal tell us that daily applications lead to a quick improvement in skin health. Our latest cream, Dr. Pickart's Diabetic Skin Therapy Cream, is a welcome addition to our copper peptide product line designed specifically for the treatment of diabetic skin issues.

Treating Skin After Burns, Radiation Treatment, and Chemotherapy

Burns caused by thermal injuries, radiation treatment, and chemotherapy heal quite slowly. After the burn, a "zone-of-stasis" often grows around the inflamed tissue, turning it into an oozing sore or skin ulcer. Under these circumstances, the body does not receive the proper signals to heal the skin. This inability to repair can result in scarring and permanent damage. Chemotherapy also slows skin repair and increases the development of sores.

If your skin has been injured by any of these treatments, I recommend you apply BioHeal after the burn has scabbed over (about a week post-burn) or after treatment has finished. Use a light coating of BioHeal every day in the morning and evening as needed.

"A PATIENT OF MINE HAD A CHRONIC SORE FOR FOUR MONTHS ON HER CHEST AFTER SURGERY AND RADIATION THERAPY FOR BREAST CANCER. NOTHING SEEMED TO HEAL THE SORE SO I TRIED THE BIOHEAL AROUND THE PERIPHERY OF THE SORE AND IT HEALED OVER IN ABOUT THREE WEEKS. I HAD HER CONTINUE TO USE THE CREAM ON THE SKIN AREA FOR ANOTHER TWO WEEKS AND THE HEALING HAS BEEN COMPLETE." -J.D., NEW YORK

Treating Allergies

Approximately 25 percent of people are allergic to nickel, and many more are sensitive to plants such as poison ivy and poison oak. Many cosmetic ingredients such as fragrances and plant essential oils can cause skin rashes and allergies as well. For example, in Europe cosmetic manufacturers now list on the package 26 common allergens found in plant essential oils if they are present in the formulation. This measure was introduced due to many complaints from customers who developed rashes, skin redness and other problems after using products with those substances. BioHeal works well in these situations and is much safer than cortisone and other corticosteroids. Corticosteroids (including cortisone) stop the inflammation but produce damaged and thinned skin (often 50 percent thinner) by inhibiting the natural repair process. Overuse of corticosteroids can promote diabetic conditions, thymus involution, immune suppression, the spread of cancers, bone damage, and cataracts.

In one study, BioHeal both accelerated the recovery of skin after injury and had an anti-inflammatory action on the skin of nickel-allergic subjects who were exposed to nickel salts. (See references in Chapter 18). Many of our clients have also reported rapid healing of insect bites after using BioHeal.

Because allergies are so diverse, I recommend that you first test BioHeal on a small area of skin. If your skin responds well, apply a light coating once or twice daily until the allergy is resolved.

"Dear Skin Bio,
I am writing to tell you that your product BioHeal® took away my poison ivy. I have a history of problems with poison ivy since 1975. It is always treated in the same way, first soaps, then cortisone creams in increasing strength. This does not work. It keeps spreading and getting worse. I develop an allergenic reaction to it and end up on prednisone. The prednisone is very hard to take. Last summer I needed to be on the medication for three weeks and suffered through some difficult side effects.

I can't stay away from gardening. I got it about two weeks ago on my hands. It was suggested that I try some Protect and Restore®. I did and it took away the itch immediately and the blisters that were developing never did [develop]. Thank you! I only hope that others that suffer from poison ivy can know about Protect and Restore® and what it can do for them." -*Allergic*, Minnesota

Treating Contact Dermatitis

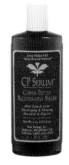

Contact dermatitis is an inflammation of the skin caused by direct exposure to an irritating substance. A corrosive chemical agent (an irritant) such as acetone or sodium lauryl phosphate, damages skin cells causing their membranes to break down, which in turn triggers an inflammatory response from the skin's immune cells. With repeated exposure the condition may become chronic. Healthy skin does not allow entrance to irritants, but as soon as there is some damage to the barrier, there is a high possibility of dermatitis.

This is why contact dermatitis often occurs after we shave or wax our face, arms or legs, because when we run a razor blade over the skin or pull out hairs with a waxing strip, we remove some of the skin's protective barrier. These hair-removal methods not only make the skin more prone to dermatitis, but they also allow bacteria and viruses to invade and thus infect our skin. Since viruses can cause warts, we often get these growths in frequently shaved areas, including the legs of women and the beard area in men. The more rapidly we heal our skin barrier, the better we can protect it against viruses and bacteria.

Another common culprit is nail-polish remover, which contains acetone or acetonitrile. This flammable solvent extracts skin fats, damages the skin on the fingers and cuticles, and often produces hangnails, skin flaking and increased incidence of dermatitis.

If you suffer from contact dermatitis, applying BioHeal or CP Serum to the affected area may help healing, as the following letter demonstrates:

"In researching contact dermatitis around the eyes, this was the ONLY site on the Web describing the condition. I ordered some CP Serum (already had Squalane) and Emu Oil-S. I have a cabinet full of oils that I purchased to get rid of this condition. Only the CP Serum and Emu Oil-S or Squalane helped heal it. I wasn't even able to wear makeup...I can now use Super CP and all my makeup. My eyes are looking great." -*J.B.*

AIDS and Skin Health

Persons with AIDS and HIV face a constant battle to maintain their dermal health. Small abrasions and cuts heal at a snail's pace due to their depressed immunity. Skin infections pose a never ending threat that can rapidly turn into annoying exudative lesions and mycotic infections. The SRCPs in products such as BioHeal and CP Serum have been shown to restore normal skin repair and hair growth in immunosuppressed animals: their immune systems were suppressed by pretreatment with cortisone or chemotherapeutic drugs (See references in Chapter 22). However, neither product has been approved by the FDA for use on open wounds or skin ulcers.

"Your copper blue cream really helps with my multiple skin annoyances associated with living with HIV for 14 years and AIDS now for 5 years. BioHeal is wonderful for my face to keep down the usually exudative type mycotic lesions and infectious irritations which are gone now after the Bioheal cream." -V.F., California

Treating Psoriasis

Five million people in the United States suffer from psoriasis, a skin condition that produces inflamed, itchy, thickened, and cracked skin. Many Skin Biology clients have reported that daily applications of BioHeal alleviate the problems associated with mild psoriasis outbreaks. In 1996, Professor DiJun Rong of Shanghai Medical University wrote Skin Biology: He claimed that after treating his psoriasis patients with BioHeal, he observed lesions and itchiness reduce and quality of skin improve. Copper peptides lower Tumor Nerosis Factor alpha (TNF alpha) a protein that may trigger psoriasis outbreaks. See Chapter 22, The Science Behind SRCPs. Here's another letter describing the positive effect SRCPs have on psoriasis.

"Hello there, Dr. Pickart!

I wanted to let you know that P&R [Protect & Restore, another SRCP product] has virtually eliminated my mother's psoriasis. It is truly amazing—she had a large patch on her right forearm that was constantly irritated from rubbing against the armrest of her wheelchair, and nothing was helping, so I gave her a tube...It showed immediate improvement, so when she finished one tube, and the psoriasis was diminished by about 50 percent, we got her another tube right away. Once that one was finished, there was just a light trace left, and we ordered a 4-ounce tube. She's barely gotten started on that one, and it's practically gone!... She will never be without your product again!" -D.H., Texas

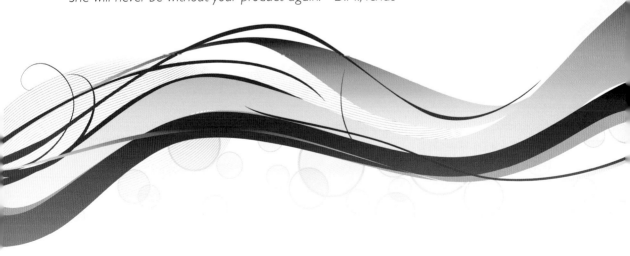

SRCPs Plus Emu Oil-S

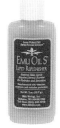

To enhance the benefits of BioHeal, Super GHK-Copper, or CP Serum to better treat eczema, psoriasis and other skin conditions, I suggest you follow these SRCPs with Emu Oil-S. The fatty acid composition of human skin oil shares a similar profile with emu oil. This similarity may offer one of the factors that enables emu oil to demonstrate such positive actions (Zemtsov et al 1996).

Numerous studies have shown the effectiveness of emu oil. A study by Lopez and colleagues found strong anti-inflammatory effects of topically applied emu oil after skin was exposed to a very strong irritant (Lopez et al 1999). Politis and Dmytrowich found that if emu oil was applied two days after injury, it aided the healing process. Researchers at the University of Texas Medical School found emu oil at up to 100 percent concentration in lotions to be non-allergenic, non-comedogenic, bacteriostatic, and to have low irritation potential (Politis & Dmytrowich 1998). Throughout history, emu oil has been used to help alleviate the discomfort of skin conditions such as arthritis, shingles, eczema, psoriasis, and other inflammatory conditions (References in Chapter 22).

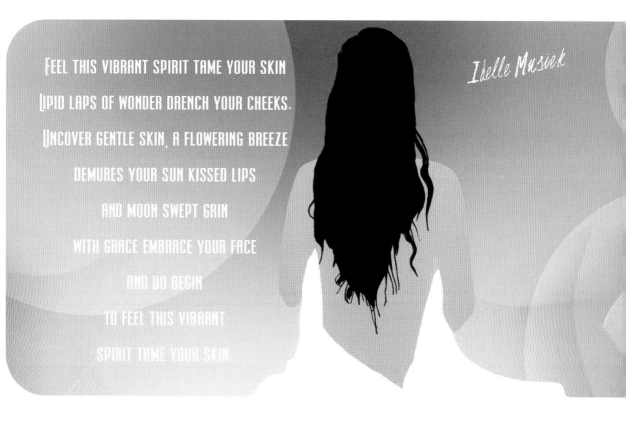

FEEL THIS VIBRANT SPIRIT TAME YOUR SKIN
LIPID LAPS OF WONDER DRENCH YOUR CHEEKS.
UNCOVER GENTLE SKIN, A FLOWERING BREEZE
DEMURES YOUR SUN KISSED LIPS
AND MOON SWEPT GRIN
WITH GRACE EMBRACE YOUR FACE
AND DO BEGIN
TO FEEL THIS VIBRANT
SPIRIT TAME YOUR SKIN.

Idelle Musiek

KEEPING YOUR SKIN YOUNG & BEAUTIFUL
WITH COPPER PEPTIDES

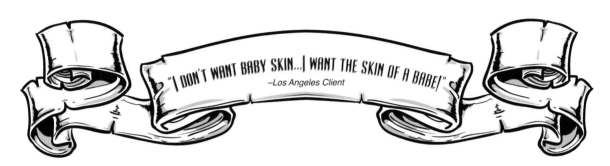

"I DON'T WANT BABY SKIN...I WANT THE SKIN OF A BABE!"
–Los Angeles Client

I s beauty only skin deep? Beauty may radiate from within but it begins with the skin... the skin of a baby. As a baby cries out and gurgles for attention, we experience her inner innocence and charm. At the same time, we are also drawn to the baby's skin, luring us to nurture this exquisite beginning of life. In every culture, the most coveted complexion can be observed on a young person between the age of 10 and 20, often admired for having skin like a baby. People with young, clear, blemish-free skin possess the power to impact others. Psychological studies covering 170 human cultures have found beautiful skin to be the number one factor in interpersonal attraction.

Beyond the musings of poets, gorgeous skin can be characterized as follows:

- ✔ · A clear, vivid look

- ✔ · A firm, elastic tone

- ✔ · Smooth and free of defects

- ✔ · Often has some lingering traces of "baby fat"

- ✔ · Free of skin breaks and cracks

- ✔ · A reddish tint (regardless of skin color) from profuse blood circulation

Biologically, these characteristics translate into healthy skin as follows:

✔ · A healthy acid mantle and strong protein/lipid skin barrier

✔ · A rapid turnover of skin cells

✔ · Collagen and elastin fibers in excellent repair

✔ · A constantly renewed blood circulation, ensuring an adequate flow of nutrients to the skin

✔ · Ample levels of water-holding molecules proteoglycans and glycosaminoglycans

✔ · The ability to heal itself rapidly after injury

✔ · High antioxidant levels (and anti-inflammatory proteins superoxide dismutase and decorin)

✔ · Adequate but not excessive natural skin oils

✔ · A high level of subcutaneous fat cells

With the proper skin-care regimen, beautiful skin is within your grasp. In this chapter, you will learn about many of the components of healthy skin and what you can do to keep your skin young and beautiful.

QUOTABLE QUOTES: *The skin of a delicate woman is an example of softness and smoothness united.*
—Uvedale Price

THE PROTECTIVE SKIN BARRIER
Research shows that with healthy skin we resist the damage and irritation which can age our complexion. The ability of the skin to resist environmental assaults depends on the integrity and reparative functions of the protective skin barrier.

This barrier has three lines of defense: 1) the acid mantle on the skin's surface, 2) the hard outer skin proteins of the stratum corneum tightly glued together by lipids and 3) the neuro-immune network of the epidermis.

When we compromise the barrier, we leave our skin vulnerable. This makes us susceptible to warts, moles, bacterial and viral infections, allergic responses, inhibited skin repair, more rapid aging, blotches or rashes. Since a healthy barrier waterproofs the skin, any breach in this fortress also increases water loss. Fortunately, we often don't even notice when we break our skin barrier because of excellent repair mechanisms. However, if the assaults to the barrier are too frequent or too severe (or if the reparative skin mechanisms are broken) the skin quickly becomes dehydrated, wrinkled and dull looking. Many so called anti-wrinkle creams do nothing more than add a bit of moisture to your skin, which instantly brings it back to life, erasing wrinkles and brightening complexion. But since those creams do not repair the barrier, the effect is very short lived and you have to reapply the cream to maintain the result. This is why it is essential to understand what makes your barrier strong and how to take care of it.

The First Line of Defense – The Acid Mantle

One way to preserve your protective skin barrier is to maintain a healthy acid mantle. The mantle, composed of sebum (oily fats) and perspiration, constantly secretes these products to cover the dermal surface. Normal skin pH is somewhat acidic in the range of 4.2 to 5.6. It varies from one part of the body to another and, in general, the pH of a man's skin is lower (more acidic) than that of a woman's.

The acid mantle benefits your skin in many ways. First of all, it has strong antioxidant properties. An antioxidant is a chemical that prevents the oxidation of other chemicals and in some cases helps the body fight infection. The sebum is rich in antioxidant vitamins such as vitamin E. Another antioxidant substance in the sebum is squalene, which in young healthy skin constitutes up to 12% of sebum lipids. If the acid mantle's antioxidant level is depleted (for example, if there is not enough squalene or vitamin E), the excessive oxidation of skin lipids can lead to the buildup of reactive oxygen species (free radicals that contain oxygen) and subsequent damage to underlying skin barrier structures.

The mantle also repels water. Your acid mantle behaves like a duck out of water, fending itself from environmental pitfalls. The fats in the mantle repel water much as the oil on a duck's feathers wards off water. This keeps water from loosening and damaging the skin's outer layers of hard protective proteins and lipids. It also renders the mantle less vulnerable to damage and attack by environmental factors such as sun, wind, and dehydration.

The mantle inhibits bacterial growth. The acidic pH of the mantle inhibits bacterial growth on the skin, especially the growth of foreign pathogenic bacteria and fungi. As a result, the skin remains healthier and has fewer blemishes. Also low pH supports the growth of beneficial skin bacteria such as lacto-bacteria that protect the skin from pathogenic invaders. Be aware that overuse of antiseptic skin soaps, astringents and hand-sanitizers can deplete beneficial bacteria on the skin and open the gate to the dangerous pathogens.

In addition to the low pH, your acid mantle has one more surprise for the omnipresent pathogenic microorganisms—antimicrobial peptides! They are just like natural antibiotics with the difference that they do not have any side effects and are very efficient in eliminating viruses, bacteria and fungi.

𝕿𝖍𝖊 𝕾𝖊𝖈𝖔𝖓𝖉 𝕷𝖎𝖓𝖊 𝖔𝖋 𝕯𝖊𝖋𝖊𝖓𝖘𝖊 – The Epidermal Barrier

The acid mantle covers the skin surface. But even more skin barrier structures lie beneath it, in the upper layers of the epidermis. This epidermal barrier is built from hard keratin proteins glued together by lipids. Today it is known that these lipids have a highly organized structure resembling liquid crystals. Once the structure is disrupted, the barrier becomes much more permeable to water and toxins. To maintain barrier structure, the skin needs a good supply of essential fatty acids, in particular linoleic and gamma-linolenic acids. Harsh soaps and aggressive cleansers containing alcohol and acetone can disrupt the crystallic structure of the skin lipid barrier, increasing water loss and making skin more vulnerable to infection.

Keratin must maintain an acidic pH to keep the protective proteins tightly bound together and to maintain its hardness. More alkaline pHs weaken the lipid glue which thereby softens and loosens the fibers of keratin. This creates gaps in the barrier that allows allergens, irritants, bacteria and viruses to penetrate into the skin. Acne, skin allergies and other dermal problems grow more severe when the pH becomes more alkaline.

𝕿𝖍𝖊 𝕿𝖍𝖎𝖗𝖉 𝕷𝖎𝖓𝖊 𝖔𝖋 𝕯𝖊𝖋𝖊𝖓𝖘𝖊 – The Neuro-Immune Network

The third line of defense in the skin barrier multilayered fortress is a neuro-immune network formed by the sensitive nerves and reactive immune cells.

In addition to normal nerve endings that transfer the feeling of touch and temperature from your skin, the upper layer of skin is traversed by special kinds of sensitive nerve endings. Those are the nerves that make you shudder when some insect crawls over your skin, no matter how small or insignificant. They also can react to wooly clothing (remember that old sweater your grandma wanted you to wear when you had a cold?), and to caustic and irritating substances.

When the sensitive nerves of the epidermis are agitated, they secrete special chemicals (neuro-peptides) that make your skin itch and burn. This sensation makes you want to scratch your skin and remove the irritating object or substance. If an offending agent doesn't go away that easily, the sensitive nerves send a signal to the immune cells residing in the epidermis—Langerhans cells.

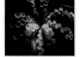

The Langerhans cells resemble little octopuses and spread their "tentacles" to the skin's surface. They can detect allergenic foreign substances, bacteria and other microorganisms. The sensitive nerves and the Langerhans cells maintain a close relationship and usually alert each other when either of them sense trouble. However, you don't want your sensitive nerves and Langerhans cells to get alerted because first, they will make your skin burn and itch and second, they can set off an alarm summoning all the forces of the immune system to fight invaders. A war is never pretty and the war inside your skin is no exception. So you better keep your first two lines of defense strong and avoid a conflict escalation.

PROTECTING YOUR DELICATE SKIN

Your skin, like a fragile flower, needs to be nurtured. The following methods will minimize damage while protecting your delicate skin.

1. Cleanse your face, hands, and bathe only as needed.

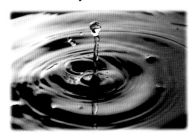

Take showers no more than once a day except for when you participate in athletic activities. When we bathe too often, we remove the skin's natural oil layer, which evaporates moisture from our skin. These oils help retain water which makes our skin supple and soft. If you want moist skin, baby it with short showers and minimize baths.

When you soak in baths, you lose precious oils and dry your skin. If your skin is dry or irritated, cleanse with lukewarm temperatures since hot water parches skin. Limit your time to 15 minutes or less in the bath or shower. Use a minimum amount of soap. Long, hot baths, although wonderfully relaxing, should be limited to once or twice a week.

Take care of your skin after cleansing. When toweling, gently rub the skin. Blot or pat the skin dry so there is still some moisture left on it. Apply a biological healing oil, such as Emu Oil-S, Squalane, CELES Oil or squalane/octyl-palmitate, after bathing. You might also want to add these oils to your baths to minimize moisture loss.

2. Use a mild gentle soap.

In order to keep your skin at the proper pH, you need to choose your soap carefully. Since each pH unit has a 10-fold difference in alkalinity, soap with a pH of 10.5 has 10 times the alkalinity of soap with a pH of 9.5. Even "mild" soaps are often quite alkaline (with a pH of 9.5 to 11) and can damage the skin by stripping away the acid mantle. Most soaps also contain a high level of synthetic detergents which loosen the protective wall of keratin proteins and lipids. Irritated and eczematous skin tends to have a more alkaline pH. When you wash with soap, you increase this alkalinity thus making your skin even more vulnerable to irritation and infection. One easy way to maintain the desired pH of the acid mantle is to use lactic acid skin care products. Lactic acid is an alpha hydroxy acid that is naturally found in the skin and it provides the safest way to boost your skin pH balance. Use Lactic Power 10 exfoliator in the evenings after cleansing your face. Apply gently to your face being extra careful around the eye areas, since they may be sensitive to the acid.

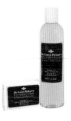

Strong soaps remove the beneficial bacteria that occurs naturally in our skin to protect us from harmful bacteria that can cause disease. I especially recommend that you avoid harsh antibacterial soaps, which not only kill friendly bacteria, but also make us less able to fend off the harmful bacteria as we grow resistant to these soaps. Limit the use of soap to areas that develop an odor, such as the armpits, genital area, and feet.

A FEW HUNDRED YEARS AGO, MARIE ANTOINETTE SHOCKED
THE FRENCH COURT BY BATHING AT LEAST WEEKLY
THE FRENCH ARISTOCRACY STUCK TO THEIR TWICE YEARLY BATHS

Make sure you rinse all the soap from your skin after washing or before you leave the tub or shower.

Skin Biology carries a cleanser in their product line specifically for sensitive and damaged skin (Dr. Pickart's Face and Body Cleanser) which I originally developed for the fragile skin of cancer patients after chemotherapy or radiation treatments. The cleanser comes in a clear, translucent bar or liquid and contains no harsh detergents, caustics or "flash" foaming agents. The pH of 7.5, ranks far below the alkalinity of other soaps. Nurses and physicians report that Dr. Pickart's Cleanser works well on sensitive and fragile skin conditions such as eczema, psoriasis, diabetes, in the bedridden and after cancer therapy. Strong soaps can literally dissolve fragile skin.

3. Saunas, hot tubs and steam baths provide blissful alternatives to bathing and showering since they cleanse without soap and can beautify your skin.

Scandinavian men and women, who take daily saunas, are famous for their sensational complexions. While dry saunas range between 160-170 degrees Fahrenheit, the skin temperature only reaches about 104 degrees due to water evaporation.

The heat generated by saunas, hot tubs and steam baths creates an almost magical effect on the body. Whereas long baths damage the skin barrier, brief exposures to hot water or steam can heal and soothe your senses. This special form of heat has been found to improve blood flow, lower blood pressure, kill disease organisms and inhibit cancer growth. Saunas can detoxify the body from heavy metals including mercury, lead, cadmium and aluminum. Some gerontologists have suggested that high heat may increase the production of free radicals. However, humans residing in warm habitats share a similar maximum life span to those in cold climates. Many cold-blooded reptiles live short lives while birds such as crows, with a temperature of 105 to 110 degrees F, can thrive for more than 90 years.

Saunas, hot tubs and steam baths soften the oils and waxes that clog our pores allowing them to function normally while removing the waxes. It's kind of like "Liquid Plumber" unclogging our pipes. Our skin, the largest organ in the body, excretes wastes as we sweat. While taking a sauna, the heat induces us to perspire and thereby clean the accumulated residue of dead cells, rancid oils, bacteria and perspiration wastes.

As exhilarating as a sauna, hot tub or steam bath may feel, please take some caution before plunging in. Let your body adapt over several weeks before you increase the temperature of the unit and the time you spend in it. Do not eat for two hours before heating your body. You should not raise your body temperature above about 105 degrees F, even after you have acclimated. After using a sauna, hot tub or steam bath, let your body cool down slowly, for the same reason as you would after vigorous exercise—to allow your vascular system to readjust to normal function.

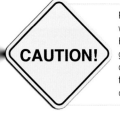

Pregnant women should exercise special caution when taking saunas, hot tubs and steam baths. However, when enjoyed properly, they can benefit greatly from their use. A study of Finnish women, of whom 98.5 percent use saunas while pregnant, found common birth defects to be among the lowest of any country in the world (Saxen et al 1982).

Never take a sauna, hot tub or steam bath if you have been drinking alcohol. Alcohol coupled with the heat can cause extreme vasodilation, and blood pressure can drop to a point where you become unconscious. Inebriated hot-tubbers have been discovered after several days of slow cooking in the tub.

4. Avoid astringents and toners, which are drying to the skin. They make the face look very clean and smooth by stripping away the top layer of oil and briefly tightening the skin. However, the skin responds by increasing oil production.

5. Many skin researchers consider pure squalane from olive oil to be the best sexual lubricant. Most skincare companies refrain from selling it because of squalane's relatively high wholesale cost.

6. There are benefits to be derived from our botanical friends. Plants do more than beautify your room. When you fill your home with plants, you provide one of the best and pleasant ways to add humidity to the air and reduce dry skin. Alternately, a water humidifier will keep indoor air at healthy humidity levels.

KEEPING YOUR SKIN IN GOOD REPAIR Have you ever wondered why some young girls can seemingly break every rule that we discussed above, alternating between cheap color cosmetics and harsh makeup removers, using astringents and alkaline soaps, eating junk food and basking in the sun for hours and still have the skin that makes you green with envy? Although, treating your skin gently and protecting it from environmental assaults is very important, it is even more important to keep it in good repair. And this is where SRCPs can do their magic again.

To preserve a protective skin barrier we need to maintain good skin cell turnover —a constant flow of cells moving outward in the skin to supply new proteins and lipids to replace the older, outer layers. As we age, this revitalizing flow slows down making skin more vulnerable to assaults and less able to repair damage. However, as we learned in previous chapters, the aged appearance of our skin can be deceptive because even in very old skin, there is still a good supply of never-aging eternally young skin stem cells residing in the lower layers of the epidermis. According to the recent studies (see Chapter 18) SRCPs can revive the skin stem cells by stimulating the synthesis of p63—an anti-senescence protein. This allows us to use SRCPs to restore proper skin turnover and to ensure speedy restoration of the disrupted skin barrier.

SRCPs also aid in dermal restoration stimulating the production and repair of the elastic strings of our skin—collagen and elastin fibers. They also ensure that collagen strands properly assemble by stimulating the synthesis of a "collagen quality control" proteoglycan—decorin. By keeping your skin in excellent repair, SRCPs not only ensure strong barrier formation, but also smooth, resilient and wrinkle-free skin. For those of you over age 30, I recommend regular use of SRCPs along with the skin's natural hydroxy acids to speed skin-cell turnover. For skin maintenance, use the following products weekly: Apply mild or moderate strength SRCPs 3 to 4 times a week and an exfoliating agent such as 7 to 10 percent lactic acid or 1 to 2 percent salicylic acid (three times weekly should suffice). Additionally, many clients use retinoic acid two to three times a week.

Manual exfoliation also works well. As we discussed earlier in the book you can use a skin brush, a pumice stone or a buffer. Some of our clients abrade with a spot scraper to "flake-off" damage. Microdermabrasion and needling can also prove successful in removing damaged skin.

YOUR ROSY CHEEKS Regardless of the skin color, young skin has an attractive reddish tint indicative of good blood circulation. When the roses and peaches of youth start to fade, which usually happens after the age of 30, many women just start using more makeup. Although makeup is easy to buy and it masks the deficiency of circulation splendidly, it is not a solution. Profuse blood circulation of 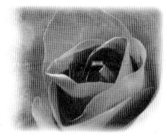 youthful skin is more than just a pretty color. It is an essential factor determining the skin's well being and its ability to repair itself. The sad examples of the grim consequences of the deficient blood circulation in the skin are bed sores and skin ulcers in elderly residents of nursing homes. You can think of it like this. Let's imagine a busy home construction site. To make the work go smoothly and without delay, you have to have a constant supply of building materials. As soon as there is an interruption or insufficient delivery of the materials, the work stalls. The same happens in your skin when blood supply is not adequate, because skin receives its nutrition and oxygen through the blood.

SRCPs re-establish new blood vessel growth in aged and damaged skin, speeding up skin's repair and restoring its youthful glow. They also dilate the constricted blood vessels, which increases oxygen perfusion of the skin. As a result, skin repairs itself more quickly and acquires this unmistakable clear and vivid look that indicates perfect health. Because of the general confusion created by many journalists who write about skin and cosmetics without obtaining any deep knowledge of skin biology, some have expressed concern that stimulation of blood flow may somehow lead to an increase of skin tumors. However, it should be pointed out that good blood circulation is found in the skin of babies and healthy, young people. It is an essential attribute of healthy skin. If it were true that excellent blood circulation itself could cause cancer, young people would get cancer much more often than older folks, which is not the case. Although it is true that tumors are notorious for their extensive circulation, it is very different from normal blood circulation that exists in healthy skin the same way as skin repair is different from abnormal cell growth that occurs in tumors.

Recently there has been a growing body of evidence that SRCPs in fact may have anti-cancer activity. According to researchers, they block the activity of some genes linked to tumor development and they increase the production of the anti-tumor

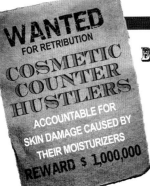

WANTED
FOR RETRIBUTION
COSMETIC COUNTER HUSTLERS
ACCOUNTABLE FOR SKIN DAMAGE CAUSED BY THEIR MOISTURIZERS
REWARD $ 1,000,000

BIOLOGICAL SKIN OILS vs. COSMETIC MOISTURIZERS

THE REAL SKINCARE SHOWDOWN

Dry, but Healthy Skin

Biological Oils Applied

Quick Fix Cosmetic Moisturizer Applied

Oils increase acid mantle. Skin surface proteins and lipids remain intact and protective.

Immediate Effect:

Skin retains internal moisture and is soft and supple.

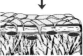

Added water and chemicals loosen skin protein/lipid barrier, penetrate and swell skin so that skin looks great for a few hours.

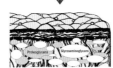

Using SRCPs and biological oils reduces water loss and increases water-holding proteoglycans and glycosaminoglycans.

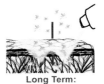

Long Term:
Viruses, bacteria, free radicals and pollutants enter the skin.

Less protective skin accumulates more moles, warts, lesions, and sun damage.

Methods of Skin Moisturization

METHOD	HOW IT WORKS	Time to be Effective	PROBLEMS	RECOMMENDED
SRCPs	Mimic natural repair, repair skin damage, and increase the skin's proteoglycans and GAGs	About 2-3 weeks	None	Protect & Restore and CP Serum
Waxes and Greases	Heavy oils such as petrolatum seal skin surface to water loss	Immediate	May disrupt the skin barrier	NO
Biological Oils	Oils such as octyl palmitate and squalane help reduce water loss. Oils similar to human skin oils: Emu Oil-S and Squalane	Immediate	Not as durable as waxes and greases but stimulates skin repair	Calypso's Oil, Octyl-palmitate, Squalane, and Emu Oil-S Lipid Replenisher
Retinol in Squalane	Increases natural skin oils	2 weeks	Avoid acne-prone areas	Retinol in Squalane
Quick Fix Cosmetic Moisturizers	Designed to improve the look of skin at cosmetic counters, mixtures of oils, water, and surface-active chemicals quickly swell the skin by rapid water uptake	5 minutes	Acts like irritant to loosen protective skin barrier, skin more susceptible to infection	NO

122

protein decorin (more details can be found in Chapter 18). The cancer incidence increases when the level of SRCPs in the organism declines, which also suggests that SRCPs play an important protective role.

KEEPING YOUR SKIN SOFT AND SUPPLE Does your skin dry as quickly as sand? No one wants quicksand hands. Not only does dry skin look and feel rough, it also loses its tone and resilience much faster than well moisturized skin. There are two mechanisms that deplete your skin from water:

1. *Damage to the skin's protective barrier, which produces excessive water loss through the skin.*

2. *A reduction in the concentrations of the skin's water-holding sugars and proteins, the proteoglycans and glycosaminoglycans/GAGs.*

In order to reverse these problems, I recommend you treat dry skin with biological healing oils such as emu oil or squalane to replenish its lipids and use SRCPs regularly to increase glycosaminoglycans and proteoglycans in the dermis.

Biological healing oils are superior to the vast array of hocus pocus lotions that promise youth in a jar. Rather than moisturize the skin, many cosmetic moisturizers often loosen the protective barrier and can actually age and damage the skin instead.

For thousands of years, our ancestors used biological healing oils to improve the health of their skin. Archaeological evidence reveals ancient peoples in Egypt, China, Assyria, Sumeria, Crete, and Babylonia were adept at extracting and blending aromatic plant and biological oils—using them as ointments, fragrances and incense for both medicinal and religious purposes. However by 1920, the cosmetic industry began advertising the idea that these oils harm the skin and merchandised the use of oil/water/detergent mixtures instead. This proves reminiscent of deceptive campaigns intended to banish women for breast feeding in order to sell synthetic infant formulas. Let us now explore how emu oil and squalane can rejuvenate your skin.

EMU OIL Australian aborigines discovered the benefits of emu oil thousands of years ago. This intensive skin moisturizer is the only easily-absorbed natural oil that molecularly mimics the oil found in human skin and all other organs of the body.

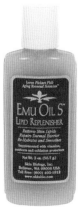

Both human and emu oil consist of monounsaturated oleic acid as the most prevalent element, followed by palmitic acid, and then by linoleic acid (an essential fatty acid required for lipid barrier formation). This high concentration of mono-unsaturated fatty acids explains emu oil's ability to penetrate easily through the skin. Emu oil performs its magic by re-balancing the lipid/fatty acid composition in dry and aging skin which can accelerate skin repair. Use emu oil to treat dry skin, eczema, burns and psoriasis.

Emu oil offers special benefits for damaged skin. A study at Texas Tech reported that emu oil applied directly to the burn reduced pain as effectively as 600 mgs of Ibuprofen taken internally three times daily. Another study, by Lopez and colleagues, found that emu oil had strong anti-inflammatory effects after skin was exposed to croton oil, a very strong irritant. Twelve hours after applying the emu oil, there was significantly less edema and swelling (Lopez et al 1999). Politis and Dmytrowich found that if emu oil is applied two days after an injury, it aids the healing process. However, they also found that when emu oil is applied immediately after an injury, it delays healing (Politis & Dmytrowich 1998). So for skin repair, first use an SRCP product to help initiate repair. Follow the SRCP with a later application of emu oil.

Skin Biology's Emu Oil-S Lipid Replenisher for Skin is a peroxide-free emu oil supplemented with Co-Q10, mixed isomers of natural tocotrienols, lutein, lycopene, and vitamin E, all of which provide powerful antioxidants. Skin Biology also makes an emu oil product for the hair, Emu Oil-S Lipid Replenisher for Hair, a peroxide-free emu oil supplemented with similar antioxidants and saw palmetto oil.

The ingredients in Skin Biology's emu oil products were carefully selected. Tocotrienols selectively accumulate in skin and serve to protect it against ultraviolet damage and oxidation. In rats it was found that UV radiation significantly reduced vitamin E concentrations after 29 minutes of UV exposure, but in skin treated with tocotrienols, the vitamin E concentrations were seven to 30 times higher after the radiation (Traber et al 1997). Lutein and lycopene are powerful antioxidants that occur naturally in the human body. CoQ-10 pumps up your mitochondria for greater energy. It also serves as a lipid-soluble antioxidant in the skin. Animals fed CoQ-10 have lower cancer rates. When using emu oil, apply a light coating to your skin or scalp. If your skin feels too oily, lightly wipe off the excess oil with a tissue (enough of the oil will stick to your skin to be effective).

QUOTABLE QUOTES: *The great hearted Odysseus was home at last. The maid Eurynome bathed him, rubbed him down with oil, and drew around him a royal cape.*
—Homer 800 B.C.

SQUALANE Squalane and squalene, the major lipids in human skin, share parallel attributes. Together they compose 15 percent of the skin fats in teenagers' skin, but decline to about 5 percent after age 50. As we lose lipids, our skin grows to be rough, dry, and vulnerable to damage.

For thousands of years, fishermen from Scandinavia, Japan, and the South Pacific have used fish fats rich in squalane/squalene for healing the skin of their faces and hands after salt water inflamed their skin. Squalane from olive oil is more commonly used today since it is less easily oxidized than squalene. Squalane/squalene serves as an antioxidant for cell membranes and within the cell. The compounds possess anti-cancer properties and promote the activity of T and B lymphocytes and macrophages (Lee & Langer 1983). Mice were protected against the toxicity and injury of radiation when fed a diet

QUOTABLE QUOTES: *Thou anointest my head with oil…My cup runneth over.*
—23rd Psalm of King David

supplemented with 2 percent squalane (Storm et al 1993). The compounds also have some anti-fungal properties and enhance the effects of Amphotericin B (Fungizone) against a variety of candida species (Masuda et al 1982).

When you apply squalane on a regular basis, your skin maintains the moisture level you experienced in childhood. Your skin appears softer, smoother and radiant. This light biological oil absorbs deeply and quickly leaving no oily film. It is especially useful on dry, scaly portions of the body. Some women prefer to use Emu Oil-S, a richer oil, at night and Squalane which leaves no oil residue during the day.

WHAT ABOUT COMEDONES?

Many cosmetic moisturizers boast "oil-free" formulations as a lure for those who are afraid of unsightly comedones. Could biological skin oils increase comedones? You may be surprised, but in a scientific study of comedogenic cosmetic products, the strongest comedone-inducing substances were not natural oils, but fatty acid esters and other chemicals that impart the soft feel to oil-free cosmetic formulations.

1. *Cleanse with Dr. Pickart's Face and Body Cleanser.*
2. *Apply Sebum Be Gone Oil Reduction Serum lightly by itself or under CP Serum.*
3. *You can also apply Sebum Be Gone at night to prevent oily sheen in the morning.*

A **comedone** is usually formed when a skin pore (which is actually an oil gland opening) gets plugged by a thick paste made from sebum and dead skin cells. This can happen when an increase in sebum production is combined with a buildup of dead cells at the oil gland opening. There are many reasons for an increase of the oil production including hormones and weather conditions (skin produces more sebum in hot, humid weather). But there is one cause that you can easily avoid, and that is skin irritation. As latest research shows, skin irritation triggers the production of neuro-peptides that stimulate oil production. Dead skin cell buildup is caused by insufficient exfoliation and by certain cosmetic ingredients that disrupt skin cell turnover.

At first, the sebum is white and the comedone is called a **whitehead**. But then the sebum can become oxidized, impregnated with melanin and other pigments that turn it an unpleasant dark color creating a **blackhead**. Excessive sebum provides a fertile breeding ground for a special kind of oil-eating bacteria—Propionibacterium acnes. Those tiny pests break down the oil releasing skin irritating fatty acids that trigger swelling and inflammation. This leads to the development of inflamed comedones or **acne**.

Acne is a dermatological condition that often requires a combined antibiotics and retinoids treatment, so if you have acne, please consult a medical professional first. However, almost everyone develops clogged pores as well as occasional blackheads and pimples from time to time. To prevent this from happening, you need to (1) avoid skin irritating comedogenic cosmetic products, (2) take care of your skin barrier structure as described in this chapter, (3) and exfoliate your skin regularly using alpha hydroxy acids—salicylic and lactic acids are the best.

SRCPs have been scientifically proven to reduce excessive sebum production in the oil glands thereby preventing comedone formation. For reducing oily sheen, use Sebum Be Gone—a light serum with SRCPs, aloe and salicylic acid.

Method to Keep Pores Open and Clean

© Loren Pickart PhD

The pore is an opening of an oil gland. When oil glands function properly, pores are not visible. Problems begin when there is an increase in sebum production that fills and enlarges the pore so it becomes visible. Bacteria can invade which feeds on sebum and changes its quality. Skin irritation increases sebum production even more, resulting in a clog of the opening. The pore plug is formed from dead skin cells that are not properly exfoliated and sebum lipids. When lipids get oxidized, the plug turns black.

In order to keep pores open and clean, several things are needed:

- **Suppress sebum production**
- **Help dead skin cells exfoliate**
- **Reduce inflammation**
- **Fight bacteria**

HOW TO AVOID: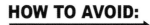

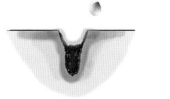

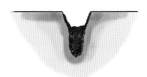

Pore is clogged
(with sebum / proteins)

Apply Exfol Serum or LacSal Serum
Leave on to loosen compacted blockage

+

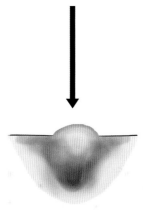

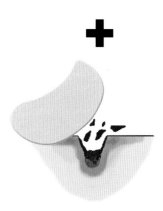

Bacteria
infects the area

Cleanse once daily
with 2% salicylic acid pads

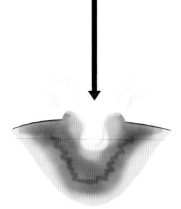

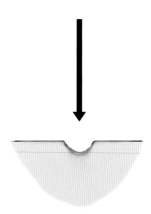

Bacteria infection
results in pimple rupture

Pores kept
clean and healthy

BUILDING UP DERMAL PROTEOGLYCANS Biological oils can restore your skin barrier, but you will also need to increase production of water-holding molecules in the dermis—**proteoglycans** and **glycosaminoglycans**. These substances act as molecular sponges taking up water and holding it inside your dermis.

The most popular glycosaminoglycan in the dermis is hyaluronic acid which is often found in cosmetic moisturizers. However, large molecules of hyaluronic acid cannot penetrate the skin. Moreover, when pure hyaluronic acid is injected into the skin, it is quickly dissolved by dermal enzymes. That is why all "wrinkle filling" products based on hyaluronic acid usually contain a chemically modified form that dissolves more slowly. It plumps up the skin, at least temporarily, but does nothing else.

Since SRCPs have been scientifically proven to stimulate the synthesis of water holding molecules of the dermis, with copper peptide based products you can avoid chemically modified skin plumpers and plump your skin with its own proteoglycans instead. Skin Signals Solution is one of Skin Biology's products specially developed to increase dermal molecules such as collagen, elastin and proteoglycans. For the best result, it should be combined with alpha hydroxy acids or microdermabrasion.

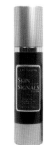

1. **Morning:** After cleansing the skin, apply a light amount of Skin Signals Solution. An adequate application should just barely cover the area without leaving it excessively wet or damp. Massage into the skin for 5-10 seconds. Can be diluted first with water if using around the eye area, or if you have sensitive skin. Afterward, apply Emu Oil-S Lipid Replenisher on top.

2. **Evening:** After cleansing the skin, apply a light amount of Exfol Serum or LacSal Serum (hydroxy acid chemical exfoliators that help break down damaged skin proteins).

3. **Finish** by applying a light amount of Emu Oil-S Lipid Replenisher, a biological healing oil, or Two Timing Tightener (a DMAE tightening serum).

REDUCING PORE SIZE As we age, our skin grows thinner and our bodies gain girth. How unfair! Most of us want the reverse. Not only that but thin skin makes pores appear more prominent. Contrary to what magazine advertisements tell you, oil removers do not reduce pore size, but rather cause the skin to produce more oil and larger pores to compensate for the removed oil.

In contrast, both retinoic acid and lactic acid reduce oil production and pore size. When you increase the rate of skin renewal, this also reduces pore size, since the firmer and thicker skin helps squeeze the pore downward and inward. Skin renewal serums and creams that increase collagen, elastin, proteoglycans and the amount of subcutaneous fat (the very thin layer under the skin) both firm the skin and increase its thickness. Our clients often tell us that Super CP Serum works well for this purpose.

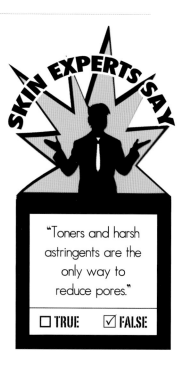

SKIN EXPERTS SAY

"Toners and harsh astringents are the only way to reduce pores."

☐ TRUE   ☑ FALSE

PROTECTING YOUR HANDS There are specific things you can do to protect the one area of your body most exposed to aging elements. Start by wearing vinyl gloves whenever you come in contact with household chemicals and other harsh elements. Wear gloves when folding laundry, peeling vegetables or handling citrus fruits or tomatoes. Purchase four or five pairs and keep them in the kitchen, bathroom, nursery and laundry areas. Have other pairs for non-wet housework and gardening. Avoid latex gloves, since many people are sensitive to them. Dry out the gloves between cleaning jobs. When outdoors in cool weather, wear unlined leather gloves to protect against dry and chapped skin. Since you can't always wear gloves, take care when washing dishes or clothes. Just say no to dish pan hands! Avoid hand-washing items if you can, and if you must, keep your hands out of the soapy water as much as possible. Using an automatic dishwasher will protect your hands and also effectively sterilize your dishes. Remove rings whenever washing or working with your hands. When you wash your hands, use lukewarm water and very little soap. Use TINPEP Hand Cream for daily repair.

SPECIAL NEEDS OF THE EYELIDS Your eyelids, the thinnest skin on the body, require special attention. Before you apply eye makeup, add a light protective layer of CP Night Eyes Premier. As your skin grows thicker and stronger, move on to CP Night Eyes Regular. If these products feel too strong for your sensitive skin, try Super GHK-Copper Serum or Super GHK-Copper Cream. These gentle products provide a protective coating with antioxidant protection. Since makeup can irritate and damage your eye area, use as little eye shadow, eye liner, and mascara as possible. You may discover "less is more" when you emerge with beautiful skin. Remove eye makeup with either Emu Oil-S for Skin or pure Squalane. Most cosmetic makeup removers are harsh and damaging to delicate skin.

PROTECT AND RESTORE As you see, keeping your skin young and beautiful boils down to one simple phrase: "Protect and Restore". It is really that simple! It is true, that you can avoid many skin problems just by keeping it out of harm's way—treating it gently, preserving its protective barrier, avoiding unnecessary assaults from the environment and unhealthy cosmetic products.

However, protection alone is not enough. You need to take special care of your skin's reparative and restorative mechanisms to ensure its speedy recovery from occasional damage and stressful influences. Remember, babies and young children are not particularly careful with their skin, and yet their skin is perfect because of excellent repair systems. If we only could retain this outstanding reparative power of our skin, we would never grow old. Today we know that the main reason why we start to lose this power is age-related depletion of central regulators of the repair process. By protecting the skin from damage while supplying it with those magical molecules, Skin Remodeling Copper Peptides, we can reverse skin aging making it radiate health and alluring beauty.

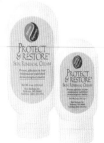

Aerobic Exercise Improves Skin Health

Aerobic exercise can imbue you with a rosy glow. It markedly improves skin quality and overall body health. Aerobics prevent bloating and puffiness, acne, and loss of muscle tone. Exercise brings more oxygen and nutrients to the skin to make it firmer and better nourished. Aerobic exercise can also slow down aging. Mail carriers, who spend their days walking, have the longest lifespan of any occupational group in the United States. Many people who live to a ripe old age walk, hike or run daily.

Physical ability decreases less with age than commonly believed; the body "wears out" faster from a lack of use than overuse.

The benefits of aerobic exercise are too numerous to list here. Exercise increases the blood capillary density in the skin and improves the nutrition of skin cells. It increases overall body metabolism and retards many of the effects of aging. In one study, healthy men in their 50's who exercised vigorously displayed a tissue oxygen uptake capacity and cardiovascular function that was 20 to 30 percent higher than sedentary young men (Paffenbarger et al 1978).

Ideally, you should get between three and five hours of vigorous aerobic exercise a week. Researchers have found that when you perform moderate work outs, you get the same health benefits as high intensity aerobics. It doesn't have to be hell to be healthy. The best forms of exercise are fun and reduce your stress level. Do what makes you happy and feel good. Golf, hiking, walking, hunting, fishing and even gardening are all good options.

Once you establish an exercise routine that works for you, keep it up! Unless you are an elite athlete, if you start skipping workouts, your aerobic capacity will rapidly decrease, dropping by 50 percent in just one week. After five to 12 days, your capillary density will decrease by 10 to 20 percent and the capacity of your heart to pump blood will also diminish. Two months of inactivity will wipe out about 90 percent of the conditioning gained through exercise (Coastal 1984).

DO YOU REALIZE THAT: The new exercise idea is that very brief periods of intense exercise (for example 30 seconds) followed by a few minutes of very light exercise, then repeated, is all you need to switch your gene output to younger-type proteins.

My List of New Exercise Goals:

PSYCHOLOGICAL STRESS DAMAGES SKIN

We all suspect that stress can age us. Just take a look at some of our past presidents after four years in office. Well, now we have proof. Psychological stress ages the skin.

A study measuring the skin barrier recovery of students before and after exams demonstrated how psychological stress adversely affected their skin. The study assessed the skin barrier recovery of medical, dental, and pharmacy students starting at four weeks

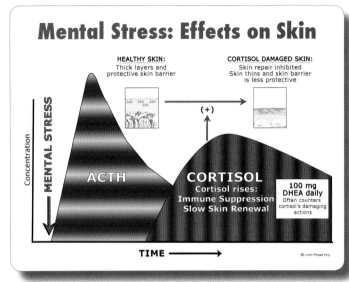

Mental Stress: Effects on Skin

HEALTHY SKIN:
Thick layers and protective skin barrier

CORTISOL DAMAGED SKIN:
Skin repair inhibited
Skin thins and skin barrier is less protective

Concentration

MENTAL STRESS

ACTH

(+)

CORTISOL
Cortisol rises:
Immune Suppression
Slow Skin Renewal

100 mg DHEA daily
Often counters cortisol's damaging actions

TIME ⟶

© Loren Pickart PhD

before final examinations through four weeks after final exams during spring vacation. There was a noteworthy decline in skin barrier protection and healing during the stressful period that they studied for exams. But during spring vacation, their skin health recovered. According to researchers of the study, "The greatest deterioration in barrier function occurred in those subjects who demonstrated the largest increases in perceived psychological stress." (Garg et al 2001).

Another study confirmed that psychological stress has a negative effect on the skin. The subjects were female volunteers who underwent a night of sleep deprivation, a three-day exercise regimen, and the psychosocial stress of an interview. The conclusion was clear: "Acute psychosocial stress and sleep deprivation disrupts skin barrier function homeostasis in women." (Choi et al 2005).

How does this happen? Acute mental stress raises the level of ACTH (called Adrenocorticotropic Hormone, also called corticotropin), the body's stress response hormone. ACTH then stimulates the secretion of cortisol which in turn inhibits skin repair.

A NOTE ON LIP CARE

PUCKER UP! Many women desire plump luscious lips. They also want to treat their dry, chapped smackers while protecting them from the elements. Our clients find that two Skin Biology products can work wonders: TriReduction with Retinol and Emu Oil-S for Skin. Female long-distance runners have reported that TriReduction with Retinol protects their lips from heat, wind and cold as they dash through the elements. Women also tell us that the SRCPs in TriReduction and the deep moisturization of Emu Oil-S plump up the lips giving a fuller appearance. Protecting your lips is certainly part of keeping your skin looking young, beautiful and kissable.

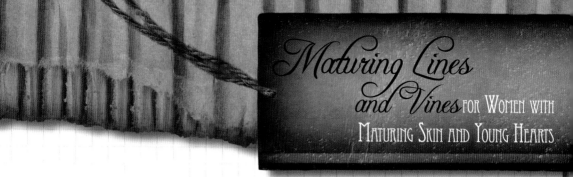
As I graze the soul of time,

maturing skin like vintage wine,

So young at heart yet sweet and deep,

our golden years enrich the vine.

While young grapes fall

before their time

still half asleep go undefined.

Nurture maturing skin

for a grape bouquet bonanza.

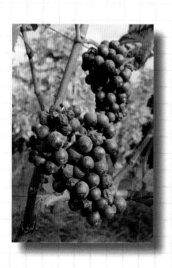

Full of grace,

let young hearts shine.

Wry wine will ripen senses.

Fine line and wrinkled glances

delight the mindful heart.

Idelle Musiek

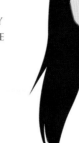

"LONG LET ME INHALE, DEEPLY THE ODOR OF YOUR HAIR, INTO IT PLUNGE THE WHOLE OF MY FACE, AS A THIRSTY MAN INTO THE WATER OF A SPRING, AND WAVE IT IN MY FINGERS LIKE A SCENTED HANDKERCHIEF, TO SHAKE THE MEMORIES INTO THE AIR." –CHARLES BAUDELAIRE

(12)

HEALTHY HAIR GROWTH
Strengthen, Thicken, Lengthen from Root to Tip

Give me a head of hair... a crowning glory to frame thy rosy complexion. Now ponder this: no matter how much we baby our skin, we may not look our best without our lustrous luminous hair. Simply put, a good skin day does not make up for a bad hair day. So let us now explore how to enjoy good hair days for all the days of our lives.

Our hair, like skin, starts its journey renewing itself with youthful vigor. When we are young, we flaunt our thick, well-pigmented, and fast growing hair. But the passage of time takes a toll, and our hair begins to thin or vanish, grow more slowly, and turn gray. While the search for methods to restore healthy, younger hair is ancient, the reality is that, even today, in the era of Rogaine® (minoxidil) and Propecia® (finasteride), the therapies that profess to restore hair health give a marginal result at best.

While far from a miracle therapy, research on SRCPs has uncovered an unexpected benefit: they stimulate hair follicle growth and function. More and more, SRCPs are being used to improve hair growth and condition, with promising results.

Why the Big Apple is a Bad Hair Town
The effect of the hair-care industry on hair health has been disastrous according to many scientists, including Russian Physician George Michael. Dr. Michael immigrated to New York City with his family after the 1917 revolution and later set up a medical practice. Despite the city's abundance of beauty salons and other businesses that cater to hair, Michael was immediately struck by the poor quality of women's tresses. He reminisced that, in the Russia of his youth, many women in their 60's and beyond displayed healthy, well-pigmented, waist-length locks; whereas in New York City the

women had difficulty growing their hair longer than six inches. Dr. Michael concluded that the excess of dyes, cutting, blow drying, and relaxers, was damaging the women's hair. He went on to emerge as the guru of long-hair care, opening a chain of Long Hair Clinics and working with famous long-haired beauties such as Crystal Gayle. (For more information on Dr. Michael, visit Jennifer Bahney's www.longhairlovers.com).

WHY MEN GO BALD AND WOMEN GET THIN HAIR No matter how bitterly women complain about hair loss and thinning, they do have to admit that a woman who goes completely bald is a rare sight, one that is usually associated with certain medical conditions. The long known fact that so many men go bald, while women do not, prompted scientists to suspect that baldness is caused by male sex hormones, or androgens. Eventually the male hormone testosterone was established as the main culprit in male pattern hair loss. However, further research revealed a much more complex picture and even now there is still no complete clarity on why people lose their hair.

Each hair follicle goes through the three distinctive phases of growth and decline. The phase of hair growth is called **anagen** and it lasts for several years. Then a hair follicles enter the short phase or **catagen** (about two weeks), during which the follicle shrinks and pushes hair out. The resting phase, during which hair follicles are not producing hair, is called **telogen** and it lasts for several weeks. Then the whole cycle is repeated.

Testosterone that is found in blood is a weak androgen and has little effect on hair growth. However, in hair follicles testosterone can be converted into a much more potent form—dihydrotestosterone or DHT. Normally, DHT stimulates body and facial hair, but has no effect on scalp hair follicles because they lack specific DHT receptors.

Normal Aging and Other Damaging Actions

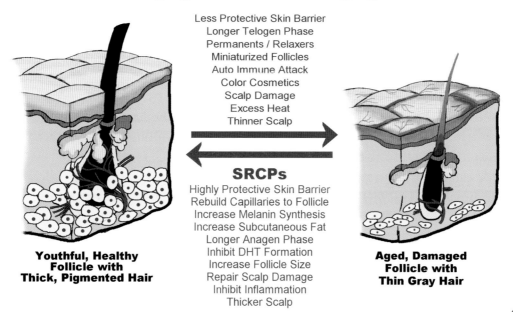

Less Protective Skin Barrier
Longer Telogen Phase
Permanents / Relaxers
Miniaturized Follicles
Auto Immune Attack
Color Cosmetics
Scalp Damage
Excess Heat
Thinner Scalp

SRCPs
Highly Protective Skin Barrier
Rebuild Capillaries to Follicle
Increase Melanin Synthesis
Increase Subcutaneous Fat
Longer Anagen Phase
Inhibit DHT Formation
Increase Follicle Size
Repair Scalp Damage
Inhibit Inflammation
Thicker Scalp

**Youthful, Healthy
Follicle with
Thick, Pigmented Hair**

**Aged, Damaged
Follicle with
Thin Gray Hair**

The problems begin when certain scalp hair follicles start responding to DHT (develop DHT receptors). In this case, DHT shortens their growth phase (anagen) and eventually causes miniaturization (progressive shrinkage) of the hair follicles. As a result, with each hair cycle, the hair grows thinner and thinner until the follicles start producing thin, barely visible vellus hair instead of thick, beautiful terminal hair.

Men usually have DHT sensitive hair follicles all grouped together, typically on the forehead and on top of the head. These are the areas where hair loss is often profound and noticeable ("male pattern baldness"). In some cases, every single one of the hair follicles on a man's head can be DHT sensitive, eventually resulting in complete baldness.

Women on the other hand, have diffuse distribution of DHT sensitive follicles. That is why women rarely go completely bald and may just develop thinning hair instead. Since the degree of DHT-dependent hair loss is determined by DHT sensitivity of hair follicles, it is quite possible for a man to have a full head of hair regardless of a high level of DHT.

An enzyme that converts testosterone into DHT is called 5-alpha-reductase (5AR). Normally skin and hair (as well as the liver) contain 5-alpha-reductase Type I, while the prostate contains 5AR Type 2. However, it was found that hair follicles in a balding scalp often contain both types of 5AR—Type I and II. That explains why male pattern hair loss can somewhat be reduced by a drug finasteride—or selective inhibitor of 5AR Type II. Unfortunately, finasteride has little effect on female hair loss.

Yet, while the DHT role in hair loss may seem so well established, recent studies have proven that it is not the whole story (Ellis et al 1998). Today other factors such as follicle inflammation, poor circulation and disrupted skin remodeling have started to come forward as true forces behind the age-old hair loss problem.

WHAT IS BEHIND HAIR LOSS? The causes are far more diverse than many people realize. The following is a description of the factors that can inhibit hair growth.

Hair Loss and TGF-beta. Miniaturization of the hair follicles is the most distinctive finding in individuals experiencing balding or thinning hair. So it is natural to assume that DHT is the cause of it. However, some researchers now believe that DHT causes miniaturization of hair follicles *indirectly*, and that its main action is to raise the level of TGF-beta (a scar promoting and pro-inflammatory cytokine). In turn, TGF-beta causes inflammation and accumulation of excessive collagen around hair follicles, restricting their growth and impeding circulation. It has been demonstrated that miniaturization of hair follicles is usually associated with inflammation, increased level of TGF-beta and accumulation of fibrose tissue around the follicle (Uno 1988).

Inadequate follicle microcirculation. The blood flow of older follicles slows down as we age which diminishes synthesis: the formation of necessary compounds. As a result the follicles shrink in size and function. The synthesis of new hair necessitates a very high nutrient flow to the follicle bulb. Morphological studies, which measure structures of aged follicles, often observe a markedly diminished capillary blood supply in aged, miniaturized follicles. This alone may be the cause of follicle miniaturization and inadequate hair synthesis (Stenn et al 1991).

Decreased subcutaneous fat layer. The layer of fat at the base of the skin, known as subcutaneous adipose tissue or "baby fat", diminishes with age. Researchers have noted that fat accumulates around the healthy follicles that vigorously grow hair. In contrast, they observed a lack of fat around dormant follicles. They postulate that these fat cells serve a supportive function for the hair follicle. Conditions that inhibit hair growth, such as chemotherapy and starvation, also decrease the subcutaneous fat layer (Stenn et al 1991).

Supplements of MSM may greatly help me to grow out my hair!

Lack of sulfur donors. Hair is composed of 35 percent sulfur-containing amino acids. Only bird feathers can boast a similar level of amino acids. Nutritional sulfur supplements, such as methyl sulfonyl methane (commonly known as MSM), have long been shown to beautify the manes of racehorses; and my clients rave about how MSM adds health and luster to their hair.

Damage from relaxers, excessive heat, coloring agents, and dyes. As we discussed, an array of razzle dazzle hair products, designed to beautify can inflict more harm than good as they damage the scalp and frazzle the follicles. Relaxers, permanents, color cosmetics with their organic dyes and metallic salts, and excessive heat from blow dryers and hot oil treatments can literally boil the follicles and also damage the hair shaft's hard outer layers of keratin. When we combine these treatments, it's like adding oil to a fire as these procedures ravish hair follicles and reduce hair growth. This follicle onslaught is most noticeable when some women lose their eyebrows and eyelashes by age 40. Such self-inflicted damage can also result in hair loss via excessive breakage, when hair shafts get so badly damaged they break, leaving only short stumps much like those in a heavily logged forest. This form of hair loss can often be reduced by a regular use of a good, well formulated conditioner. But avoiding the damage in the first place would be a much better strategy.

Excessive hair cutting. If long, lush, healthy locks are what you crave, I have good news for you. According to Dr. George Michael, long hair is healthier than short hair. He contends that the longer you grow your hair, the stronger your roots. It is possible that the hair follicles thrive from the tension produced by the weight of a heavy hair shaft in the same manner that muscles and bones respond to exercise. So cut your hair less and get more out of your hair.

ESTROGENS AND HEALTHY HAIR Estrogens are female hormones that inhibit the growth of facial hair (with the exception of eyelashes) and body hair (with the exception of underarm and pubic hair), while stimulating scalp hair. Estrogens counteract the effect of androgens. That is why a hormonal shift can have a profound effect on a woman's hair:

Extreme exercise. Severe exercise tends to reduce estrogen and raise testosterone. This hormonal shift can stop the menstrual cycle. It may also lead to brittle bones and hair thinning or loss. While there are many positive aspects of exercise, there can be too much of a good thing.

Sudden hormone shifts. Hair loss can intensify after a woman gives birth or discontinues oral contraceptives. In these cases, I recommend a brief therapy with hair stimulators; they can usually restore hair to its previous condition. Such hair stimulators include SRCPs, and other supplements such as MSM, and Flaxseed Oil.

Effect of menopause. Pre-menopause and menopause is associated with a progressive decline of estrogen level, which can result in hair loss. In this case, herbal supplements containing phytoestrogens such as red clover, soy, flaxseed, pomegranate and others can be recommended.

Using SRCPs to Stimulate Hair Growth—A Hair Raising Discovery

One of the most exciting discoveries from stem cell researchers, truly hair raising, reveals that hair follicles provide the source of stem cells for skin. This vital finding links hair follicles with skin repair. However, long before this discovery I observed that, after applying GHK-Cu to a wound, hair follicles enlarged dramatically at the edge of the wound.

Since then, SRCPs have been proven to:
- Increase hair growth in humans
- Increase hair follicle size in humans
- Improve the "take" of transplanted hair plugs
- Reduce hair loss caused by chemotherapeutic drugs
- Increase the recovery of hair loss caused by chemotherapeutic drugs

An in-depth discussion of the above actions can be found in Chapter 18, "The Science Behind SRCPs".

IMPROVING HAIR VITALITY WITH SRCPS While recent studies hold promise, SRCPs are not the panacea for hair loss. A more important future use of SRCPs may be as a regular scalp treatment or hair tonic, used once or twice weekly, for the enhancement of hair and scalp health. SRCPs have numerous actions that may improve the hair and scalp. These include:

Reducing DHT formation in hair follicles. An enzyme which converts testosterone to DHT, (5-alpha reductase (5-AR)), damages hair growth. It exists in two forms: type 1, which functions in hair follicles, and type 2, which acts in prostate tissue. Follicle-damaging DHT is produced in the hair follicles. Propecia (finasteride), a prescription treatment for hair loss in men who have male pattern baldness, inhibits 5-AR throughout the body and improves hair growth. But it works best on the type 2 form and is better suited for controlling prostate enlargement. It also must be administered by pills that spread the drug throughout the body. A superior way to inhibit the type 1 5-AR that damages hair growth may be to increase copper ions in the skin. Sugimoto et al found that copper (II) ions could give up to a 90 percent inhibition of type 1 5-AR. At 1.2 micrograms copper ion per milliliter, type 1 5-AR activity reduced by 50 percent, but copper (II) ions were 10-fold less active on inhibiting the type 2 prostate form. Thus, copper ions are more specific inhibitors of 5-AR than Propecia. Human transdermal studies have found that concentrations of up to 0.50 micrograms per milliliter of copper ion can be introduced into the skin with SRCPs without irritation. For comparison, the blood plasma copper level is approximately 1 microgram per milliliter (Sugimoto et al 1995).

Blocking TGF-beta Formation. SRCPs block production of TGF-beta, a cytokine closely involved in the processes that lead to miniaturization of hair follicles. Copper peptides inhibit TGF-beta directly by stimulating the production of decorin —a molecule that also inhibits TGF-beta production (see Chapter 18).

Improving microcirculation to hair follicles. Hair follicles have extreme rates of metabolic activity. However, morphological studies of aged follicles often find an inadequate capillary circulation. As a result, some researchers have suggested that the reduced nutrient flow may cause hair shafts to thin as we age. SRCPs have angiogenic activity (growth of new blood cells from pre-existing vessels) that may correct this problem. See Chapter 18 which goes into more depth about the science behind SRCPs.

Protective anti-inflammatory actions. The final event in the sequence of degenerative changes produces non-functional hair follicles which have involuted, (rolled inward). These changes cause tissue damage, auto-immune inflammation and free-radical reactions around the follicle. SRCPs reduce inflammation and free radical formation in hair follicles since they block the inflammatory actions of both interleukin 1 and Transforming Growth Factor beta 1. Also during tissue injury, the release of ferrous iron from ferritin increases the formation of tissue-damaging free radicals, but SRCPs block the release of iron from ferritin. Finally, only about 50 percent of copper zinc superoxide dismutase is activated due to a lack of copper in the protein. SRCPs can supply additional copper to zinc superoxide dismutase and increase its antioxidant effectiveness as well. Autoimmune damage causing hair loss exists in conditions such as alopecia areata, diabetes, vitiligo, certain types of thyroid disease, and pernicious anemia.

Physicians normally treat these conditions with a short course of any cortisone-type drug, which often restores hair growth. However, when we inject cortisone into bald spots, the hair regrowth is temporary. Here's the problem: corticosteroids inhibit skin repair, thereby producing thinner, less functional skin left unable to support hair follicle functions. In studies on nickel allergic patients, Zhai et al wrote that SRCPs were effective in reducing redness and inflammation after allergic reactions while also stimulating skin repair. See Chapter 18 for details.

To take care of the health of my hair, I first need to take care of my scalp!

Enhancing the skin's subcutaneous fat layer and thickening of the scalp. Newborns and small children have ample padding of subcutaneous fat underneath scalp skin, which protects their little heads from injuries. As we age, some of us grow stubborn and thick headed while our scalps get thinner. None of us mind a thin waistline—but a thin scalp? The scalp becomes thinner in part because the subcutaneous fat layer that surrounds hair follicles diminishes with age. Pathologists have noted that large subcutaneous fat cells are associated with large, healthy hair follicles and have postulated that the fat cells provide nutritional support to the follicles. Conditions that cause hair loss, such as cancer chemotherapy, are associated with a sharp decrease in the volume of subcutaneous fat cells. SRCPs increase both hair follicle size and the amount of subcutaneous fat.

SRCPs also help increase skin thickness by boosting the dermal levels of collagen, elastin, and the water-holding proteoglycans (carbohydrate molecules linked to protein) and glycosaminoglycans (unbranched polysaccharide molecules composed of many carbohydrates). See Chapter 18 for further information.

Reviving hair follicle stem cells. SRCPs have been shown to restore the vitality and reparative ability of skin stem cells (see Chapter 18 for more details). Since hair, just like skin, requires an adequate supply of stem cells in order to grow, stem cell health is an important attribute of long and lustrous hair.

Repairing damaged scalp. Women often lose hair as a result of numerous assaults inflicted by relaxers, permanents, coloring chemicals, and excessive heat from blow dryers and hot oil treatments. SRCPs work wonders to speed up the repair of scalp damage after various hair procedures.

Reducing graying of hair. Hair grays with age, but the speed at which this occurs may depend on the availability of copper in the scalp. Melanin and other hair pigments are produced from the amino acid tyrosine by the action of tyrosinase, a copper-containing enzyme. Additional scalp copper might slow the graying process. Skin Biology clients often report the re-pigmentation of gray hair after using SRCP products.

USING FOLLIGEN TO IMPROVE HAIR HEALTH My research in the 1980's led to my earlier inventions with products such as Tricomin™, which was demonstrated to increase hair growth in humans, and GraftCyte™, which was proven to increase hair transplant success in humans. For more specifics, see Chapter 18. My latest inventions, a line of Folligen products, takes hair repair to the next level. Folligen began as an SRCP skin repair cream that was tested in the Dermatology Department at the *University of California San Francisco*. A 41-year-old woman with severe hair loss tried the skin repair cream on her head because nothing else had worked to restore her lost hair. Over the next two-and-a-half months, she regained all of her lost hair. Word spread and other people began using the skin repair cream to counter hair loss. In time, Folligen emerged as a distinct product designed to repair hair. Folligen's biological effect is similar to the results achieved by my earlier line of hair products; however this new generation appears more effective as demonstrated in my basic tests on hair function.

Skin Biology offers three forms of Folligen: Folligen Cream, which works well on hairlines; Folligen Lotion, a more liquid solution suitable for dense hair; and Folligen Solution Therapy Spray, a fine mist to be sprayed on the scalp. Skin Biology also offers a Folligen shampoo and conditioner, described at the end of this chapter.

Many clients use Folligen products to calm scalp tissue irritated by other hair growth stimulators, such as minoxidil and retinoic acid. When you rub on Folligen to calm your scalp, start with a light application. If your scalp is irritated, Folligen can cause a brief stinging, but as your scalp repairs itself, it will become more protective and less sensitive to irritation by minoxidil, retinoic acid, and other products.

My Hair Regrowth Recommendations

I recommend the following products and procedures, based on reports from our clients, to help restore lost or thinning hair. Women often lose hair as a result of stress or hormonal shifts caused by menopausal changes or after they discontinue birth control pills. Another frequent cause of hair loss is extreme dieting that can result in hormonal shifts (sometimes to the point of even disrupting the menstrual circle) and essential nutrient deficiency. Fortunately for women, their hair loss is easier to reverse than for men.

1. Apply an SRCP product such as Folligen Lotion, Folligen Cream, Folligen Solution Therapy Spray, Hair Signals Cream or Hair Signals Therapy Solution. The recommended frequency is four to five times a week applied as a light coating before bedtime. Clients usually report that Folligen markedly reduces hair loss in about three weeks, improves scalp health, reduces irritation, and results in a thicker head of hair in about four months.

2. Apply Emu Oil-S for Hair. The combination of Folligen's SRCPs and emu oil often produces drastic reductions in hair loss and increases hair growth. Recently, Dr. Michael Holick of Boston University Medical Center reported a clinical study that found emu oil accelerated skin regeneration and also stimulated hair growth. He wrote, "The hair follicles were more robust, the skin thickness was remarkably increased...Also, we discovered in the same test that over 80 percent of hair follicles that had been 'asleep' were awakened and began growing hair."

3. For added stimulation, apply minoxidil (2 to 5 percent). Start by using 2 percent minoxidil and progressively increase to 5 percent. At times minoxidil can irritate the scalp. If this occurs, stop using the product and only use Folligen until your scalp health is restored. Then, resume the use of 2 percent minoxidil, and eventually 5 percent if your scalp remains healthy.

Hideo Uno, who wrote the textbook on Rogaine®, found that both SRCPs and minoxidil work synergistically to improve hair health. While minoxidil primarily stimulates new vellus hair growth, SRCPs prove more effective in thickening the hair shafts.

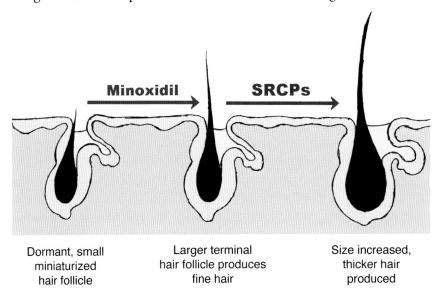

| Dormant, small miniaturized hair follicle | Larger terminal hair follicle produces fine hair | Size increased, thicker hair produced |

4. Retinoic acid (0.01 to 0.05 percent) also stimulates hair follicles. Retinoic acid helps produce thicker hair shafts when combined with minoxidil, but this combination may irritate the scalp. When used lightly, Folligen can greatly reduce the irritation.

5. If your hair thins or falls out as the result of low estrogen caused by menopause or other hormonal shifts, you may benefit from estrogen supplements. However, be mindful that recent studies have shown that there is a link between hormone replacement therapy and certain cancers, so make sure you talk to your doctor first (Sugimoto et al 1995). Phytoestrogens such as soy isoflavones or red clover may soften the sharpness of estrogen decline and reduce hair loss. Since subcutaneous fat becomes an important site for estrogen synthesis in pre-menopause and menopause, steer clear from extreme dieting and consider keeping a few extra pounds instead of trying to slim to the bones.

6. For those who prefer an all-natural approach, there are several non-drug DHT blockers. These include saw palmetto oil, pygeum and nettle root extract, the soybean isoflavones genistein and daidzein, ginkgo biloba, and gamma linoleic acid.

Saw palmetto oil has been used for more than 400 years as an herbal treatment for enuresis, nocturia, atrophy of the testes, impotence, inflammation of the prostate, and as a mild aphrodisiac for men. Women used the berries to treat infertility, painful periods, and problems with lactation. Extracts of two plants, pygeum bark (Pygeum africanum) and nettle root (Urtica dioica) are widely used to treat prostate hyperplasia.

Isoflavonoids, such as genistein and daidzein, are weak estrogens and may lessen the risk of osteoporosis and heart disease. Several studies have found that isoflavones can protect against the development of cancer. The Chinese report that daidzien exhibits hair-growth and hair-color-promoting activity.

Ginkgo biloba is a popular herb used worldwide to improve cerebral blood flow and general blood circulation.

QUOTABLE QUOTES: *And Delilah made Samson sleep upon her knees; and she called for a man, and she caused him to shave off seven locks from Samson's head; and she began to afflict him, and Samson's strength went from him.* —Capture of Samson, Judges 16

Getting Rid of Any Green

No one wants to hear "the dye is cast" if it means turning blond hair green. Blond hair may pick up a green tint when exposed to Folligen, resembling the green chlorine that is cast by a dip in a swimming pool. In order to reap Folligen's benefits without tinting hair, be careful to keep the products on the scalp and off the hair. If you notice a green hue, blend a solution of one part lemon juice and four parts water to remove the green color. A tin-peptide product (such as Folligen for Blondes) presents no color problems and often works to reduce hair loss.

FOLLIGEN SHAMPOO & CONDITIONER   Folligen Therapy Shampoo and Folligen Therapy Conditioner are relatively low pH products. I designed them to clean hair with the minimum amount of damage and then tighten up and re-seal the hair shafts. I added SRCPs to enhance the vitality of the hair follicles and scalp.

Hair contains a high sulfur content from the amino acid cysteine and can easily form cross-links to other cysteines in the hair molecule. These bonds keep the hair tough and strong and thus able to resist abrasion. The cross-links hold the hair fibers together. As long as this organization is not disrupted, the fiber remains robust and appears "healthy".

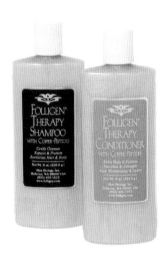

Shampoos with a high alkaline pH may work better to clean the hair and scalp, but they also strip away too many natural scalp oils and extract the "glues" that help hold the hair shafts together. Folligen Therapy Shampoo does not contain "flash-foamers" or foaming chemicals that add lather (which does nothing for the hair and damages the hair shafts and scalp).

Folligen Therapy Conditioner is formulated to re-acidify the hair after shampooing. When you restore this natural acid environment to the hair and scalp, you keep your hair proteins hard and thereby prevent the growth of foreign bacteria. The conditioner contains the highest-quality amino acids and pantothenic acid (vitamin B-5) to re-seal the hair cuticle. It is designed to help de-tangle the hair and add a lustrous shine. SRCPs are added to help enhance the health and vitality of the hair, scalp, and hair follicles.

Overwashing my hair can cause more damage than it may help!

Because Folligen Therapy Shampoo and Folligen Therapy Conditioner are concentrated, you may want to mix the products with a small amount of water to make them easier to use.

"I HAVE BEEN USING THE FOLLIGEN SPRAY FOR ONLY ABOUT A WEEK NOW ALONG WITH EMU OIL...I CANNOT BELIEVE IT, BUT I AM ALREADY SEEING NEW BABY HAIRS IN ONLY ONE WEEK...I'M CONFIDENT THAT WITH BOTH OF YOUR PRODUCTS ALONG WITH THE MSM I'VE BEEN TAKING, I WILL BE ABLE RE-GROW MY HAIR FASTER AND HEALTHIER THAN ANYTHING I'VE USED SO FAR. I CAN'T WAIT TO BE ABLE TO TELL YOU THAT IT'S ALL FILLED IN AGAIN. I WILL KEEP YOU UPDATED. AND THANKS AGAIN SO MUCH FOR EVERYTHING." —C.C.

"I have been using Folligen Spray (applied with a dropper), Emu Oil for hair and Folligen Shampoo for the last 3 and 1/2 months. I was applying the Folligen Spray every day until SkinBio reported better results with every other day application. Since then I am following their recommendation...The reason I started using CPs on my hair was to get a healthier scalp, not for baldness. But the hair on the top of my head was less thick than the rest of it. So, after more than 3 months I am noticing a lot of new growth. It is quite visible since I had a tuft of white hair and the new growth is dark and shorter...It is a lot of fun to see all those new hairs, and dark too! I also notice my hair grows faster; I need to have a hair cut more often." —M

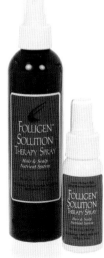

One client has had great results using Folligen Spray, MSM, and Minoxidil to enhance beard growth as the following testimonial and pictures demonstrate.

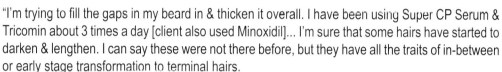

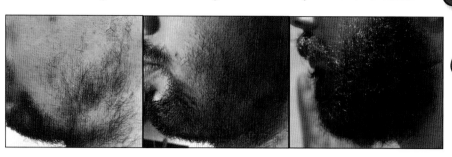

"I'm trying to fill the gaps in my beard in & thicken it overall. I have been using Super CP Serum & Tricomin about 3 times a day [client also used Minoxidil]... I'm sure that some hairs have started to darken & lengthen. I can say these were not there before, but they have all the traits of in-between or early stage transformation to terminal hairs.

I use large doses of Super CP Serum on the face and have found no irritation or side effects. I use up to 2ml per dosing. I have also used Folligen as well in a similar dosage. I have no solid reports to give any comparison between the two, but I do feel personally that the Super CP is more effective, although i did see similar effects from both... Oh, may I add that I have found any product applied to the face has effect in the scalp as well through systematic absorption. I do not suffer from MPB (male pattern baldness) and my father's pattern at age mid 50's is a general overall thinning rather than frontal loss.

But application to a non scalp area (cheeks) has had a noticeable positive effect on my overall scalp strength & density in which scalp growth and density has been improved/boosted and sustained at an increased level to normal through systematic dosing." -C.R.

HAIR GROWTH TESTIMONIALS

"Update on my husband. He was, and still is, using minoxodil 5%, and introduced diluted CP Serum about three months ago, switching to Folligen and also adding nizoral twice a week in the last month. He has new growth along the hairline, and in some spots the hair is black at the roots and grey at the tip. My kids were amazed with that...He is very impressed." -K

"I have NEW hair!! LOL, I was looking in the mirror yesterday and noticed I had new hairs growing around my hairline. They are about one inch long, yippee...I've been using Folligen Cream sporadically and then more consistently for the last 3 weeks or so. About three weeks ago I started using some minoxidil sort of regularly about the same time I started using the Folligen more regularly. I'm excited! Just last week I ordered the Folligen Shampoo and Conditioner and now I'm really motivated to be good about using everything on a regular consistent basis and see what happens." -S

"For about three weeks I have been using a dilution of 50% Folligen Spray/50% purified water which I apply with a bottle dropper on parted hair at top of my head and rub in with Q-tip. I started slowly and built up to it over a week to 10 days which allowed me to stop using minoxidil at night. Result: my hair has stopped falling out and for days at a time no hair at all has fallen out. And no more flaking scalp or irritation and dryness. My regimen: 5% minoxidil full strength in am @16 drops and Folligen 50% dilution in am @/16 drops. I have very light blonde hair chemically processed every 2 months. I have not had any color from the Folligen stain my hair at all and I use it every night. I will keep you informed about my progress. My background as you know is as a product formulator with years in the chemical business and in healthcare products development. The science and research studies in your book and on your website really convinced me to try your copper peptide formulations for my hair, face and body and so far they all really work." -AC

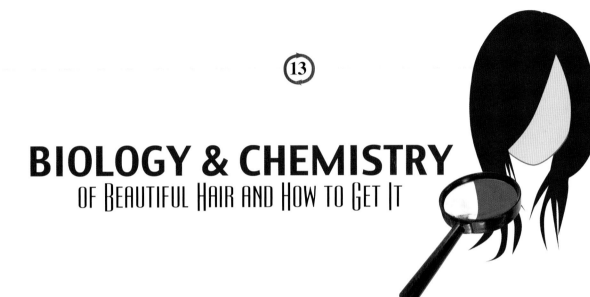

BIOLOGY & CHEMISTRY
OF BEAUTIFUL HAIR AND HOW TO GET IT

Long locks of hair unlock the key to a man's heart... Throughout history, women have woven a tapestry of desire with their alluring tresses. Legend has it that mermaids and sirens lured sailors to their deaths while combing their long lustrous curls. Australian aborigines saved their wives' hair clippings as a prized possession. Even today, some orthodox Jewish women only allow their husbands to see this most enticing treasure... their crowning glory.

In this cultural tapestry of diverse hair styles, the esthetic for what makes beautiful hair can vary greatly. Although different cultures desire different qualities in hair, most people are attracted to lush, thick, long locks, especially in women. The barometer for a beautiful head of hair is youth. Just as a child's skin radiates with newborn freshness, young hair reigns supreme as the ideal crown to frame our dewy complexion. Sadly, our hair moves away from that ideal as we watch it grow thin, lose pigment and get more and more damaged over mother time. However, proper hair care can reduce, and in some cases even reverse, the effects of the passing years.

WHAT IS HAIR? What if I told you that nails, scales, feathers, horns and claws are skin? Would that surprise you? Well, that's just the hairy truth. You see, hair is a specialized form of skin. Although the hair on our head generally invites the most attention, hair grows over a large percentage of the human body serving to protect, send sensory signals and sexually attract potential mates.

I can't count the number of times I've heard my clients say: Give me a head of hair...long beautiful hair. The question is how many beautiful hairs does it take to make up one head of hair? Well, a single hair has a thickness of 0.02 to 0.04 millimeters, so it takes 20 to 50 hair fibers stacked next to one other to span about one millimeter. We have about five million hairs on our bodies, with about 450,000 of them found above the neck. Now that's a whole lot of hairs isn't it? Most people have about 150,000 hairs on their head and normally shed 25 to 100 a day while growing an equivalent number of new hairs. Another 30,000 hairs reside in men's mustaches and beards. Blondes usually have more scalp hair than those with dark or red hair.

Mature hairs are filaments composed primarily of proteins (88 percent) which form a hard, tough, fibrous type of protein known as keratin. Proteins are composed of a long chain of amino acids that link together. The keratin found in human hair also forms a major protein in fingernails. Hair contains a tough outer coating, the cuticle, which consists of overlapping scale-like bits of hard keratin. Inside the hair shaft, or cortex, resides a core of softer protein filaments.

Hair proteins have a high sulfur content from the amino acid cysteine, which forms cross-links in the hair proteins that are responsible for the hair's toughness and abrasion resistance. You would never guess when looking at all the hairs that collect in your brush, but human hair is as strong as a wire of iron. Nevertheless, it rips after being damaged or stretched 70 percent beyond its original length.

QUOTABLE QUOTES: *If a woman has long hair, it is a glory unto her.*
—St. Paul, 1 Corinthians

HAIR'S MANY HUES The sumptuous shades of human hair are too vast to count. This colorful rainbow ranges from black, brown, red and blond with subtle variations like burgundy, strawberry blond, and copper brown. This rich feast treats our eyes with a smorgasbord of endless hues.

As in a rainbow where light bounces all around us, light bounces off the hair proteins and this partially influences hair color. However, it is the type and amount of pigment within the hair shaft center that primarily determines the tint. Eumelanin is the pigment found in black and brown hair and to a lesser degree in blonde hair. Pheomelanin produces red hair, while a mix of eumelanin and pheomelanin produces the blonde-red combination known as strawberry blonde. The greater the amount of pigment, the darker the hair color. As the amount of pigment decreases, the hair color turns from black to brown and then reddish or blond. When pigment drastically diminishes, the hair appears gray, and when absent, the hair looks white.

As we age, our hair color generally changes. Many "towheaded" children who have blonde-whitish hair as youngsters turn into brunette adults and eventually gray or white-haired elders. Swedes, famous for their blond hair, often grow into brunette adults. Ingmar Bergman, a famous Swedish director, paints his young innocent blond characters to grow up as dark, somber and reflective. So could the transition from blond to brunette provide him with a useful metaphor?

Under some circumstances, the hair can lose its color prematurely. Severe stress can turn hair white overnight. Legend has it that Marie Antoinette went "white" the night before her execution. In the trench warfare of World War I, there were cases of young men whose hair turned gray within two months after prolonged episodes of severe fighting and artillery bombardments. Malnutrition can also cause hair to prematurely turn gray or white. A lack of sufficient dietary copper can cause the hair to lose its color. Excessive dietary zinc from supplements may drive out the copper needed to synthesize hair pigments and turn hair gray.

HAIR LENGTH AND GROWTH Hair grows faster in the spring and summer. Advertisers often manipulate this fact to "prove" that certain hair-growth remedies work wonders. In actuality, one's age, health, diet or genetics determines the rate at which the hair grows. The length of time your hair follicles stay in the anagen (active growing) phase determines the maximum length your hair will grow. On average, waist-length hair takes about five years to grow out from a short haircut with periodic trims included. The following list illustrates the average lengths and growth rates of the hair on the head and body.

HAIRS:	Average Length (cm)	Growth Rate Per Day (mm)
On the head	70	0.35
Eyebrows	1.0	0.15
Mustache (beard or whiskers)	28	0.4
Armpit hairs	5	0.3
Pubic hairs	4	0.2

FACTORS THAT DAMAGE HAIR Many factors damage hair fibers including environmental elements (such as prolonged exposure to sunlight or wind) plus chemical and mechanical injuries (such as tight hairstyles, hot rollers, hot oil treatments, and harsh use of hair dryers). The chemicals we use to alter our hair come with a price. Bleaches, dyes, relaxers, and perming agents, all cause varying degrees of damage. Some cosmetic products partially repair damaged hair, but a good quality of hair will return only after new hair grows in.

The Damaging Things We Do to Our Hair

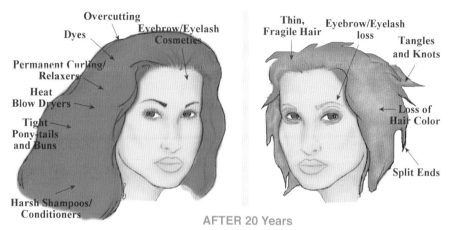

AFTER 20 Years

Choosing the Right Shampoo

When we wash our hair excessively, we shampoo out more than grime. We also wash out natural oils which protect our scalp. As a result, too much shampooing damages hair shafts. It is important to choose shampoo carefully. The best shampoos are around pH 6.0, at the high end of the slightly acidic pH of the scalp (4.5 to 6.0). Maintaining the natural acid environment of the hair and scalp keeps the hair proteins hard and prevents the growth of foreign bacteria. Thus, by using the best shampoos and not over washing, we preserve the hair and skin oils that benefit our scalp.

Shampoos with a higher pH have a negative impact on the hair for several reasons. While more alkaline shampoos work better to clean the hair and scalp, they also strip away many of the hair's natural oils and the "glues" that help hold the hair shafts together. A high pH shampoo may make hair look great for a few weeks, but eventually it will lead to dry brittle hair and increase breakage.

Don't be fooled by baby shampoos that claim to be gentle to your hair and eyes. Many baby shampoos have a high pH that can strip hair and are thus not at all gentle. Also be cautious with "clarifying shampoos." Formulated to remove buildup of gels, mousses, pomades and other products that weigh down your hair, they can also remove color and perms. Some hair experts recommend using a combination of plain baking soda and your normal shampoo to remove build-up. Other ingredients to avoid include flash foamers, chemicals that enhance the foaming of shampoo, and added fragrances, neither of which have a positive effect.

Choosing the right shampoo is especially important for those with an oily scalp. Greasy hair is more difficult to manage than normal or dry hair and is often tough to comb. Oily hair is covered with sebum from the sebaceous glands of the hair follicle. While frequent washing with a stronger, more-soapy shampoo may help remove oil, it can also damage the hair. Some Skin Biology clients use retinoic acid to reduce oil production. Retinoic acid should be used sparingly, as overuse can irritate the scalp.

Avoid selecting a shampoo based on its high price tag. Costly shampoos are not a head above the rest. A shampoo's price is generally related to the cost of its advertising. If the label on a shampoo bottle tells you to wash your hair twice, ignore it; the manufacturer is simply encouraging you to use more of the product. Always use a minimum amount of shampoo. Some shampoo manufacturers recommend that you comb through wet hair to distribute the shampoo evenly. But wet hair is more easily broken, and you will only end up with damaged hair.

When you are done washing your hair, the shampoo should be completely rinsed out to help bring the pH back down to its natural level. If your hair is very dry, only shampoo every three days. Our ancestors went months between hair washings, one of the reasons their hair was so healthy.

Choosing the Right Conditioner

The outer layer of hair called the cuticle is somewhat like fish scales made of hard keratin. The cuticle is held together by disulfide bonds plus small amino acids. In healthy shiny

INSIDE:
Cortex is the soft center of hair shaft.

Cuticle is the outer hard, overlapping scales of protein.

hair, the outer layer of scales lies flat which allows for combs and brushes to smoothly glide through it. Hair with a damaged cuticle appears dry, drab, split, brittle, or frizzy.

Quality conditioners add amino acids, peptides, and pantothenic acid (vitamin B-5) into the cuticle to help glue the scales tightly to the hair shaft. If the cuticle stays open, it can start a tear in the hair shaft which leads to breakage of the shaft. This is why it is important to use a conditioner separately.

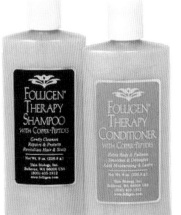

Conditioners that strengthen the hair have a low pH of about 4.0 to 4.7. The hair proteins remain hard and strong at a low pH. Some conditioners contain a small amount of fat to give the hair a better shine. The best products are sold in successful hair salons. These salons need happy, repeat customers and usually do not advertise their products. The longer you leave the conditioner on your hair, the better it works. Some manufacturers recommend leaving conditioner on the hair for only a few seconds, but longer is generally better (one to two minutes).

Is It Important to Use Both a Shampoo and Conditioner?

WHY YOU SHOULD NEVER USE A 2-IN-1 SHAMPOO/CONDITIONER

1.

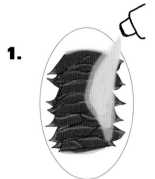

Damaged hair has an open cuticle that causes ripping, tearing, and breakage. Use a mild shampoo and <u>rinse well</u>.

2.

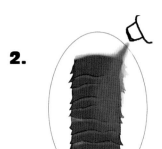

Follow with an acid conditioner to harden and flatten cuticle and apply protective nutrients.

3.

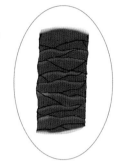

Over a period of time, hair shaft lies flat providing sealed hair shaft with protective protein that prevent growth of bacteria, split ends, help detangle, and add a lustrous shine to the hair. *SRCPs also help calm scalp irritation.*

TIPS FOR LONG, HEALTHY HAIR In the last chapter I told you about George Michael (now retired), who became famous for helping women grow their hair to extraordinary lengths. As I mentioned, Dr. Michael believes that longer hair is healthier hair, or as he puts it, "The longer the hair, the stronger the root." Many women are taught that by age 30, their hair should be no longer than shoulder length. Dr. Michael feels the contrary is true. He believes long hair majestically frames a mature woman's features—that it downplays wrinkles and makes her look younger.

When counseling women on how to grow long hair, Dr. Michael taught them that it is important to have hair of one length, without bangs or layers. According to his findings, the body tries to equalize uneven hair by excessively shedding strands.

LONGER HAIR REDUCES SHEDDING - STUDIES BY DR. GEORGE MICHAEL	
Hair Length - Inches	Number Hairs Lost Per Day
4	87
12	26
Waist Length	16
Floor Length	2

When working with long-haired clients, Dr. Michael utilized many methods to protect the hair. He set hair dryers at only about 10 degrees F higher than body temperature (most blow dryers reach temperatures of up to 260 degrees and damage hair follicles). When curling the hair, he used large rollers of soft mesh or plastic rather than rollers that grab the hair and can tear it. He took special care to protect the ends of the hair when rolling or setting. Shampoos were kept to a minimum. He recommended vitamin and mineral supplements. Dr. Michael also advised women to cover their hair at all times when exposed to direct sunlight. (See www.longhairlovers.com).

HAIR EXPERTS' 17 SUGGESTIONS
WHAT WORKS FOR
LONG, HEALTHY HAIR

1. Cut dry hair for best results.

2. Detangle dry hair before washing. Detangle the ends first and work your way up. Do not try to remove kinks from top to bottom since this may pull out hair. Before entering the shower, give your hair a few strokes with a comb or brush. This aligns the strands and helps prevent tangles.

3. When shampooing, use water at room temperature. The lower the temperature, the better it is for your hair. Warm water opens the hair scales, making the hair shaft more vulnerable to damage.

4. When preparing to wash your hair, bring the hair in front of your face before wetting it and leave it there. Let your hair hang down in front during shampooing. Try not to move your hair while you wash it. This keeps the hair strands in position so they won't move upwards and wrap themselves around other strands, resulting in tangles.

5. Don't try to overwash your hair. The purpose of shampoo is to remove dirt from the top layers. Just let the shampoo penetrate the lower layers briefly as it flows over your hair.

6. Make sure to wash out all of the shampoo. When you think the shampoo is gone, allow another half-minute of constant water flow to ensure the removal of residue. For a final rinse, immerse in cool or cold water.

7. Use an acidifying conditioner with peptides to re-glue the protein scales of the cuticle. Put extra conditioner on your hair ends to prevent split ends. Give the conditioner at least a minute to glue into the hair. For a final rinse, use cool or cold water.

8. Air-dry your hair whenever possible.

9. When you must blow-dry your hair, first wrap it in a special, highly absorbent towel to remove water. Blow-dry the hair for a few minutes, and then let it air dry. A cool setting on the hair dryer helps "set" the hair.

10. Never use a heavy-duty reconstructor on your hair. It does more harm than good.

11. Avoid excessive sunlight and tanning beds which harms the hair.

12. Apply a non-alcohol hair spray since alcohol dries the hair.

13. Use wide-toothed combs and picks.

14. Only use coated or snag-free elastics and hair fasteners.

15. Think of your hair as a silk garment and treat it accordingly. Both silk and hair are protein fibers. You wouldn't wash a silk garment with a cheap detergent in a washing machine at a high temperature with a high agitation cycle and then dry it in a dryer at a high temperature.

16. Many hairdressers only "cut" hair. For long healthy hair, tell them to keep trimming to an absolute minimum.

17. If someone criticizes your hair, IGNORE THEM. Hair arouses many emotions and jealousies, so arrange your hair in a fashion that pleases yourself.

CHANGING THE LOOK OF YOUR HAIR

You can dramatically alter your hair's appearance by changing its shape through permanent waving or straightening. However, both of these procedures cause damage to the scalp and hair. This damage might include breakage, thinning, lack of growth, scalp irritation, scalp damage, and hair loss. If the damage becomes excessive, serious hair loss may occur. Before undergoing any hair treatment, especially one that introduces powerful chemicals to your hair, you owe it to yourself to be well informed about the following procedures.

Permanents

Permanents add depth and richness to limp or frizzy hair. However, they can also be quite harsh. Permanents break the disulfide bonds in the proteins that hold hair together during the process of wrapping hair around a roller to form it into a new texture. As a result, the disulfide bonds are chemically reset and the new, curly texture locks into place. However, when the perming solution is left on too long, is too strong, or when applied to hair damaged by dye, bleach, or an earlier perm, the hair and follicles can get severely damaged. If this happens to you, rub Folligen Lotion into your scalp for three to four nights following the procedure to restore scalp health.

PERMANENTS
STRAIGHTENING
RELAXERS
FLAT IRONS
CURLING IRONS
HAIR DYES

Hair Straightening

Many women love the look of straight locks of shiny hair. Thus, straightening is an increasingly popular option. During the procedure, an alkaline-reducing agent breaks down disulfide bonds that keep hair curly. Hair relaxers, typically creams or cream lotions, contain about 2 to 4 percent of strong bases such as sodium hydroxide, potassium hydroxide, and lithium hydroxide or 5 percent calcium hydroxide plus a solution of up to about 30 percent guanidine carbonate. The pH is around 12. Some relaxers contain about 4 percent ammonium thioglycolate as the active ingredient.

Before the straightening procedure, you apply a petroleum-base cream to help protect the scalp. Then rub on the chemical relaxer and gently comb the hair straight. After a period of time, remove the relaxer with warm water and a neutralizing formula. Finally, apply a conditioner to restore some of the natural oils and proteins removed by the chemical.

As with perms, the harsh chemicals in straighteners can cause severe damage to the hair. I suggest you follow the procedure with applications of Folligen Lotion to restore scalp health.

Only employ a hair-care specialist with a record of success in chemical straightening. I strongly recommend that you obtain professional conditioning treatments before and after the process.

Alternatively, you can apply intense heat to reset bonds which straightens curls. Some use a flat styling iron. Others boldly flatten their hair with a clothing iron over an ironing board covered with a smooth towel. And for many years people have used "hot combs" to press out the hair by running a metal comb (heated either electrically or manually) gently through the hair. However, it is important to note that extreme heat can severely damage the hair. So caution is needed with whichever method of straightening a person may individually decide to use.

Chemical Hair Relaxers

Sit down and relax to the hair raising story of hair relaxers. It began early in the twentieth century.

His name was Garrett Augustus Morgan, and he was born the seventh of eleven children of former slaves. He is best known for his invention of the automatic traffic signal and gas mask. Around 1910, while attempting to invent a new lubricating liquid for the sewing machine, Morgan wiped his hands on a wool cloth and found that the wooly texture of the cloth "smoothed out." He experimented on his curly haired Airedale dog and successfully duplicated the effect. Morgan called his discovery a "hair-refining cream" and patented the first chemical hair relaxer.

Today Morgan's discovery, lye (sodium hydroxide), is still a common ingredient in chemical relaxers because it provides the strongest and most dramatic effect. However strong drain cleaners also contain this harsh chemical. Try visualizing drain cleaner on your scalp. Not a pretty picture!

Guanidine hydroxide, another chemical commonly found in hair relaxers, is often promoted as the "no-lye" relaxer. However, do not let the name fool you. It still contains strong chemicals. Although this type of relaxer can inflict less damage than its counterpart, your hair and scalp should still be in top condition before you attempt the procedure.

How Chemical Relaxers Work

How can chemicals "relax" or straighten hair? Both lye and no-lye relaxers contain harsh chemicals that work in the same manner: they both alter the basic structure of the hair shaft. The chemical penetrates the cortex or cortical layer and loosens the natural curl pattern. However this inner layer of the shaft not only gives curly hair its shape, it also

CORTICAL LAYER

MEDULLA

MELANIN

CUTICLE

provides strength and elasticity. Once you perform the straightening process, the result is irreversible. Although you end up with straighter hair, you are now left with much weaker strands susceptible to breakage.

It is easy to "over-process" hair by using excessive relaxers or by applying more chemicals to hair already processed or relaxed. This over processing illustrates the most typical misuse of hair-relaxing chemicals. Once you apply the initial relaxer to "virgin hair", perform touch-ups over new growth no more than every six to eight weeks.

HAIR REMOVAL 101

Hair Removal Techniques for Women and Men

Fess up women... It's hair confession time. How many of you have bleached or waxed hair from above your lips or other parts of your body? Surveys indicate that 80 percent of women and more than 50 percent of men have unwanted hair in various areas of their bodies. Much of this excessive hair is genetic, but sometimes it results from other causes, such as testosterone treatment. Those looking to get rid of unwanted hair have several options as follows:

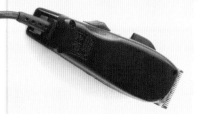

- **Depilation:** The removal of the visible portion of the hair: Shaving, chemical or mechanical depilation. Hair grows back fast and must be removed regularly.

- **Epilation:** The destruction or removal of the entire hair <u>with</u> its roots: Tweezing, waxing, electrolysis, laser hair removal. Hair grows back slowly and it is usually thinner and lighter. Some methods allow permanent hair removal.

Keeping It Simple — Shaving 101

The most popular form of hair removal by far is shaving. However, since shaving must be repeated often to maintain a smooth appearance, the proper technique is vital. Before you start, wash the skin to exfoliate it and lift the hair away from the follicle; this softens the hair and prepares it for the shave. Be sure to shave in the same direction each time (down rather than up); this helps train the hair to grow out straight, making hair removal easier.

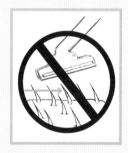

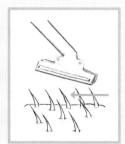

You may notice small bumps appear not long after you shave. These razor rashes may become further irritated, resulting in redness, itchiness, discoloration, or infection. The medical term for bumps is pseudofolliculitis barbae commonly referred to as "ingrown hairs" or "razor bumps." Many people have found they decrease ingrown hairs by using an electric razor although the shave may not be as close as that of a blade. Exfoliate and cleanse your face before shaving to obtain the best defense against ingrown hairs and razor bumps. I recommend the following agents to exfoliate your skin: Skin Biology's LacSal Serum or LacSal Cream. When you gently cleanse your skin and keep it smooth and supple, you moisturize follicles. As a result, the follicles grow in the right direction to prevent razor bumps.

Chemical Depilatories

This type of depilatory contains the harsh chemical calcium thioglycolate that literary dissolves the hair shaft. The partially dissolved hair then can be removed with a sponge and warm water. Since the root remains intact, hair grows back promptly. Chemical depilatories are found in the form of creams, lotions or sprays. Many modern formulations also contain additives to soothe irritation or slow down hair growth.

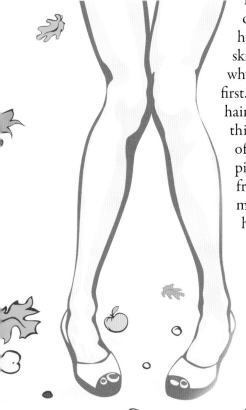

However, if your hair is thick and the skin is sensitive or damaged, painful irritation may develop earlier than the hair will finish dissolving. The result will be red, inflamed skin covered with the remains of the unwanted hair. That is why it is always important to test this method on a small area first. Harsh chemicals that are strong enough to dissolve your hair will not be so gentle on skin either. Those with sensitive thin skin should be especially careful with this method of hair removal. Since skin irritation leads to increased pigment production, it is important to protect your skin from UV rays immediately after depilation, otherwise it may develop pigmented spots. Also make sure to apply healing products that calm down irritation and facilitate recovery post hair removal.

Tweezing

Hair on small areas such as eyebrows can be plucked out with tweezers. This method works well for shaping eyebrows or removing hairs remaining after other methods of hair removal such as waxing. Tweezing does damage hair roots and eventually the hair grows back thinner and lighter. However, this method causes frequent damage to hair follicles and may lead to inflammation and the development of red bumps. If freshly plucked skin is exposed to sunlight, unwanted pigmentation may also develop.

Waxing

For eons, hair waxing has been used by Asian women for hygienic, cultural and esthetic reasons. Modern chemistry in many cases brought modifications to this method; however the basic principle remains the same—extraction of the hair from its root with the aid of a sticky substance. The best waxes are those that do not stick as much to the skin as they do to the hair, thus ensuring a relatively painless and complete hair removal. Sadly, the majority of hair waxing products grip the skin as well, pulling it and stripping away thin layers of the stratum corneum. This results in irritation, damage of skin elastic fibers, and disruption of the skin barrier. Those treated with systemic retinoids such as Accutane should not use waxing methods because their skin will be fragile and more easily damaged. Additionally, waxing should not be used on anyone with damaged skin, warts or moles.

Electrolysis

This is a slow and often painful procedure, but it is the only FDA approved method of permanent hair removal. An electric current is delivered to the hair follicle via a very thin needle that has to be precisely situated in the follicle. If the esthetician misses the follicle, the hair will grow back and the procedure has to be repeated. Since actively growing hair is the most sensitive to the procedure, it takes many sessions (15-30) to target all the hair. Although with patience and time (not mentioning money) hair can be permanently removed using this method, the damage to the skin and hair follicle can result in keloid formation, warts, and skin discoloration.

Laser Hair Removal

The laser hair removal technique utilizes the process of light absorption by the dark hair pigment—melanin. When high energy laser irradiation is absorbed by melanin, the hair heats up, burning the hair follicle just as a metal rod in the fire burns the hand that holds it. The result is severe damage to the follicle which stops hair growth. However, the skin also contains melanin which can absorb laser energy and heat up, burning the surrounding areas. Therefore the more pigment in the hair, the less in the skin, the better. So those with the contrast of black hair and very light skin have the best chance for successful hair removal with minimal skin damage.

Lasers have revolutionized hair removal allowing fast, relatively painless elimination of hair from large areas. But this is still a method that you should be very cautious about. The intense heat delivered straight into the hair follicle incinerates not only the unwanted hair but often your skin's gold reserve as well—we are talking about your stem cells located in the "bulge area" of hair follicles. You know the saying that you cannot make an omelet without breaking a couple of eggs? Well in this case, you simply cannot burn down the hair follicle without damaging your stem cells as well. Make sure that it is a price you are willing to pay for smooth, hairless skin.

Although lasers are considered "safe" under the direction of a skilled expert ("safe" in that there may not be any visible or immediate complications), they can turn into a weapon of skin destruction if used improperly. Dermatologists often see disfigurement, burns, scars, and skin discoloration in those who didn't spend enough time researching the credentials of their laser hair removal specialist. Remember though that even if no visible complications are present, the skin rarely emerges from such a procedure intact, and therefore needs your special attention to recover.

 HOW TO REDUCE ANY SKIN DAMAGE AFTER HAIR REMOVAL:
1. USE BIOHEAL COPPER-PEPTIDE CREAM TO REPAIR IRRITATION
2. FOLLOW WITH EMU OIL-S LIPID REPLENISHER TO SOOTHE AND MOISTURIZE

IMPORTANCE OF SKIN HEALING AFTER HAIR REMOVAL
All hair-removal methods (tweezing, shaving, waxing, electrolysis, lasers, pharmaceutical creams, and so on) cause skin damage that allows viruses and bacteria to penetrate into the skin. For example, warts seem to develop from injured or broken skin. In adults, warts tend to grow where hair-removal procedures have damaged the skin, such as the beard area of men and the legs of women. To restore the skin after shaving, many Skin Biology clients apply BioHeal. The cream closes the skin's surface to viruses and bacteria to help heal the skin.

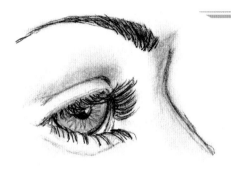

Longer Eyelashes, Thicker Eyebrows The loss of eyebrows and eyelashes often results from long-term use of cosmetics. However, some have reported a reversal of this effect through the light use of an SRCP product. We recommend trying a light application of Folligen Cream followed by Emu Oil-S.

This regimen often helps restore the lost hairs in about two months. For eyebrows: each day apply Folligen Cream followed by Emu Oil-S for Hair. For eyelashes: Each day apply a light coating of Folligen Cream and Emu Oil-S for Hair to the skin below or above the eyelashes near the "eyelash bed" (where the eyelashes would protrude from).

Testimonials:

"I put some Folligen on my eyelashes, because I seem to lose a few every week, and after 2 weeks, they are much longer and thicker and curling upwards... I started applying Folligen, because I used to lose a lash or two each week, not that it was noticeable, but just found them on my cheek. Since I started applying Folligen, none have fallen out...I am using a tiny amount, by the way, just enough to be able to spread across the lash line. I do both upper and lower...Mine are definitely longer, not just thicker, and in just 3.5 weeks I would say at least 10-20% longer." — D

"I have been using copper-peptides for 4 months now and I too have noticed my eyebrow hair thickening. In fact they are wrapping around thicker all the time. So not only is my skin younger looking but my eyebrows are younger looking also." — GH

"I use the Folligen on my eyelashes (upper and lower) in the morning. At night I use [a cosmetic product for eyelash growth], but find that [the other product] helps only in length but not strength or thickness. Folligen improves strength and thickness.." — J

"I've been using CP Night Eyes, CP Serum, Exfol, and P&R for about one month...I did notice about two weeks ago when I put on Mascara that WOW my lashes were looking very good! The mascara was the same as always so I can only assume that the lashes are changing. I have noticed more length and possibly thickening. In any case, I certainly like this added benefit." — BRG

"Must say my eyebrows & lashes are looking so much thicker I am very happy about that." — MY

"My light eyebrows are definitely getting darker! I am elated!" — JN

"After many years of using eye makeup and eye makeup remover I've noticed that my lashes are no longer as thick as they once were. I have been using the follicle cream and emu oil [Folligen Cream and Emu Oil-S for Hair] on my lashes... it seems that my eyelashes are thicker. I believe that I am no longer losing lashes like I use to. Also, my husband has a little bald spot the size of a nickel. The loss of hair was due to stress and has never grown back. I am applying the creme along with the emu oil on it nightly. So far it appears that thin blond hairs are starting to grow...We're both really impressed with your products." — NL

Metallic UFOs Have Landed in My Eye Shadow

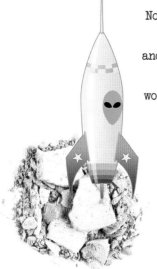

No these are not friendly green Martians abducting my makeup.
This alien brew of chemical dyes, metallic salts,
and optical diffusers unleashes venom while abducting its prey.
Women apply foreign chemical critters and
wonder why their eyebrows fall out or their skin turns sallow.

Well, it's the Invasion of the Hair Snatchers.

These alien thugs damage hair follicles and
rob us of our beautiful eyebrows.
For years, I painted my eyebrows, not because I needed to,
but I wanted to enhance them.

Now I have no choice but to paint what meager brows
that remain because the aliens preyed upon my vellus follicles.
And these are the very follicles that produce stem cells for new skin.
And so now, I've not only lost eyebrows, I've aged my skin as well.
What's a poor girl to do? Just take it from me ladies,
it's best to use as few color cosmetics as you can,
especially when they have a list of alien ingredients
that you can't even pronounce.

• •

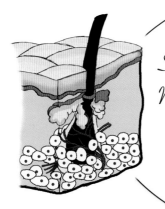

Feisty Follicles

Say Hi to follicles oh feisty molecules on top of copper

My uncut locks so rich and wicked plush lush and thick

My hair affair flow flower pot with roots

so deep to sprout the vine

Oh suave fair let hair strands shine.

Idelle Musiek

(14)

NAIL RENEWAL
Restore Health for Nails that Grow Stronger

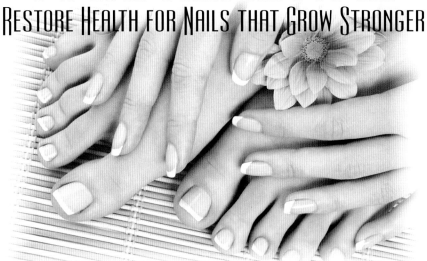

Lengthy exquisite fingernails have been the envy of women throughout the ages. While nail fashions may change from one century to the next and even from week to week, the desire for long strong nails has spanned many epochs. In ancient China, women of high status grew their nails long and painted them with gold lacquer indicating they never had to toil. Yet in other eras, nails were used as weapons. You have no doubt heard the saying, "I'm going to claw your eyes out." Nails are vestigial remnants of defensive weapons of our distant ancestors. In humans, nails evolved as aids for picking up small objects, for scratching and for taking revenge on two-timing beaus. Today women make a fashion statement with these functional, yet oh so expressive, appendages. One season, women may wear square-cut nails. A few months later, they re-shape these beauties in stylish oval. From white-tipped French manicures, shocking crimson lacquer to naked nails in the buff, your fingernails make a personal statement about how you care for yourself and who you are. In this chapter you will learn how to protect, renew and beautify one of the most expressive parts of a woman's body.

SRCPS, HORSE HOOVES, AND FINGERNAILS Skin Remodeling Copper Peptides increase the proliferation of the keratin-producing cell, the keratinocyte. Keratin is the protein that makes up our outer protective skin layer and our nails. In animals it is what composes their horns, claws and hooves.

Throughout the course of prolonged water rains in Washington State, horses often develop severe irritations and infections in their lower extremities—especially where the hair-covered lowerleg joins the hooves. During experiments to heal their inflamed skin above the hooves, copper peptide creams were generously applied to their legs, but due to the movements of these feisty horses, much product ended up on the hooves. It was no surprise to observe how rapidly the copper healed their skin. However, we were both delighted and amazed to see that the damaged hooves also improved. Later, we experimented with more controlled applications of copper peptide creams into cracks in badly damaged hooves. We found that the copper peptide cream usually produced a remarkable healing in the hooves and closure of the cracks.

Since the hooves of horses and nails of humans are biochemically similar, we experimented with applications of copper peptide creams to damaged human fingernails and toenails. We observed that as in the horses, human nails grew healthier and stronger than we could have ever imagined. Such types of copper peptides, when applied to the nail matrix and nail bed area, enhance the process of nail growth resulting in stronger, thicker, and smoother nails.

In an informal study on nail growth in humans, the fingernail growth rates of the index fingers were used as a measurement. In some experiments CP Nail Renewal was applied to the index fingernail and cuticle on the right hand while the left hand nail was untreated and used as a control. In the second set of experiments, the CP Nail Renewal was applied to the index fingernail and cuticle on the left hand while the right hand nail was treated with a placebo cream. After four weeks nail length was measured from the end of the nail bed to the tip of the nail at the center. The effect of nail growth stimulation was similar if either the right or left hand treated group was used.

Components of a Healthy Fingernail

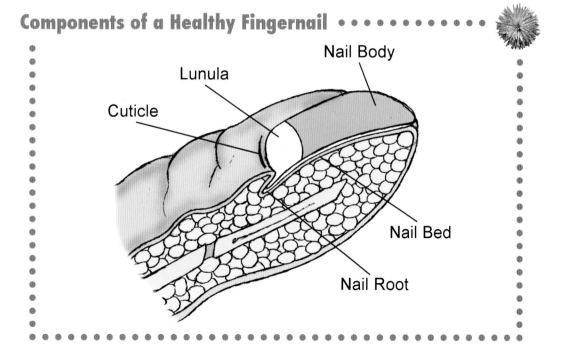

TIN PEPTIDES vs. **COPPER PEPTIDES**   But a problem arose since copper peptides often stain nails with a greenish tint. Later I found that tin-peptides, a complex of ionic tin (2+) and peptides, do not tarnish nails and are more effective than copper peptides on nail growth. Tin-peptides also work better than SRCPs in our test systems for hair growth. While tin-peptides lack the wound healing actions of SRCPs they work better at producing keratin, the major protein in nails and hair.

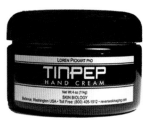

Tin-peptides beautify more than your nails. They also rejuvenate hands and hair. Our clients tell us that tin-peptides make their hands appear younger and repair damage caused by gardening, washing clothes, and other forms of physical labor.

Nail Growth and Health

While the fingernail resembles hair and shares similar attributes, it does not undergo the hair cycle of growth and non-growth. Healthy nails grow continuously throughout your life. They grow approximately

Client feedback on TINPEP Hand Cream: "I started 3 days ago the [TINPEP Hand Cream]. It is phenomenal at softening and reducing irritation. When I use it in the night, since during the night I usually do not scratch at all, it has an effectiveness in reducing irritation that is almost comparable to steroid lotions. Really impressive. [TINPEP] also smells fantastic." —R.

one-half to one millimeter weekly. It takes five to seven months for the nail to grow completely and replace itself from the time it forms at the root until it reaches beyond finger tip.

Toenails grow at a snail's pace, about a third to half the growth rate of fingernails. Like hair, nails grow more during the summer. The middle finger nail grows fastest, with the growth rate progressively decreasing on the fourth, second, fifth fingers and finally the thumb.

When a nail gets injured and falls off, a new nail grows in at the normal rate. With a damaged matrix, the new nail may grow, but in a distorted form. However, if the matrix gets destroyed, the new nail will not grow in any form. In today's life style, we expose our nails to many stresses such as detergents and hot water that damage the matrix, making nails thinner and weaker and less able to grow. To better understand the condition, of your nails, refer to the diagnostic chart on the following page.

Nail Renewal Cream

Just as SRCPs can renew damaged skin and hair, copper peptides also repair and strengthen nails, enabling them to grow faster and stronger than ever before.

Skin Biology has launched Tin Peptide Nail Renewal Cream which effectively rebuilds, strengthens and thickens nails and smooths out the cuticles. You can help your fingers feel smooth and nails grow stronger and faster with this new nail renewal cream! Once or twice daily apply a light amount on your nail bed and cuticle.

Nail Diagnostic Chart

Use this diagnostic chart to look at and understand the condition of your nails:

DESCRIPTION	POSSIBLY Due To...
Splitting, Brittle Nails	Irritating substances such as harsh detergents or nail polish remover; or silica deficiency
Longitudinal Nail Ridges	Aging, inadequate absorption of vitamins and minerals, kidney failure, or thyroid disease
Horizontal Nail Ridges	Nutrition problem, injury, or infection
Discoloration	May be an indicator of anemia
Purple or Black	Typically due to trauma, or may be sign of vitamin B12 deficiency. Also a streak (black or brown) from the base of the nail that extends all the way to the tip may be an indicator of melanoma. See your medical provider.
Yellow Color	Fungal infection, psoriasis, diabetes, heredity, or use of tetracycline
Red / Dark Pink	May indicate poor peripheral circulation
Half Pink and Half White	Fungal infection or kidney disease
Blue	May indicate that blood is not receiving enough oxygen due to a respiratory disorder, cardiovascular disease, or lupus erythermatosus
Large Moons	Possible overactive thyroid, genetics, or trauma
No Moons	Possible underactive thyroid, or genetics
Soft Nails	Malnutrition, contact with strong alkali substance, endocrine problem, or arthritis
White, Soft Nails	Fungal infection
Thick Nails	Poor circulation, fungal infection, or persistent nail trauma which may cause hardening
Loose Nail Plate	Injury, psoriasis, fungal or bacterial infection, side effects of medication, chemotherapy treatments, thyroid disease, Raynaud's Syndrome, or Lupus
"Pitted Nail" (Yellow/Brown spots)	Possible eczema, psoriasis, or hair loss condition
Spoon Shape	Possible thyroid disease or iron deficiency
Club Shape	Cirrhosis of the liver, or chronic respiratory or heart condition
Wasting Away of the Nail	Injury or disease
Infected Nail: Red/Tender/Swollen	Yeast infection or bacterial infection
Complete Loss of Nail	Trauma

SUPPLEMENTS FOR NAIL HEALTH

Biotin - Biotin can strengthen brittle nails and bring them back to health and luster. Take (2.5 mg a day) but do not take biotin if you are pregnant. In one placebo-controlled, double-blind clinical study, 60 patients who had poor nail quality but had no overt biotin deficiency were treated for 6 months with 2.5 mg of biotin per day. The improvement in nail quality was measured by (1) the resistance of the nails to swelling after incubation with an alkaline agent (NaOH), (2) the rate of water loss through the fingernail (transonychial water loss), and (3) the separate judgments of nail health by the clinical investigator and by the patient. All measured parameters showed improved nail quality (Gehring 1996). A Swiss study veterinary report described the treatment of biotin for horses' cracked hooves which are biochemically similar to fingernails (Scher 1994).

MSM - Supplements of sulfer-rich MSM (2-4 grams daily), have been shown to strengthen fragile nails. MSM also encourages your fingernails, toe nails, and hair to grow faster because you have more sulfur in your finger nails and hair than any other cells of your body. According to one of our clients:

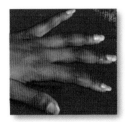

" I take MSM, 4-6 grams daily, and have noticed amazing improvements in my hair growth and nail growth. My nails are stronger, break much less often, and I can prove it!...I can tell how much faster they are growing because I have to cut/clip them so much more often. I can't wait to start using the New Tin Peptide Nail Renewal also!" —C.M.

Gelatin - Gelatin is a protein source of nine essential amino acids, histidine, lysine, leucine, tryptophan, valine, phenylalanine, methionine, threonine, and isoleucine, as well as other amino acids—all building blocks of protein. An article "Gelatin-cystine, keratogenesis and structure of the hair" in Boll Soc Ital Biol Sper (Morganti et al 1983) states that the oral ingestion of gelatin significantly increases the degree of hardness of finger and toe nails.

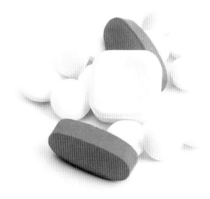

PROTECTING NAILS Like hair, nails are usually healthiest in their natural state. While nail polishes and cosmetic nails may improve your appearance, they tend to degrade nail health.

If you can avoid repeated wetting and drying of your nails, you will minimize brittle nails, chipping, splitting and breaking. Also try to avoid alkaline detergents, soaps and cleaners. Instead use cleansers with a slightly acid pH to prevent loosening of the protein fibers that form the nail.

In recent years, salons say that more nail damage is caused by cosmetic/beautifying procedures than ever before. Cosmetics such as nail polishes and artificial nails generally degrade nail health. Give your nails a break from cosmetic polishes and artificial nails for one to three months per year to allow the nails to recover. Treatments such as nail strengtheners and hardeners can help to protect nails from breakage, but polish removers weaken nails. When applying coatings of nail strengtheners and hardeners, apply them as subsequent layers over the previous treatments rather than removing earlier coatings.

Cotton lined rubber gloves are best for nails and should be used during household or job-related work that involves getting the hands wet. You can also minimize damage inflicted by environmental onslaughts and artificial treatments by applying Tin Peptide Nail Renewal Cream to restore the health of your nails.

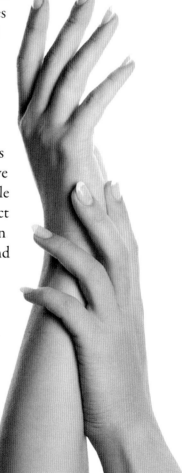

Restoring Cuticle Health and Hangnails

Since the cuticle skin is especially thin, dermatologists recommend you take special care not to damage this sensitive area. Doctors recommend that you do not cut or nip the cuticle since it acts as a protective barrier against bacteria. An intact cuticle helps to prevent infection of the nail. Ragged cuticles can deform the shape of the growing nail. Some people have found Tin Peptide Nail Renewal Cream and cuticle oils help to keep the cuticles soft, supple and healthy.

Hangnails produce small tears or splits in the nail plate or surrounding tissue. They often result from dry skin or injury. When hangnails tear, they can cause chronic pain and infect the area. BioHeal works very well on hangnail problems.

Cosmetic Nails

In the late 20th century, a wide variety of artificial nails have increased in popularity. Women use them in conjunction with natural nails and not as a replacement.

They can elongate or beautify nails. They also camouflage discolored, thickened, or malformed fingernails. Unfortunately, the glues used to fasten the artificial nails may cause both allergic contact dermatitis and nail damage.

The pre-formed plastic nail is the most popular type of artificial nail. Some come pre-glued as in press-on types while others require one to apply glue separately. The acrylic glues typically contain methacrylate, a chemical which can cause allergic contact dermatitis. There are stronger adhesives that provide better bonding, but these can cause the nail plate to separate from the nail bed or cause the biological plate to split into layers. Preformed cosmetic nails are not recommended for people with weak nails.

Sculpted Nails

These custom-made artificial nails sculpt to fit exactly over your natural nails. Sculpted nails fit extremely well and you may have a difficult time differentiating this custom nail from a natural nail. This 'nail sculpture', made from acrylic polymers, requires more care than natural fingernails. Although they can look like art on your fingers, you may pay a cost for their enhancement. After two to four months of wear, the natural nail plate may turn yellow, dry out and thin. For this reason, you should not wear sculptured nails for more than three consecutive months before allowing your natural nails a break of at least one month to improve their health. Sometimes silk or linen cloth wraps, combined with nail sculptures, can strengthen the artificial nail.

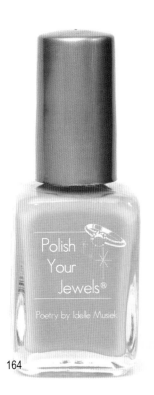

Your nails are **jewels** – not tools,
Tough as nails though they be,
Protecting the **fingers**
like hard shells at sea,
Covering **delicate** nail moons
With hair shining glances
Refueling pink **painted** pinkies
And tip toed nail dances.
Do care for your jewels with
true **love** and garnish.
But refrain from rough tough
chemical varnish.
So **treat your nails** kindly
with each lacquered coat.

Bedazzle
Be noticed
Wave fingers
Curl toes!

IT WORKED FOR THEM — IT CAN WORK FOR YOU!

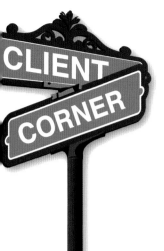

"I've been using the Tin Peptide Nail Renewal for 2 weeks and my nails have never been longer or stronger! I rub the cream into my nails and hands before I go to bed at night." -C.P.

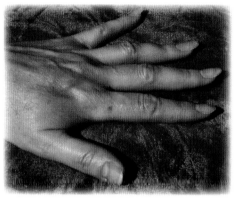

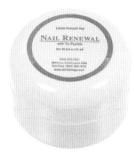

Apply Tin Peptide Nail Renewal to the nail and cuticle. Rub into the nail/cuticle area for 5-10 seconds. Use once or twice day.

"I started using the original CP for nails [CP Nail Renewal], sample size, about a year ago to strengthen my nails. Then I changed to the Tin Peptide for nails when it was given as a tester. Now, besides having much stronger nails, in the process, a very deep verticle grove that extended the length of my nail is gone. I find that remarkable, because I never expected the cream to completely remodel my nail. Also, a year ago, I lost my big toenail. Today, with the addition of mostly Tin Peptide and occasional TriReduction and CP, my toenail is good as new. I'm sold on CP's and Tin Peptide. They all work. Just give them time... I used all of them. Seriously, I used P&R Classic, TriReduction with Retinol, CP Serum, Super CP and Super Cop 2X, just whatever I had on hand...I was religious morning and night with the Tin Peptide and my nails are harder and less likely to chip or split... It takes months for the damage that we don't see under the epidermis at the base of the nail to improve, before the nail starts growing out normal. It took a year for a completely new, perfect nail using mostly tin peptides because I was using them to build stronger, healthier nails never imagining I would get rid of the ridge also. In other words, I'm now thinking (after reading Dr. Pickart) that it was the CP's that did most of the work with the remodeling. I will add that an experienced pedicurist told me my toenail would never be good when it grew out and they were wrong about that. That was a combination of Tin and CP's also." - SS

"My nails are by nature prone to peeling, and they are very soft and rip easily. I could not grow the white tips any longer than 2-2.5 millimeters without them ripping. A few months ago I got into french manicures, and I was painting my nails a couple times per week. As a result, my nails were completely trashed. Almost every one of them was peeling. Then I turned to SB's Tin Peptide, and the results have been truly amazing. At first, the peeling got a little worse as the top layer of the nail got stronger, but I kept with it and they are now incredibly strong, stronger than they have ever been!! Every nail is at least 3 mm long (I have filed them back to get rid of the remnants of damage and for shaping). I can't bend my thumbnails at all. I recently picked up a little nail buffer, and I buffed them to a high shine, and I love them so much I can't stop looking at them! I apply the cream when I think of it, 0-2 times per day, probably averaging 1x/day. Thanks so much, SB!" - RL

"I received a sample of this product a few months back. (THANK YOU). I wear acrylic nail overlays over my natural nail, have done so for years. My natural nails are thin, but grow fast. (they were this way even before arcrylic use, I also have fine hair). I have started using the Tin Peptide [Nail Renewal] daily, even over my overlay, rubbing the cream into the cuticles and under the cuticle into nail base. I also rub it around the edges of the acrylic. This has helped my nails stay flexible (which helps them adhere to the overlay better with less lifting) and also has lessened overlay separation and nail peeling. I do my acrylics myself, and am quite careful of the products used, avoiding the detrimental prep products etc. So even though I do wear acrylics, my nails are actually in quite good shape. But the Tin Peptide is a wonderful addition into my nail care, and a good option I think even for acrylic wearers." - TL

"I, too, have been using the nail cream. My splitting nails are a thing of the past. My thumb nail, in particular, used to split down to the nail bed. It was so frustrating. My nails are finally healthy. The only change I made was using the cream. Thank you!!" - LH

"I have only been using the tin peptides on my cuticles for seven days but I swear!! There is a difference. I have such thick cuticles I can pull at them...They are so smooth and normal now after seven days. I am totally hooked." - PH

"I really like the tin peptides nail cream. Now that winter is coming my cuticles have a tendency to get all jagged and painful, not to mention the cracks in the corners of my thumbs. This cream heals the hang nails virtually overnight. I hope you'll be selling this all the time because I never want to be without it. This stuff works better than any other nail treatment I've tried. Thanks SB!...I am more than happy with the tin peptides... Not only is the Tin Peptide Nail Cream great for nails but it is also an excellent hand cream. My hands were at their winter worst recently, cracking and even bleeding a little. I thought hey this works so good on the cuticles why not give it a try it on my hands as well. I always put it on my nails last thing at night and one night I used a little extra on my hands. They immediately felt refreshed and by the next morning the difference was dramatic...I love SB products." - DS

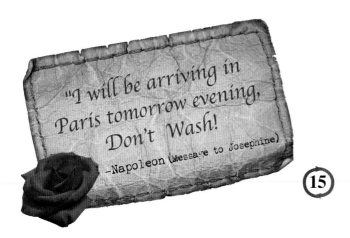

"I will be arriving in Paris tomorrow evening, Don't Wash!

—Napoleon (Message to Josephine)

(15)

THE FORMULA OF LOVE
Sniffing Out Social and Sexual Signals

What is the formula of love? Can we seek and sniff out Mr. Right? Imagine yourself sipping an espresso at a local cafe, reading the paper and minding your business. Suddenly a young person enters the room and you are immediately struck with cupid's arrow. You not only sense a chemical attraction, you smell it. Cupid has just struck you with pheromones, the 'smellprints' that evoke the chemistry of attraction. The aroma of coffee fades as pheromones brew up the scent of passion. Such is the power of pheromones. These intoxicating chemicals are given off by humans, animals and plants and serve to attract and stimulate others. Research shows that human pheromones may stir up a host of behaviors, ranging from mothers kissing their children to men being attracted to large-breasted women.

Raging hormone and sizzling pheromone levels peak at around age 18 and then slowly decline throughout our lives. When we enter a room at age 40, our pheromone signal no longer excites others as it did when we were 18. When we gaze amorously at a young beauty, we tend to assume that our eyes incite the chemical amalgam that causes our hearts to flutter. As a result, we fail to consider how scents also activate our senses. As we age, our lack of appeal may be in large part due to our drop in pheromones. As a result, the most effective way for aging individuals to attract attention may be to enhance their natural pheromone signal with supplemental pheromones, just as we take supplements of antioxidants to keep healthy and ward off disease (Kohl & Francoeur 1995, Cutler 1996, Pickart 2005).

THE TWO TYPES OF PHEROMONES

While pheromones produce less obvious reactions in humans than in other animals, they strongly shape our behavior. As pheromones move among us, they activate pre-coded genetic programs.

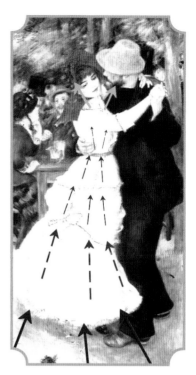

Pheromones fall into two categories, 'signal' and 'primer', that attract us to each other in different ways. Signal pheromones move through the air. These airborne particles ascend on their airy journey after the body's heat evaporates them. When you wear clothes, your body heats the air, causing it to rise toward the highest opening. As the heated air rises, it picks up the pheromones secreted from your skin. When the air emerges around your face, it causes people to notice you. It takes about one second for smells from your face to reach someone 50 feet away in still air. In addition to making others aware of our presence, signal pheromones also cause immediate changes in behavior by activating certain areas of the brain.

The primer pheromone, a heavy protein, passes directly by kissing or skin-to-skin contact. When a mother kisses her baby, it increases mother-baby bonding. The first romantic kiss provides a perfect opportunity to check out pheromones. These bonding signals may explain why kissing occurs in all human cultures; as a way of passing pheromones. Priming pheromones increase the production of many hormones that effect development, metabolism, and mating behavior. These pheromones can take time to weave their special links. Consider how at times, fertile women find it difficult to conceive. In married couples, it takes an average of six months to get pregnant. Perhaps the woman's body must slowly adjust to her husband's pheromones before becoming receptive to pregnancy. Women love to cuddle and snuggle—something that a new husband quickly learns will help him have a smooth relationship with his wife.

Why Women Call Men "Pigs"

In pigs, deer, goats, sheep and some other animals, males compete for females on the basis of pheromone strength rather than physical strength or beauty. The animals with the strongest pheromones exude confidence and display threat without giving signals of fear. This reduces the incidence of actual physical combat for females, especially among deer and moose. The male pig that signals the strongest pheromones causes a psychological castration of his competition. It's the survival of the fittest pig! Now does this make for a chauvinist pig or just an animal driven by hormonal instinct? I'll let you decide.

This type of pheromone dominance may also apply to us humans. Many believe that the pheromone response in humans and pigs is similar. As hard as this may be on the ego, it's probably true. Before we protest with a squealing 'oink-oink', consider how truffles entice both pigs and humans—and no, I'm not talking about how chocolate truffles release pleasure hormones in women. Chocolate truffles derived their name from the highly prized truffle mushroom, a fungus that grows underground near oak trees in France and Italy, has long been prized as a human aphrodisiac. Pigs, too, passionately lust for truffles and pigs used to sniff out and locate the precious fungi. Now here is some more amusing food for thought. Why do women often call men pigs when men rarely use this term for women? Could it be that ever since wild pigs were domesticated 7000 years ago, women intuitively knew that many male human hormones resemble those of pigs? So if you are a man, your pheromone scent may affect females more strongly than your good looks, money, or wit.

QUOTABLE QUOTES: *The truffle is not exactly an aphrodisiac, but it tends to make women more tender and men more likeable.*
—French gastronome Brillat-Savarin

The key pheromone in pigs, androstenone, gives boar urine its characteristic odor and also accounts for some of the odor in human male urine. Both women and female pigs respond to the smell of androstenone in their male partners. Pig breeders spray androstenone from aerosol cans on the backs of female pigs to determine whether the female is ready for breeding; if the sow arches her back, she is sexually receptive.

SMELLS AFFECT OUR EMOTIONS During the Middle Ages, a man would wipe his brow after dancing and present the cloth to his lady as a love token. He may not have consciously realized that his smell would remain with her as a momento. The wives of Welsh miners put their husband's nightshirts on their pillows in order to smell their men who spent nights away in the mines. Even today a lady might wear her beau's unwashed T-shirt. Aah! The compelling force of pheromones.

QUOTABLE QUOTES: *The purest union that can exist between a man and a woman is that caused by the sense of smell and is sanctioned by the brain's normal assimilation of the animate molecules emitted by the secretions produced by two bodies in contact and sympathy, and in their subsequent evaporation.* *—Auguste Galopin*

Current theories postulate that smells affect the brain's emotional control areas by activating nerves in the vomero-nasal organ (VMO) in the nasal septum. To understand how the sense of smell influences the brain, it helps to understand how the brain works. The brain consists of three areas. The lower part of the brain, the brain stem, controls functions such as breathing and heartbeat. The central area called the limbic system, generates emotions. Some limbic areas promote feelings of peace, contentment, and attraction, while other areas cause feelings of anger, rage, hostility, loneliness, and so on. The conscious brain, where thinking occurs, occupies the topmost and outer area of the brain. However, the conscious mind does not emit emotions. The reason we love someone has more to do with how one smells to the limbic system than what we consciously think. Smell signals are sent directly to the limbic system where emotions arise.

QUOTABLE QUOTES: *Her breasts, like lilies, 'ere their leaves be shed;*
Her nipples, like young blossomed jessamines;
Such fragrant flowers do give most odorous smell.
But her sweet odour did them all excel. —Edmund Spencer

Pheromones affect how we feel about and react to others from the moment we are born. Newborn infants follow the breast odors emanating from their mother's nipple/areola region. These odors exert a pheromone effect that guides the infant to nurse at his mother's nipples. Within minutes of birth, the mother's breast odor causes the baby's head to turn and helps guide the baby to successful suckling of milk. These nipple pheromones may also explain the irrational obsession of men with women's breasts (Winberg & Porter 1998, Porter & Winberg 1999, Schaal et al 2003).

Since smells have such a powerful impact on our emotions, it should come as no surprise that a lack of smell limits our ability to emotionally bond. Approximately 1.3 percent of the population is born with a total lack of smell, known as anosmia. Persons with anosmia often complain about a lack of libido. While they may marry, emotional distance remains a problem. Likewise, the decline in sex drive with aging coincides with the decline in smell.

PHEROMONES ACT EVEN IF YOU CAN'T SMELL THEM
While many pheromones give off distinctive odors that evoke emotion, they may be too weak to consciously detect. For example, a male dog can respond to pheromones from a female dog at a distance of up to three miles, at a concentration too faint to consciously smell. Humans also respond to pheromone levels that are too low to smell. At Stanford University, Sobel and colleagues found that an airborne fragrant pheromone (oestra- 1,3,5(10),16-tetraen-3yl acetate) activated brain centers even when present at concentrations below a threshold of conscious detection (Sobel et al 1999).

Bathing and the Decline of Bonding
As our culture advances, we tend to bathe more and bond less. This suggests that washing removes skin pheromones and weakens interpersonal bonding in families and between couples.

The tie between washing and the decline of chemical attraction is present throughout history, from ancient to modern times. In the Roman Republic, family ties were very strong. However, as this society evolved into the wealthy Roman Empire, with its adequate water supplies and free municipal baths, personal bonds grew weaker, divorce became common, and social disorganization increased. With the rise of Christianity and its dislike of nudity and bathing, family ties began to strengthen.

In the USA, California led the way in personal cleanliness. By the 1940's, many Californians bathed or showered daily, washing away their personal pheromones in the process, while most of the USA stuck to weekly bathing. California soon led the nation in divorce rates and family breakdown. At about the same time, Scandinavia led Europe as a hallmark for personal cleanliness and soon it also experienced family breakdown. Swedes often complained that they felt cultural isolation. Both California and Scandinavia, with their immense social programs, prosperous economies, and basic friendliness have not solved these problems.

WHY EXPENSIVE PERFUMES DON'T WORK Studies by Alan Hirsch and Jason Gruss (Smell and Taste Treatment Research Foundation, Chicago and University of Michigan) found that expensive perfumes are less effective than many essential oils and common foods. They studied the effects of several different scents on sexual arousal of males and females by comparing the subjects' blood flow in sexually aroused tissues (penile or clitoral blood flow) while wearing scented masks and while wearing non-odorized, blank masks. Expensive perfumes increased blood flow by only 3 percent in men. In contrast, the combined odor of lavender and pumpkin pie produced a 40 percent increase in men. Many other scents also worked better than the perfumes. While these results pertain to men, the researchers reported that women also responded poorly to expensive perfumes and positively to other smells.

Hirsch suggests that certain scents may increase sexual arousal by acting on the brain in three different ways: by reducing anxiety, which inhibits natural sexual desire; increasing alertness and awareness, making the subjects more aware of sexual cues in the environment around them; and acting directly to the septal nuclei, a portion of the brain that induces sexual arousal (Hirsch 1998).

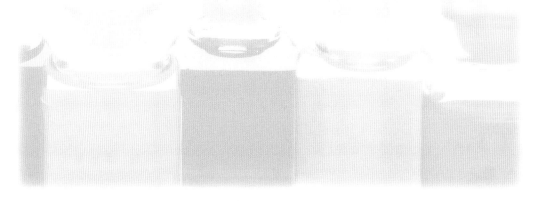

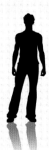

MEN: Effect of Perfumes and Scents on Blood Flow in Male Sexual Tissue

ITEM TESTED	Median % Increase in Penile Blood Flow
Lavender & Pumpkin Pie	40
Pumpkin Pie & Doughnut	20
Orange	19.5
Black Licorice & Cola	13
Black Licorice	3
Lily of the Valley	11
Vanilla	9
Pumpkin Pio	8.6
Lavender	8
Musk	7.5
Peppermint	6
Cheese Pizza	5
Roasting Meat	5
Rose	4
Strawberry	3.5
Oriental Spices	3.5
Expensive Perfumes	Averaged 3.0
Chocolate	2.8

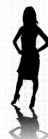

WOMEN: Effect of Perfumes & Scents on Enhancement of Clitoral Blood Flow

ITEM TESTED	Median % Increase
Cucumber and Licorice Candy	13
Baby Powder	13
Lavender & Pumpkin Pie	11
Charcoal Barbecued Meat	Inhibited: Anti-arousal
Cherries	Inhibited: Anti-arousal
Expensive Men's Colognes	Inhibited: Anti-arousal

Above Chart based on publications of Alan Hirsch and Jason Gruss

SOCIAL PHEROMONES Have you ever entered a crowded room and felt anxiety and agitation? Or how about road rage? You're stuck in traffic not going anywhere with drivers honking and cursing. What can you do?

Although most research has focused on sexual pheromones, there are aromatic oils that also boast harmonizing properties that change behavior patterns, reduce mental stress, and improve social interactions.

These "social pheromones" include many long established pure essential oils that have been used for thousands of years in social events, weddings, and spiritual gatherings. For example sanatol, one of the active ingredients in Sandalwood Oil and Asian Oud, has harmonizing and anti-conflict properties. When mice are caged together, this leads to conflict and fighting. Exposure to the smell of sanatol reduces the conflict among the mice. Ylang Ylang has similar anti-conflict properties.

Lavender Oil reduces perinatal discomfort in women following childbirth and the pain of patients in intensive care units. Remaining still inside a cramped magnetic resonance scanner often causes anxiety and claustrophobia. Whiffs of heliotropin, a vanilla-like fragrance, before the procedure reduced patient anxiety 63 percent. Some oils are considered to have a mild aphrodisiac effect (jasmine, ylang-ylang, rose, sandalwood, vanilla) but this may be due to their calming and stress reducing actions.

These social pheromones can calm the worst of moods and decrease conflict in social situations. Ylang Ylang is just one of several pheromones that has been shown to lessen conflict and aggressive behavior. Sandalwood Oil also has a calming affect by reducing anxiety. And if you are under mental stress at work or school try Lavender Oil, which can calm you down so that you can focus and be more alert.

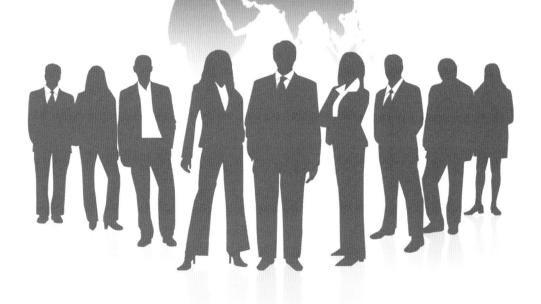

EFFORTS TO CREATE AN EFFECTIVE PERFUME Several companies have been set up to develop romantic pheromones for consumers, based on "the" human pheromone, but most have failed to deliver results.

For me, the use of aromatic plant oils as body perfumes was just an idea. Women who had been buying my experimental cosmetics with copper peptides kept asking me about perfumes, so I read everything that I could find. My conclusions were:

1. If pheromones are species-specific, humans shouldn't be able to detect animal-derived pheromones. But even if they could, what reactions might we expect? Taking into account that many animals become more dangerous during mating periods, humans shouldn't be attracted to the smell of a ready-to-mate boar; they should feel fear or aggression.

Androstenone triggers both sexual attraction and aggression in boars. In mice, certain pheromones cause male mice to kill other male mice (male odors increase attacks, female odors decrease attacks). Male lions and bears will kill the offspring of a female in order to mate with her. If purely sexual human pheromones, similar to pig androstenone, were discovered, they couldn't be used in perfume. If humans followed the urge for pheromone-induced mating, people would get arrested!

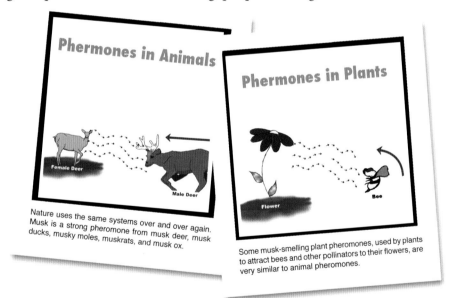

Nature uses the same systems over and over again. Musk is a strong pheromone from musk deer, musk ducks, musky moles, muskrats, and musk ox.

Some musk-smelling plant pheromones, used by plants to attract bees and other pollinators to their flowers, are very similar to animal pheromones.

2. Human interactions are complex, and the social element is very important. There could be 100 human pheromones that affect different aspects of behavior.

3. Some musk-smelling plant pheromones, used by plants to attract bees and other pollinators to their flowers, are very similar to animal pheromones. Nature uses the same systems over and over again. For example, musk is a strong pheromone from musk deer, musk ducks, musky moles, muskrats, musk ox, and musk beetles. However similar pheromones exist in musk melons, musk hyacinths, musk cherries, musk thistle, musk rose, musk plums, and musk wood.

Brain research suggests that calming oils may improve sexual function. Neuroscientist Gert Holstege (University of Groningen), using positron-emission tomography, found that to achieve a human sexual climax, the amygdala (the brain's center of vigilance and fear) is silenced while activity in brain areas that are involved in judgement and reflection are greatly reduced. This occurs in men and even more so in women. He commented "Fear and anxiety need to be avoided at all costs if a woman wishes to have an orgasm" (Holstege 2005).

4. When creating pheromone perfumes, most companies just use the molecule with the chemical smell rather than the original essential oil. But we don't know which component of the complex mixture is able to communicate with our brain, and it might even be an odorless component. By throwing away everything but the part that the nose can smell, these companies might also be throwing away the magic.

5. Historically, many of the traditional mood-altering essential oils have also been used for skin care. Patchouli has long been used as an anti-inflammatory and aid for dry, cracked skin. The oil of lavender soothes skin and was applied to wounds in ancient Greece and Rome. It is still used today. Sandalwood is used for skin regeneration and to treat acne, dry skin, rashes, chapped skin, eczema, itching, and sensitive skin. It also has anti-skin cancer actions (Kaur et al 2005, Dwivedi et al 2003, Dwivedi & Zhang 1999). Ylang ylang is used to treat eczema, acne, oily skin, and irritation associated with insect stings or bites. With so many ways to benefit from essential oils, it is difficult to find a reason not to use them.

QUOTABLE QUOTES: *Thy God hath anointed you with the oil of gladness.*
—Saint Paul

FROM THEORY TO PRACTICE   At Skin Biology, I experimented with a variety of expensive human pheromones from other companies and gave them to volunteers for testing plus various pheromones from the essential oils of plants. The volunteers were asked to wear each of the pheromones and record people's reactions. In every case, the test subjects found few positive responses to the human pheromones. Conversely, all of them reported positive responses to at least some of the plant pheromones, such as people were more friendly, talkative, and/or affectionate. Based on client responses, the most effective plant pheromones were reported to be the essential oils of *jasmine*, *ylang-ylang*, **nutmeg**, **sandalwood**, *Asian oud*, **patchouli**, and *lavender*.

BODY PERFUMES WITH PLANT DERIVED PHEROMONES

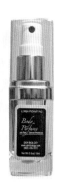

Based on our experiments, we created pheromone products that have won rave reviews from clients: Body Perfumes with Plant Derived Pheromones, Romantic Oils, and 4 Sensuous Scents Oil. There are several different scents to choose from, including patchouli (good for attracting women), ylang ylang (good for attracting men), musk, sandalwood, and jasmine (all universal attractants). A full list is available online at www.skinbiology.com. By using an appropriate version of our perfume oils, you can strongly modify your personal "odor signature" in a positive way.

Think Torso and Legs, Not Wrists and Earlobes

For thousands of years, people would apply perfumes to the torso and legs. The heat of the body would evaporate the pheromones and scents in the oil and blend them into a person's individual odor signature. This signature brew is made up of a complex mixture of pheromones, body oils, fatty acids, sweat, and hormones such as androsterone secreted onto the skin from the apocrine glands. In addition, the 40 million skin cells that you shed each day add to your odor signature.

The modern method of applying perfumes to the wrists and earlobes only reflects the ignorance of the modern cosmetic industry. It is best to apply body perfumes after a bath or shower. Dry yourself, and then spray pheromone products on to your body, especially on large, heat-producing areas such as the chest, breasts, and legs. If you bathe at night, the oils should be applied to your dry skin in the morning.

Finding the Body Perfume with Plant Derived Pheromone that best complements your unique odor signature and attracts the type of people that you desire may take some trial and error. Work your way through the oils one by one until you find the one that is most effective. Apply the oil, and then dress normally and go about your daily routine. If the oil is working, responsive people will unconsciously notice you from three to five feet away. Watch for people who unexpectedly turn and smile or extend conversations. Using plant-derived pheromones is a little like trolling for salmon while testing different lures; it takes some time, but keep trying and eventually you'll find the right lure (scent).

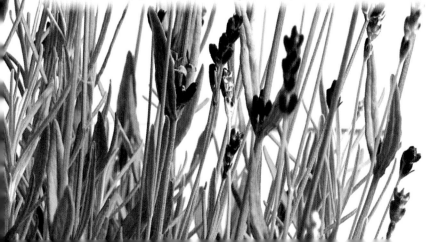

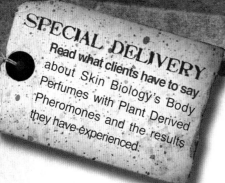

SPECIAL DELIVERY
Read what clients have to say about Skin Biology's Body Perfumes with Plant Derived Pheromones and the results they have experienced:

2011

JUST
IN

"I've been using either the jasmine or the stealth version before company meetings with male executives. Now that I use the oil, they very often agree with me. Their aggression level seems to drop when I have Calypso's Oil on...I will just keep this method secret."
—*Anonymous client from New York*

"Whenever I use ylang ylang and nutmeg oil, I always get compliments, such as 'What are you wearing? I really have to know.'" —*K.S.*

"I am 60 years old, and the oil is working better than Viagra for me. I prefer the oils with ylang ylang and jasmine. My wife agrees." —*K.S.*

"I love the stuff. I got the jasmine-scented one with the pheromones. It's not oily at all...a little goes a long way and soaks right in. I put it on my neck and shoulders, and not two minutes later my husband was kissing my neck." —*L.E.*

"I tried the ylang ylang, nutmeg, and SB-74. I rubbed the oil on my upper body and breasts in the morning, and then went about my usual day. I was amazed at the number of men who started friendly conversations with me. It's great!" —*F.H.*

"I would just like to add another affirmation of these Body Perfumes. They are definitely winners. I've been wearing them since my last order a few months back, and I can assuredly say that they are quite addictive. They kind of have a bit of an aromatherapeutic lift for me in addition to their powers of attraction...Great job, Skin Biology!" —*K.*

BEST SELLING FRAGRANCES:
Ylang-Ylang/Nutmeg
Jasmine

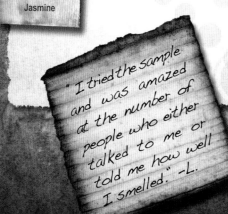

"I tried the sample and was amazed at the number of people who either talked to me or told me how well I smelled." -L.

Plant Derived Pheromone Chart

Note: These are general comments from our clients. Responses may vary widely among individuals.

Mood Enhancer	Mood Effects	Effects on WOMEN	Effects on MEN	Traditional Uses
LAVENDER	Calming Relaxing Soothing	STRONG	STRONG	Skin healing, beneficial for acne, burns, wounds, rashes, psoriasis, PMS, stress, tension, and muscle cramps
JASMINE	Erotic Very Pleasant	STRONG	MODERATE	Aphrodisiac: Said to increase arousal, attractiveness, and appeal. Emotionally produces feelings of optimism, confidence, euphoria, reduces tension, anxiety and depression, relieves menstrual cramps and pain
ASIAN OUD	Calming Erotic	STRONG	STRONG	A historical favorite in Arab countries, produced by a fungus that lives on trees
YLANG YLANG	Erotic Relaxing	MODERATE	STRONG	Strong aphrodisiac: said to increase arousal and attachment. Traditionally spread on the marriage bed in Bali
SANDALWOOD	Erotic, Musk-like, Relaxing	MODERATE	STRONG	Scent is very similar to musks from animals such as deer musk, civitone musk from civit cats, and castorium from beavers which are traditional aphrodisidacs for both men and women
NUTMEG	Energizing	STRONG	STRONG	Very stimulating, helps with frigidity, impotence, neuralgia, and nervous fatigue. Used for better circulation, arthritis, gout, muscular aches and pains
PATCHOULI	Mildly Erotic	STRONG	LOW	A favorite of women: erotic for women probably not on men

(16)

GLOWING GOOD HEALTH
Better Suntanning with Less Skin Damage

Hundreds of years ago Copernicus proclaimed the sun to be the center of our universe. Throughout thousands of orbits, humans have worshiped the sun's warmth and power. Primitive societies believed in a sun god that warmed their bodies, souls and brought in the harvest. They praised the sun for its power to heal certain illnesses. In the early 20's, tanning became a fashion statement when Coco Chanel obtained a suntan while cruising from Paris to Cannes. The tanning trend continued for several decades. It wasn't until 1979 that the FDA concluded that sunscreens could help prevent skin cancer and developed the first rating system for SPFs.

Today, the media hypes the dangers of tanning and encourages us to slather on tons of sunscreen even if we are only in the sun for a short period of time. This media frenzy scares us silly.

But is it really healthy to avoid the sun? Consider the following: Humans evolved in the presence of abundant sunlight. Geneticists and archaeologists calculate that our ancestors lost their body hair 1.2 million years ago but only started wearing clothes 72,000 years ago. So for more than 1,128,000 years, our forebearers lived in splendid nudity and flourished.

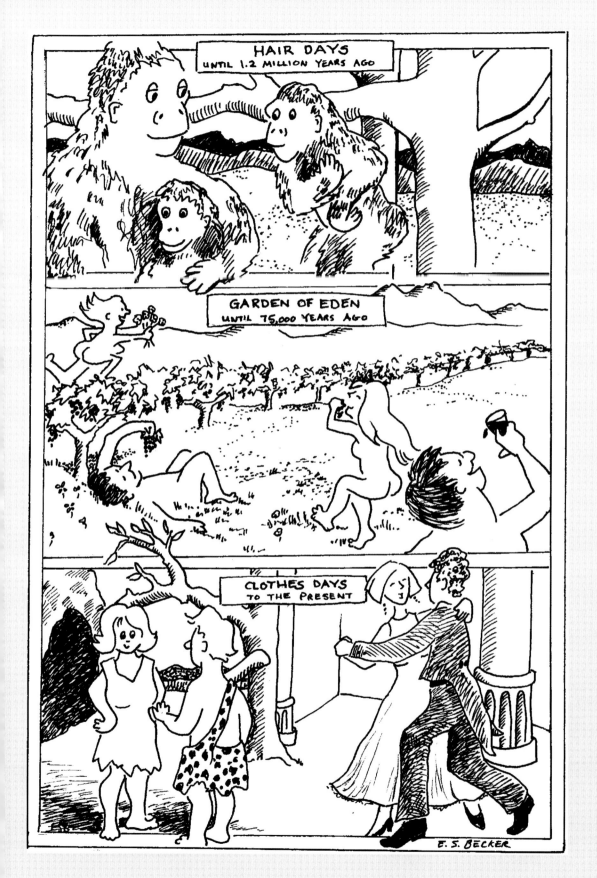

Additional evidence that human skin thrives when exposed to sunlight (Hobday 2000, Holick 2003).

- In the United States, people in professions with high sunlight exposure (such as farmers and mail carriers live the longest.

- Cancer rates are the highest in northern states with the least sunshine.

- Rates of the major lethal cancers are drastically lower in people who get more sunshine.

- Sunlight-associated cancers increased most in locations where sunscreen was most heavily promoted.

- Sunlight improves the moods of those with seasonal affective disorder (SAD).

- Psoriatic skin lesions are reduced by sunlight.

- Sunlight raises testosterone levels in males.

- Sunlight exposure may reduce the incidence of schizophrenia.

- Sunlight improves bone health.

- Sunlight decreases auto-immune diseases such as multiple sclerosis, Type 1 diabetes, and rheumatoid arthritis.

Old Fashioned Sunscreens

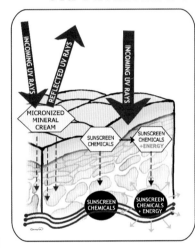

SUN SCREENS with MICRONIZED MINERALS

Can penetrate and accumulate in lower layer of skin

UV ABSORBING SUNSCREEN CHEMICALS:

As much as 35% of sunscreen chemicals enter the blood stream

SUNSCREEN CHEMICALS + ENERGY:

Once sunscreen chemicals combine with energy they can enter the blood stream and damage the DNA

Healthier Sun Protection

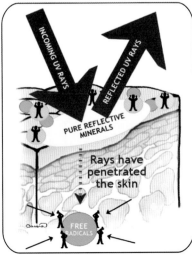

PROTECTIVE CREAM on skin
ANTIOXIDANTS & Pure Reflective Minerals
Topically protect skin from Free Radical formation:

SRCPs
Vitamin E Family
Tocotrienol Family
CoQ10
Lycopene
Lutein

 = PROTECT

= BREAK DOWN

PROTECTIVE ANTIOXIDANTS within SKIN
Fight off Free Radical formation:

Superoxide Dismutase
Vitamin E Family
Tocotrienol Family
CoQ10
Lycopene
Lutein
Vitamin C

= FREE RADICALS

= PURE REFLECTIVE MINERALS

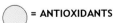 = ANTIOXIDANTS

SUNLIGHT AND GOOD HEALTH

A certain amount of sunlight is necessary for good health. Suns[...] a gene called pom-C, which in turn helps create melanin that determines [...]. This beneficial gene enhances sex drive (the endorphins or "happiness hormones"), as well as leptin, which helps burn fat and keep you thin.

Sun also promotes health and beauty by triggering the skin to produce vitamin D. Vitamin D refers to two very similar molecules: vitamin D3 named cholecalciferol which is created in the outer skin's keratinocytes (remember GHK-Cu increases keratinocyte proliferation) in response to UVB light and vitamin D2 called ergocalcifcrol produced in plants. Then, within the body, both of these types are converted into vitamin 1,25D, the active form of vitamin D.

This essential nutrient helps build strong bones and muscles which may contribute to beautiful smiles and sculpted bodies. Furthermore, vitamin D strengthens immunity and reduces breast cancer which can promote longevity. Deficiencies of vitamin D increase bone fractures, susceptibility to infection, and auto-immune diseases.

When a bikini-clad woman with a white complexion basks in the summer sun, her skin generates 10,000 units of vitamin D in as little as 10 to 15 minutes! However, less is more since additional exposure does not increase vitamin D. During winters in Northern Europe, where sunlight is sparse, 92% of adolescent girls and 37% of older women were found to be deficient. Conversely, in climates with long sunny seasons, skin with higher levels of melanin synthesizes much less vitamin D. Caucasian skin absorbs approximately twice as much vitamin D as African skin. Those with darker complexions are at serious risk for vitamin D deficiencies. Topical sunscreens can reduce vitamin D production by more than ninety-eight percent.

Persons who have more sun exposure have much lower rates (reductions of 40 to 80%) of major internal cancers that cause 99% of cancer deaths (breast, colon, prostate, ovarian). This appears to be linked to low vitamin D. A three-year study of 1,179 women in Nebraska found daily supplementation of 1,100 units of vitamin D3 and 1,400 mgs of calcium lowered cancer risk 77%.

While many of the sun's healing benefits are attributed to an increased production of vitamin D, the sun's actions are likely to be far more complex. Sunlight generates many other molecules in the skin, perhaps dozens or hundreds more. Some of our clients who suffered from seasonal affective disorder (SAD) during dark winter months have told me that extra vitamin D (400 to 1,000 units per day) failed to alleviate their depression, whereas a brief sojourn in a UV tanning booth every week did relieve their mid-winter depression.

Your skin maintains UV anti-oxidant protection under full sunlight for approximately 45 minutes, but ultraviolet tanning booths produce 10 times the UV intensity of full sunlight. So the time using tanning booths should be quite brief—2 to 4 minutes.

As for the mixture of vitamin D and sunlight, the best answer may be to use vitamin D supplements (1,000-2,000 units daily, there is no consensus about the optimal dosage) combined with 10 to 15 minutes moderate sunlight several times weekly on areas of your body that rarely are exposed to sunlight.

While sunlight promotes good health, the ultraviolet (UV) rays do cause skin damage. The question is, how can we find methods that will provide adequate sun exposure while reducing sun damage (Drug and Cosmetic Industry 1997, Podda et al 1998, Steenvoorden & Beijersbergen van Henegouwen 1999, Hobday 2000, Lee et al 2000, Granstein et al 2001, Morganti et al 2002, Gonzalez et al 2002, Heinrich et al 2003, Holick 2003).

Many dermatologists advocate the use of chemical sunscreens to prevent skin cancer. Yet epidemiological studies have failed to demonstrate that these sunscreens prevent cancer. In 1998, epidemiologist Marianne Berwick of the Sloan-Kettering Cancer Center analyzed 16 studies with mixed results. She reported that four studies suggested sunscreen protects against skin cancer; five studies found no effect; and seven studies found a higher rate of cancer with sunscreen use. Her conclusion was that "Sunscreen may not protect against skin cancer" and "We don't really know whether sunscreen prevents skin cancer" (Fackelmann 1998).

> You might be tempted to reach for any old bottle of sunscreen on the grocery store shelf to protect yourself from the sun. DON'T! Chemical sunscreens contain oily chemicals that strongly absorb the energy in light photons and can cause more harm than good.

In the opinion of ultra-marathoner Dr. Gordon Ainsleigh, sunscreen use might actually increase the number of cancer deaths. After analyzing a 17 percent rise in the breast cancer rate, he stated that the increase could be the result of sunscreen use. Dr. Ainsleigh also concluded that there are 2,200 sunlight-associated cancer deaths annually in the U.S., versus 138,000 for sunlight-inhibited cancers. Worldwide, the greatest rise in melanoma has occurred in Queensland, Australia, where sunscreen use is heavily promoted. Most Australians grew up hearing the slogan "Slip, Slap, Slop" with regard to sunscreen. They were told the more sunscreen they used, the better (Garland et al 1992, Ainsleigh 1993, Garland et al 1994, Larsen 1994, Farmer & Naylor 1996).

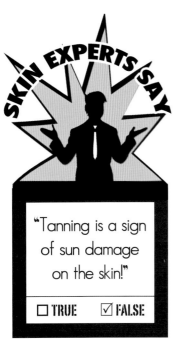

"Tanning is a sign of sun damage on the skin!"

☐ TRUE   ☑ FALSE

Is ozone depletion, rather than sunscreen, the culprit in rising rates of skin cancer? Not likely. Johan Moan of the Norwegian Cancer Institute found that from 1957 to 1984, the annual incidence of melanoma in Norway had increased by 350 percent and 440 percent respectively, but concluded that "ozone depletion is not the cause of the increase in skin cancer" (Moan & Dahlback 1992).

Sunless Production of Melanin

After topical SRCPs were sealed on the leg for a week, the cup was removed leaving the skin tanner by naturally increasing the production of melanin.

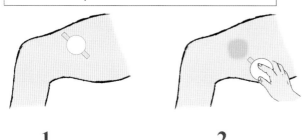

1.   **2.**

Sensible Suntanning

Does the idea of obtaining a healthy tan sound like an oxymoron? It may if you have spent years avoiding the sun. While too much sun can damage the skin, a low dose of golden rays can enhance your mood and health. Now that's good news isn't it? You can obtain the life enhancing effects of sunlight and still keep your skin healthy and attractive. The basic strategy is to increase melanin production. Many of you may not be aware that melanin helps block UV damage by serving as a free radical scavenger. Sensible suntanning is a balancing act since too much sun can damage the skin. Sun-induced skin damage and tanning (melanin production) are two separate biochemical processes and are not linked.

YOUR GUIDE

HOW TO GET A BETTER TAN WITH LESS SKIN DAMAGE

3 Days Before	Take supplemental anti-oxidants: vitamin C, Co-Q10, alpha lipoic acid, vitamin E, beta carotene, or antioxidant loaded whole vegetables.
BEFORE Sunning	Apply Copper Sun Tanning & Firming Lotion: Helps moderate UV rays and diffuses light, supplies copper to assist melanin production for a natural, perfect tan
Tanning Times	Mid Morning (around 10:30 am) or Afternoon (around 3:00 pm) Tan in natural sunlight for 20-30 minutes
AFTER Sunning	Apply Protect & Restore Body Lotion: Helps to repair possible skin damage from exposure

MELANIN = GOOD

DAMAGE = BAD

In spite of what you may have heard, a tan does not damage your skin. In human safety studies of SRCPs, the testing lab observed strong melanin production in human skin in the total absence of light when small cups of strong SRCP creams were taped to volunteers' skin for five days.

So go ahead! Have fun in the sun. Just go slow. Your key for achieving a fabulous tan is to sunbathe sensibly in stages and not overdo it. For most, I recommend suntanning a maximum of 20 to 30 minutes a day to produce the best results. Whole-body suntanning, the most efficient and safest method, permits maximum sunlight exposure in the shortest amount of time since the sun reaches a large area of the body. On the other hand, children generally need less sun than adults; most have thin skin that burns quickly and should not be exposed to sunlight for more than five to 10 minutes at a time. Infants under age 1 should be protected from intense sunlight at all times.

When you tan sensibly, your skin's natural protective system can defend you. This protective system includes defenses against oxygen radicals, such as vitamin E and beta-carotene, as well as copper-zinc superoxide dismutase, which detoxifies oxygen radicals and reduces skin damage.

In addition to monitoring how much time you bask in the sun, you may want to adopt protective measures when you take tropical vacations or spend longer periods enjoying the sunshine. I suggest you take the following steps before sun exposure:

1. Prior to suntanning, apply a thin coat of Skin Biology's Day Cover or Copper Sun Tanning & Firming Body Lotion. Both products contain SRCPs to remodel skin. They also include titanium dioxide, which scatters UV, along with high levels of anti-oxidants. A small amount of water may be used to help spread the creams. Recent studies suggest that GHK, my earlier generation SRCP, may prevent UV damage. However, further studies will be needed before making absolute claims. I will discuss this exciting new research later in the chapter.

2. If you burn easily or plan to extend your stay in the sun, apply a reflective sunblock over the Day Cover or Copper Sun Tanning & Firming Body Lotion. See the paragraph Pure Reflective Sunblockers for more information.

3. After suntanning, apply Protect & Restore Body Lotion. Suntanning produces damage to the skin barrier that must be promptly repaired to reduce peeling. Skin Biology's SRCP creams help the process of remodeling the skin barrier.

4. Three days prior to tanning, take a daily supplement of Vitamin C (1 g), Co-Q10 (30 mgs), alpha lipoic acid (100 mgs), Vitamin E (400 units), and tocotrienols (35 mgs). Several skin researchers have recommended beta carotene (30 mg), mixed carotenoids from algae (50 mg), Vitamin E (400 units), and Vitamin C (1 g). Also, consume many antioxidant loaded whole vegetables.

5. Wear UV sunglasses that absorb ultraviolet light to protect your eyes. Also wear large hats and protective clothing during times of prolonged sun exposure.

6. When you sunbathe in a swimsuit, or better yet in the nude, as did our ancestors for millions of years, you obtain the maximum sunlight benefits with minimum skin damage.

FDA required warning: "These products do not contain a sunscreen and do not protect against sunburn. Repeated exposure of unprotected skin while tanning may increase skin aging, skin cancer, and other harmful effects to the skin even if you do not burn."

But for how long per day should you expose your nude or semi-nude body to sunlight? The answer may lie in our special tie to the sun which spans thousands of years. Given the life-giving force of the sun, it is not surprising that our ancestors soaked up healing rays to reap its medicinal powers. Greeks believed in the therapy of sunbathing called "heliotherapy" that could cure certain illnesses. And medical literature dating back to 1500 BC from India mentions treatments of natural sunlight for skin conditions. During the past century, many European clinics nestled in mountain regions offered whole body sunlight treatments to heal skin wounds and infections. Physicians prescribed 15 to 30 minutes of sunlight twice daily and were warned not to start sunlight exposure too rapidly.

Wrinkle-Free Sunshine

Perhaps like many of us, you relish the sun as it warms your skin and nurtures your senses. Yet you fear that a blazing sun will sizzle your skin, turning you into a wrinkled prune.

So what is the key to wrinkle-free sunshine? Moderation and enjoyment is the key. Reduce exposure to no more than 10 to 15 minutes a day in the morning or afternoon sun when UV rays are less damaging. However, do enjoy yourself while basking in the beauty of your favorite landscape—perhaps at sea or pruning your rose garden. The secret is to wear minimal clothing so you can expose most of your body to the healing rays. Also you will want to wear a sunblock on more wrinkle-prone areas such as the face, neck, hands, and chest. After 15 minutes, apply sunblock to the rest of your body—then continue to reflect on nature as reflective sunscreens protect your wrinkle-free skin.

Too Much of a Good Thing

While moderate sun exposure benefits the skin, too much of a good thing can overwhelm the skin's protective system. Lester Packer (University of California, Berkeley) found that as the dosage of UV radiation increases, the skin's antioxidant defenses get overwhelmed. As a result, free radicals form and cause cellular damage, such as lipid peroxidation and oxidative modification of proteins and cellular DNA. As little as 45 minutes of noon-day exposure can reduce the skin's protective vitamin C levels by 80 percent and lower other skin antioxidants. It takes the skin's melanocytes two to fives days to produce protective melanin. In contrast, a severe burn can occur in just a few hours (Podda et al 1998).

The bottom line is: You can't rush a sensible suntan. It takes a minimum of one to two weeks to develop a healthy tan. As you expose your body to the sun, the skin thickens and increases your resistance to burning.

Be careful about sun exposure if you take medication such as tetracycline, antihistamines, "sulfa" drugs, diuretics, and some oral contraceptives that can make your skin more sensitive to light.

Pure Reflective Sunblockers

If you plan to spend hours basking on the beach and want UV protection, use a pure reflective sunblocker. These products contain inert minerals such as titanium dioxide, zinc oxide, red petrolatum, and talc and work by reflecting (rather than absorbing) ultra-violet rays.

Choose a pure product with an appropriate sun protection factor (SPF) based on how much time you plan to spend in the sun. An SPF of 15 will provide 15 times the amount of protection you would get without using anything. So if 10 minutes in the sun is enough to turn you red, a sunscreen with an SPF of 15 would allow you to stay out for 150 minutes before burning.

The best reflective sunblockers consist of non-micronized titanium dioxide and zinc oxide. These minerals, usually white in color, are safer than transparent micronized products that can penetrate the lower skin layers. A pasty hue is the price we pay for safe fun in the sun. Micronized or nanoparticles are coated with silicone or other chemicals to make them transparent. These tiny molecules have the potential to inflict DNA damage in human cells.

Some feel that heavy use of zinc oxide increases facial pore size. If skin acids release ionic zinc from zinc oxide, this may enter the skin and inhibit the skin repair actions of ionic copper. Therefore, titanium-dioxide is my preferred sunblock.

QUOTABLE QUOTES: *L'assaut au soleil des blancheurs des corps de femme...*
The assault on the sunlight by the whiteness of women's bodies...
—Arthur Rimbaud 1854-1891

Chemical Sunscreens Aren't the Answer

Chemical sunscreens strongly absorb UV radiation, however they also have a dark side... and no, I'm not talking about blocking the dark side of shade! UV absorbers should never have been used for sunscreen protection. When I was a college student performing chemical syntheses, we would mix UV absorbing oils into batches of chemicals that needed free radicals to start the chemical reaction. We would then flash the mixture with a UV light, and the reaction would commence—sort of like putting a match to paper. For fifty years, chemists have known that UV absorbing oils and UV radiation generate a huge number of free radicals.

The same free radical damage occurs within human skin. The sunscreen oils do not just sit on the skin's surface and stop UV radiation. As much as 35 % of a sunscreen chemical can pass through the skin. But the story is more complicated. Sunscreen chemicals, even "stable" ones, breakdown after absorbing UV energy. These rarely studied breakdown products, which are toxic to cultured cells, then penetrate the skin. The toxic chemicals and their breakdown products then pass the outer layer of dead skin and come into contact with living tissue. Recent studies led by Kerry Hanson from UC Riverside found that when UV radiation hits the sunscreen chemicals (such as octylmethoxycinnamate, benzophenone-3 and octocrylene) within the skin, these oils generate copious amounts of free radicals that injure cell walls, lipid membranes, mitochrondria, and DNA which produce skin damage and visible signs of aging. The authors state that, under some conditions, "the UV filters in sunscreens that have penetrated into the epidermis can potentially do more harm than good." (Hanson et al 2006).

Terge Christensen, a biophysicist at the Norwegian Radiation Protection Authority found octyl methoxycinnamate (OMC), a major sunscreen chemical, to kill 50% of cultured mouse cells at 5 parts per million, a dose far lower in sunscreen products. If the cells were also exposed for two hours with simulated daylight, the OMC and light doubled the toxic actions. So, such "protective" chemicals, may actually increase your risk of sun damage. As another example of a harmful sunscreen chemical, consider psoralen used with UV light to treat psoriasis. Psoralen is similar to sunscreen chemicals, and the rate of skin cancer in patients treated with psoralen is 83 times higher than among the general population (Stern & Laird 1994).

Many sunscreen chemicals also have strong estrogenic (estrogen-like) actions that may cause problems in sexual development and adult sexual function. These include an increased rate of cancer, an elevated rate of birth defects in children, a lower sperm count and smaller penis size in men, and a plethora of other medical problems. The effects are similar to those of many banned chemicals, such as DDT, dioxin, and PCBs.

Margaret Schlumpf and her colleagues (Institute of Pharmacology and Toxicology, University of Zurich, Switzerland) have found that many widely used sunscreen chemicals mimic the effects of estrogen and trigger developmental abnormalities in rats (Schlumpf et al 2001).

Expected Effects of Estrogenic Chemicals in Humans

In Women	Endometriosis
	Migraines
	Severe PMS
	Erratic Periods
	Increases in Breast and Uterine Cancer
	Fibrocystic Breast Disease
	Uterine Cysts
In Men	Lowered Sperm Count
	Breast Enlargement
	Smaller Than Normal Penis Size
	More Testicular Cancer
	Undescended Testicles
	Loss of Libido

QUOTABLE QUOTES: *Estrogenic sunscreen chemicals might explain most of the social changes in California over the past 30 years.*
—A California customer

What About Micronized Sunscreens with Nanoparticles?

In an effort to avoid the "pasty white" look of sunscreens containing large particles of zinc oxide or titanium dioxide, sunscreen manufacturers have reduced the particle size of these UV-absorbing molecules to the "nanoscale", meaning that the lotion or cream is more transparent and cosmetically appealing.

Manufacturers know that today's consumers prefer invisible sunscreens and would be more likely to apply such a product multiple times during the day, which would result in big profits for cosmetic companies. But does this nano-techonology used in the development of these sunscreens mean that they are safe?

A recent study performed on a lotion containing nanoscale zinc oxide isotope particles applied twice daily for a five day period found very interesting results. Participants had their skin studied and their urine and blood samples collected. Upon examination, the team detected the isotope in ALL of the participants' samples. Although the person who conducted the study added, "I've tried to make the point that the amount we actually saw in the blood was quite tiny", the point is that it was found in all the volunteers' samples indicating that it was absorbed into the skin. The real question is: If this is what was found after only five days of usage, what would have been discovered after 100 days? Or after years of usage?

A safety study in rats found that zinc oxide nanoparticles (in levels used in sunscreens) applied over a period of 28 days, resulted in skin collagen loss.

Along the same line of thought, scientists at the University of California at Los Angeles also found that nanoparticles in sunscreens can enter and "wander throughout the body, potentially disrupting body funcions on a sub-cellular level". The University Women's Hospital in Basel, Switzerland investigated this phenomenon by testing the breast milk of mothers twice a year for three consecutive years (Schlumpf et al 2010). The participants' usage of various sunscreens were carefully logged. What did they find? That 85% of the human milk samples that were tested contained UV filters! Although very little is known about the significance of infants taking in milk contaminated with UV filters, the team leader confirmed that "human milk was chosen because it provides direct information on exposure of the suckling infant and indirect information on exposure of the mother during pregnancy".

There is no denying that suncreen chemicals can be absorbed into the body. This underscores the importance of carefully reviewing the types of products we use. Using certain products simply because they are more "aesthetically appealing" (such as suncreen oils or clear sunscreen products) does not mean that it is the healthiest option for our skin. It is the potential issues that may arise after long term use of such products that should be of concern to all of us.

AVOID SUNSCREENS THAT CONTAIN THE FOLLOWING

Para-aminobenzoic acid

Phenylbenzimidazole

Octyl salicylate

Homosalate

Avobenzone

Sulisobenzone

Oxybenzone

Menthyl anthranilate

Cinoxate

Trolamine salicylate

Padimate O

Octocrylene

Dioxybenzone

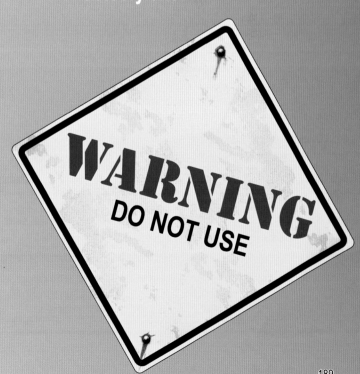

Sunscreen Chemicals Have 3 Primary Defects

They are powerful free radical generators	Their free radical generation increases cellular damage and changes that lead to cancer
They often have strong estrogenic activity	They increase risk of cancer and other medical problems
They are synthetic chemicals that are alien to the human body and accumulate in body fat stores	The human body is well adapted to detoxify biologicals that it has been exposed to over tens of millions of years. But it has often had difficulty removing non-biological compounds such as DDT, Dioxin, PCBs, and chemical sunscreens

How Chemical Sunscreen Oils Damage Skin

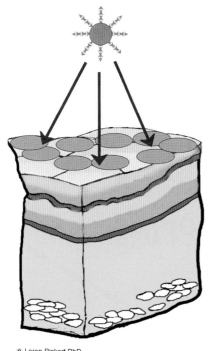

Sunscreen Oils on top of skin absorb UV rays and protect.

However,
when they enter the skin it causes damage.

Up to 35% of applied sunscreen enters the skin.

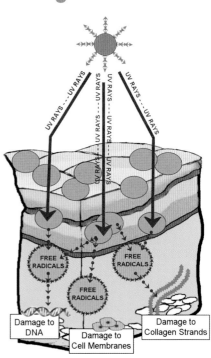

c Loren Pickart PhD

APPRECIATING YOUR NATURAL SKIN COLOR

Today's media tries to convince women that their natural skin color is not aesthetically beautiful. Dark-skinned women can become a target for skin lightening cosmetics, while fair-skinned women are pressured to tan. This can be very dangerous.

The beauty of dark skin lies in its ability to produce abundant melanin, which gives it an excellent, natural defense. Darker skin tones are more resilient and are able to withstand intensive UV irradiation for longer periods of time. When we try to prevent this skin type from producing melanin, in essence we violate it, destroying its fortress of protection.

On the other hand, fair skin often produces little melanin. It evolved in Northern areas where the most important task for skin health was to ensure vitamin D production; UV light defense was not as much of an issue. So this type of skin should not be pushed or forced into wild melanin production. It should naturally be kept fair and exposed to sun only during morning hours for a limited period of time. Light tanning with a titanium dioxide sunscreen is best, whereas attempts to achieve an unnatural darker tan can prove quite dangerous.

My best advice would be: **Treasure and love the skin you have.** Refuse to damage it with unnatural bleaching or tanning methods. Remember, beautiful skin is skin that is healthy and youthful *regardless* of its color! Being "smart about sun" means avoiding trends pushed upon us by the media. Find beauty in your skin by not altering your natural skin type and color.

MY NOTE TO HAPPY SUN WORSHIPERS:

To all of you sun worshipers who revere the sun...go out and bask slowly. Relish the sunrise and sunset and the healing power of sunlight...in small cozy doses to warm your sun senses.

THE HIGH PRICE OF A "SUNBURN-FREE" TAN

In the early 1970s, there were 6 cases of melanoma for every 10,000 people in the United States. With the advent of sunscreens, scientists predicted a dramatic drop in the melanoma rate in the near future. Yet by the beginning of 2000s the numbers nearly tripled despite growing sun awareness and increased use of sunscreens among Americans. To understand why the rate of melanoma in the U.S. climbs despite wide-spread use of sunscreens, let's take a closer look at UV-radiation and its effects.

The term **ultraviolet radiation** refers to everything that falls within the category between X-rays and visible light spectrum. Although it has a shorter wavelength than visible light (our eyes cannot see it), we can feel its effects through a painful sunburn or see its results in a beautiful tan.

UVC-R or germicidal light has a 280-100 nm wavelength. It carries high energy and is very damaging to living tissue; however, it does not penetrate the Earth's atmosphere. This type of UV-radiation can be found in germicidal UV wands and disinfecting blue lamps in hospitals.

UVB-R (315-280 nm wavelength). Its energy is lower than that of UVC, but still is enough to induce a suntan and sunburn as well as stimulate vitamin D production. It can also damage cell DNA; however, its penetrating ability is limited to the upper skin layers, which undergo rapid renewal and can easily get rid of the damage.

UVA-R (410- 315 nm). The most dangerous type of UV-radiation. Although it has low energy and never burns the skin, it can penetrate much deeper than any other UV radiation, and therefore can damage skin collagen and cell DNA, causing premature aging, immunosuppression and in some cases, skin cancer. But it does induce a nice, long lasting tan.

There are three distinct diapasons of UV-radiation: ***UVC-R***, ***UVB-R***, and ***UVA-R***. These differ in energy level and ability to induce a tan or burn the skin. They also produce other biological effects. It is interesting to note that 98.7% of all UV radiation that reaches the Earth is actually UVA radiation. But you could call it "the most aesthetically appealing" type of UV radiation because it can result in beautiful, long lasting tans, while never sunburning.

However, according to researchers this type of tan is different from UVB induced tanning and results from a darkening of existing skin pigment, rather than an increase of melanin production. Therefore, it is less protective than UVB-induced pigmentation. Additionally, recent studies have found that this kind of radiation can penetrate deep into skin and (if given enough time) ravage proteins and DNA, accelerating skin aging.

Next, there's UVB—the kind of UV that gives you fair skinned beauties your much desired tan, or a sunburn if you are not careful. It can damage the skin, but doesn't penetrate into the deeper layers. UVB is essential for vitamin D synthesis in the skin.

Finally, UVC is a germicidal, ozone producing radiation. Very little UVC reaches our skin except in high altitudes.

Nobody likes red, swollen, peeling skin and because UVB can cause a sunburn, it has long been considered the most harmful type of radiation. Nevertheless, a sunburn (albeit painful and uncomfortable) does serve important biological functions. In short, it ensures that your skin stays protected from too much UVA as well as helps clear off any damage.

How so? First, a sunburn will naturally limit sun exposure for those with fair skin and insufficient melanin production. No matter how badly a fair skinned lady may want her tan, the red and swollen back and shoulders (not to mention a red and peeling nose!) soon forces her to flee to more shaded areas. After sunburn, damaged skin quickly peels off together with the newly acquired tan. Today scientists have discovered that not only does the skin peel after the sunburn, it also frantically renovates and remodels itself, pushing out damaged cells or forcing them to commit suicide—thereby entering a state of programmed death. So even when UVB may damage skin, this damage rarely accumulates.

Furthermore, since a UVB-induced sunburn naturally limits the amount of time one can stay out in the sun, there is less time for UVA to do its damaging work. If you do not burn, it just means you have enough melanin in your skin and may not worry about sun damage (unless you're exposed for a very long period of time). Dark skin is naturally more resilient to UV radiation because it evolved in the abundance of sun. But it still needs plentiful sunlight, since it is more prone to vitamin D deficiency.

Now let us consider what happened when the sunscreen industry shifted this natural balance. Well, it all started in 1960s when a suntan suddenly became fashionable, desirable and an indication of higher social status.

The first sunscreens (which contained a very harmful estrogenic chemical PABA—para-aminobenzoic acid) were designed not for skin protection, but merely to stop the sunburn reaction allowing tan-seekers to spend more time under the sun in order to achieve the much desired tan faster. As you probably have guessed already, this came with a price! As happy, grateful beachgoers basked under the sun for hours without feeling the sting of a sunburn, their skin received a huge amount of UVA radiation.

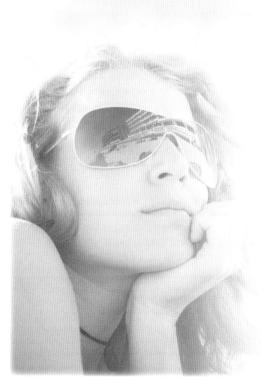

Moreover, the cells damaged by UVB (which also wasn't completely blocked by sunscreen) would not peel off—so the tan stayed, but so did the damage. Decades of such tanning practices led to the emergence of sun damaged baby boomers—men and women with deep wrinkles, and dimpled, uneven skin with broken skin capillaries.

So in the 1990s, scientists and doctors began to warn us about the danger of excessive sun exposure. However, the flourishing sunscreen industry quickly adapted to the changed rules of the game. Instead of promoting painless suntanning, sunscreen gurus started advocating sun protection, using wrinkles and skin cancer as means to justify even more sunscreen usage. Soon the sunscreen industry began to urge everyone to use sunscreens all year round, and regardless of skin color.

In addition to old-fashioned UVB sunscreens, there is now an array of UVA/UVB options that claim broad-spectrum protection. However, not every consumer knows that SPF (sun protection factor), a familiar indicator of the product's efficiency, really only refers to protection from UVB rays and tells us nothing about the level of UVA protection.

SPF is measured by evaluating skin redness after UV-radiation with and without a sunscreen. But UVA rays do not cause skin reddening and sunburn, and therefore UVA protection cannot be measured this way. Even though there is a special test that can be used to measure UVA protection (a pigment darkening test or PDT), sunscreen manufacturers were not required to perform this testing until recently.

Recent studies have found that many so called "broad-spectrum" sunscreens provide only minimal UVA protection. The only type of sunscreens that provides balanced UVB/UVA protection is natural reflective minerals such as titanium dioxide. However, chemical corporations try to convince consumers that natural sunscreens (as well as our skin's own melanin) do not provide enough UV protection. At the same time, sunscreen manufacturers push products with higher and higher SPF that are loaded with alien chemicals. To promote such products they promise such things as "all day protection" and "more time under the sun". However, starting summer 2012, sunscreen regulations are going to be tightened:

High SPF sunscreens (only achieved by the use of alien chemicals) give the illusion of protection by preventing sunburn and peeling. **Truthfully, there is no sunscreen that provides 100% protection.** Fooled by such an illusion, many beachgoers happily bask under the sun for hours without much burning or skin peeling. So now, while their skin still becomes severely damaged, the injured cells cannot peel off and may remain in the skin for decades as slow ticking time bombs until they turn cancerous.

- To be labeled "broad spectrum" products will be required to pass a FDA approved test for UVB/UVA protection.
- Only properly tested "broad spectrum" products with SPF no less than 15 will be allowed to claim that they protect against skin aging and cancer.
- SPF higher than 50 will not be allowed, so that cosmetic manufacturers will not be able to use high SPF as a marketing tool.
- Waterproof and sweatproof labels will no longer be permitted.

Indeed modern synthetic UV-filters absorb UVB so efficiently that even the palest beachgoer can safely lounge under the sun all day long. As a result, not only do the alien chemicals in their sunscreens have plenty of time to decompose under the effect of UV-radiation, releasing abundant free radicals into the skin, but they also allow the skin to receive an unnaturally high and unhealthy level of UVA exposure even with so called UVA/UVB products.

Just as with the UVB-only sunscreens of the past, if there is no sunburn, all of the damaged cells remain in the epidermis (sometimes for decades) as slowly ticking time bombs. Ironically, many sunscreen users today suffer from vitamin D deficiency because they received too little UVB. Low vitamin D levels have been recently linked to higher incidences of cancer. The price of a sunburn-free tan can be very high indeed.

"SUNSCREEN USE FOR TAN ACQUISITION WOULD THUS LEAD TO SIMILAR EXPOSURE TO UVB AND GREATER EXPOSURE TO UVA, WHICH COULD EXPLAIN THE SLIGHTLY HIGHER MELANOMA RISK OFTEN FOUND AMONG SUNSCREEN USERS." AUTIER P ET AL. CURR. OPIN. ONCOL. 2011;23(2):189-96.

"SAFETY OF SUNSCREENS IS A CONCERN, AND SUNSCREEN COMPANIES HAVE EMOTIONALLY AND INACCURATELY PROMOTED THE USE OF SUNSCREENS". BERWICK M. CLIN PHARMACOL THER. 2011;89(1):31-3.

"BLANKET ADVICE TO THE PUBLIC TO WEAR SUNSCREENS AT ANY TIME OUTDOORS IS NOT AT THIS TIME WARRANTED." BERWICK M. CANCER EPIDEMIOL BIOMARKERS PREV. 2007;16(10):1923-4.

"BECAUSE SUNSCREENS PREVENT ERYTHEMA AND SUNBURN, AND INHIBIT ACCOMMODATION OF THE SKIN TO SUNLIGHT, THEIR USE MAY PERMIT EXCESSIVE EXPOSURE OF THE SKIN TO PORTIONS OF THE SOLAR SPECTRUM OTHER THAN UVB" GARLAND CF ET AL. ANN EPIDEMIOL. 1993 ;3(1):103-10.

YOUR GUIDE

HOW TO CHOOSE SAFER & HEALTHIER SUN PROTECTION

PHYSICAL SUNSCREENS	Physical reflective sunblockers contain inert minerals such as titanium dioxide and work by reflecting the ultraviolet (UVA and UVB) rays away from the skin. 👍
CHEMICAL SUNSCREENS	Chemical sunscreens prevent sunburn by absorbing the ultraviolet (UVB) rays but may increase your risk of cancers of the breast, ovaries, prostate, and colon. Chemicals such as avobenzone, benzophenone, ethylhexyl p-methoxycinnimate, 2-ethylhexyl salicylate, homosalate, octyl methoxycinnamate, oxybenzone (benzophenone-3) are used as the active ingredients. 👎
MICRONIZED SILICONIZED PHYSICAL SUNSCREENS	Micronized or encapsulated physical sunblockers penetrate into the skin while pure titanium dioxide remains on the skin's surface - where you really want it to stay. 👎
UN-MICRONIZED PHYSICAL SUNSCREENS	Pure, non-micronized (and often pasty) minerals are better reflectors of ultraviolet light. 👍

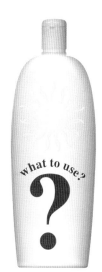

what to use?

?

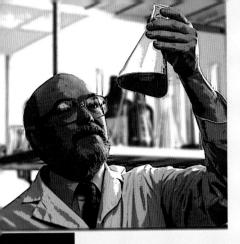

ANTIOXIDANT DISCOVERY In 1984, I observed that GHK-Cu possesses a mild antioxidant activity similar to the enzyme superoxide dismutase, which manifests itself as a calming of red and irritated skin. Steve Aust's lab at *Utah State University* discovered that GHK-Cu blocks the damage-induced release of oxidizing iron molecules from ferritin. Further discoveries followed. Vinci et al. at the University of Catalina in Italy reported that GHK-Cu blocks tissue damage by interleukin-1.

Vinci C, Caltabiano V, Santoro AM, Rabuazzo AM, Buscema M, Purrello R, Rizzarelli E. Copper addition prevents the inhibitory effects of interleukin 1-beta on rat pancreatic islets, Diabetologia, 1995; 38:39-45

Soon after, Robert Koch's lab at Stanford University reported that GHK-Cu shuts down the production, by normal and keloid fibroblasts, of the scar-forming protein TGF-ß-1. Interestingly, they also found that retinoic acid, which is thought to trigger remodeling, actually increases this scar-forming factor.

McCormack MC, Nowak KC, Koch RJ. The effect of copper tripeptide and tretinoin on growth factor production in a serum-free fibroblast model, Arch. Facial. Plast Surg 2001;3:28-32

Canapp et al. found GHK-Cu suppresses the tissue damaging cytokine TNF-alpha (tumor necrosis factor-alpha) and shifts the balance of proteases that dissolve proteins, and anti-proteases toward more anti-protease activity.

Canapp SO Jr, Farese JP, Schultz GS, Gowda S, Ishak AM, Swaim SF, Vangilder J, Lee-Ambrose L, Martin FG. The effect of topical tripeptide-copper complex on healing of ischemic open wounds. Vet Surg. 2003;32(6):515-23.

In wound healing models, biotinylated GHK increases the production of anti-inflammatory proteins such as copper, zinc-superoxide dismutase that detoxifies oxygen radicals. GHK-Cu also acts to detoxify some dangerous products of free radical reactions. Beretta et al. discovered these effects of GHK-Cu and proposed that this molecule may be useful in preventing many degenerative diseases of aging such as Alzheimer's disease, neuropathy, retinopathy, atherosclerosis and diabetes. They demonstrated that GHK binds alpha,beta-4-hydroxy-trans-2-nonenal—a toxic product of fatty acids lipid peroxidation that plays an important role in the pathogenesis of several age related conditions.

Beretta G, Artali R, Regazzoni L, Panigati M, Facino RM. Glycyl-histidyl-lysine (GHK) is a quencher of alpha,beta-4-hydroxy-trans-2-nonenal: a comparison with carnosine. insights into the mechanism of reaction by electrospray ionization mass spectrometry, 1H NMR, and computational techniques. Chem Res Toxicol. 2007 Sep;20(9):1309-14.

ARE SRCPS THE ANSWER? As I mentioned in other chapters, GHK was my first SRCP, the original skin remodeling copper peptide. GHK can provide a way to protect our skin from UV free radicals. It may provide the answer to a nagging question; how can we protect our skin without applying harmful chemicals? UV damage is mediated through molecules called Reactive Carbon Species (RCS)—a carbon equivalent of oxygen free radicals. When the UV energy transfers to the RCS molecules, they damage the components and cells of the skin.

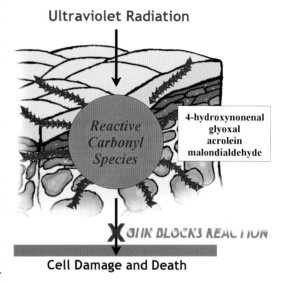

Recent studies from Lipotec, the Barcelona Bioinorganic Chemistry Department and the University of Milan, found that GHK would protect skin keratinocytes (the outer skin cells) from lethal doses of UV light. See photographs below. The GHK binds to the RCS molecules and inactivates them. They also found that GHK reduces the damaging glycation of proteins such as superoxide dismutase. The authors write: "Gly-His-Lys is able to help the natural protection of cells (Glutathione) to prevent the damage of RCS and UVB radiation and acts as a scavenger of specific RCS (HNE, acrolein) and prevents glycation of protein."

Lipotec (www.lipotec.com) sells products for cosmetic use that uses this technology.

Photographs of skin cell protection by GHK. Courtesy of Lipotec.

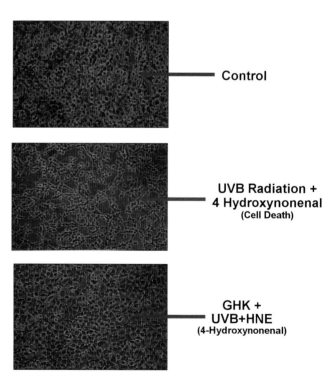

It must be emphasized that these results do not directly prove that GHK protects skin from UV damage. We performed a few uncontrolled studies with clients who had very fair complexions and sun-sensitive skin. Most reported that the SRCP creams made it easier for them to suntan and to tolerate sunlight when at the beach or skiing.

The methods that we used are detailed in the US Patent 5,698,184 by Pickart. However, given the current negative Zeitgeist concerning sunlight and skin protection, it has proven impossible to secure support to develop these observations into protective products.

(17)

NUTRIENTS THAT HELP TURN BACK THE CLOCK
Bypassing Confusion and Food Wars

THE GOAL OF THIS CHAPTER:
Making More Intelligent Nutrient Choices

The goal of this chapter is to give you a critical understanding
of current diet and nutrient research to help you make better
choices. The topics are based on commonly asked questions
from our clients. But there are no simple answers about diets. Food usage has always been
emotional and food regulations have been written into many religions and government
laws for thousands of years.

So how does what we eat affect our skin and hair? What about nutritional
supplements? In truth, there are very few studies on diet and the quality and
youthfulness of your skin. "Scientific" needs for nutrients were originally derived from
studies on the type of foods that would enable young rats to breed and have offspring.
This was then applied to humans with a few modifications.

There is less known, and more confusion, about dietary needs as we age than
is generally realized. "Great dietary discoveries" almost always fail in larger, controlled
studies. For 40 years, the dominant theories of cardiovascular disease and cancer insisted
that excessive dietary fat was a major causative factor. But the largest study ever to ask
whether a low-fat diet reduces the risk of getting cancer or heart disease, the *Women's
Health Initiative*, found that a low-fat diet has no effect. The $415 million US federal
study involved nearly 49,000 women ages 50 to 79 who were followed for eight years.
In the end, those assigned to a low-fat diet had the same rates of breast cancer, colon
cancer, heart attacks and strokes as those who ate whatever they pleased (Howard et
al 2006, Beresford et al 2006).

For all of today's focus on salt (sodium chloride) intake, which **everyone** knows
is bad, many scientists have questioned this advice. One recent seven year study of 3,861

healthy people free of cardiovascular disease, measured 24-hour sodium in urine (more accurate than a diet survey). It was found that the lowest sodium intake was associated with higher cardiovascular disease mortality (Stolarz-Skrzypek et al 2011). Another analysis of seven studies of 6,250 persons with cardiovascular disease, of whom 665 died during the studies, found no evidence that salt restriction improved survival. But in patients with heart failure, salt restriction increased the death rate (Taylor et al 2011). In studies going back 30 years, 20 grams of salt daily given to pregnant women reduced pre-eclampsia hypertension and resulted in more successful pregnancies (Farese et al 2006).

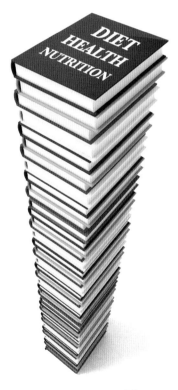

For 50 years every medical school taught about the dangers of excess vitamin D. Students were taught that ingesting more than 400 Units of vitamin D per day would cause serious health problems. But today, physicians prescribe up to 50,000 units a day for designated periods to raise blood vitamin D levels, without any ill effects. Once vitamin D levels are reached, many can continue to take 5,000 to 10,000 units to maintain optimum vitamin D levels. Before supplementing with 50,000 units, have your blood tested and retested according to your doctor's advice.

Why Is There So Much Confusion Over Diets and Nutrients?

Are you scratching your head by now asking why there is so much nutritional confusion? Over the past thirty years, advances in nutrition have seemed to explode on the front pages of health magazines, in research journals, and in numerous nutrition books. In spite of all these advances, an ongoing debate ensues over what foods make up the optimal diet. Theories abound and often conflict from high carb to low carb diets to high fat and low fat to Vegan vs Paleo. It's like riding a roller coaster, enough to make one dizzy with confusion. Perhaps we should take a breath, step back and consider how human nutrition has evolved since the time of our earliest ancestors.

There are two reasons for the confusion. First there are too many quick and sloppy studies by researchers. Academic researchers are pushed to quickly publish large numbers of articles; quality is not a serious concern. Also, research funding is increasingly controlled by "Old Boy Networks" and new ideas that contradict established ideas cannot get support. This control has made it increasingly difficult for young scientists, who develop virtually all new ideas, to obtain independent funding. Medical exploration would proceed faster if all the research money was given to the young people and let the "Old Guys" work for the young.

50,000 YEARS OF DIETARY CHANGES
The second cause is that our diet has fluctuated wildly over 50,000 years, this also leads to a conundrum that elevates confusion over the foods we choose to eat. Our human genome can only slowly adjust to such changes.

Scientists classify humans as omnivores, who are basically "opportunistic" feeders (survive by eating what is available) with anatomical and physiological traits designed to utilize a diverse diet from both animal and vegetable sources. Pure plant-eaters, such as cattle and horses, have large intestines with a large surface area designed for the extraction of energy from grasses and leaves; while carnivores (who often eat significant amounts of grass), such as lions and wolves, have short intestines that extract nutrients from easily digestible meats. But omnivorous humans have an intestine similar to omnivores, that is able to digest both plants and meats.

Humans descended from plant-eating primates that subsisted on a diet consisting mainly of plant sources (97%), especially fruits, vegetables, nuts, and roots plus about 3% meat. Then, about 50,000 years ago, humans honed their hunting and fishing skills, adding animal proteins and fats to their ration, but were most likely still consuming a large amount of vegetables and roots, except in the Arctic regions with limited vegetation. A second major change came about 10,000 years ago when grains were cultivated by early hunter-farmers. A new grain-heavy diet was born.

Dietary Changes Since the Stone Age

DIET	Stone Age	Present Day Americans	EFFECT OF CHANGE
Simple Sugars	2 lbs / year	130 lbs / year	Diabetes, tooth decay
Essential Fatty Acids	Omega-6 is about equal to Omega-3	About 14 times more Omega-6 than Omega-3	More cancer, blood clots, auto-immune disease, depression
Trans-fats Hydrogenated Fats	Very little	High in many processed foods	Damage to cell membranes, more cancer and immunological diseases
Minerals	High in mountain areas with long lifespan	Lower because of processed foods	More heart disease, cancer, and arthritis
Meat	Hunted animals were low in fat: 3% fat	Farmed animals high in fat	Heart disease, diabetes, obesity
Soluble Fiber	High vegetable fiber diet	Low fiber diet	Intestinal problems

GENERAL DIETARY CHANGES

A new change emerged within the last 400 years, when the consumption sugar dramatically increased, from about two pounds a year during the Stone Age to about 130 pounds a year today (in the USA). In the past, tooth decay was rare since simple sugars were hard to come by. In addition, alcoholic beverages became more readily available, and alcohol consumption increased by a factor of 10 to 20-fold.

The modern diet has produced or increased many contemporary degenerative diseases. Diabetes and cardiovascular disease were rare in the past. Many medical historians insist that modern heart disease only developed after approximately 1850. Ancient medical writings from China, Europe, and the Middle East, going back over 2,500 years, do not describe the characteristic symptoms of a modern heart attack, although the same ancient writings describe many other modern diseases.

FOODS & SUPPLEMENTS Essential and protective nutrients can be obtained both from foods and nutritional supplements.

When we are young, our body requires about 40 essential nutrients that we cannot synthesize on our own and we obtain many of these from plants. However, some of us have individual requirements for various biochemicals.

Roger Williams opened the door to modern nutritional supplements with his book in 1956, Biochemical Individuality: The Basis for the Genetotrophic Concept. Based on his studies on vitamins, he proposed that individuals varied widely in their nutritional needs for optimal function. For example, identical twins share the same genes, but their differing environments can result in different nutritional needs as they grow older. Some people may require 1,000 times more intake than normal of a particular vitamin to maintain their health (Williams 1956).

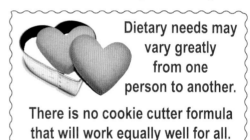

Dietary needs may vary greatly from one person to another.

There is no cookie cutter formula that will work equally well for all.

Linus Pauling later extended this idea with "orthomolecular medicine", that is, the need for the right molecules in the right concentration to maintain health. The key idea is that genetic factors affect not only the physical characteristics of individuals, but also influence their biochemical milieu.

Biochemical pathways present significant genetic variability increasing susceptibility to various diseases such as atherosclerosis, cancer, schizophrenia or depression. These diseases are associated with specific biochemical abnormalities which are causal or contributing factors of the illness (Pauling 1968).

When we supplement our bodies to correct biochemical imbalances, the effect can be life saving. Supplemental insulin was found to treat juvenile diabetics 80 years ago, and this process saved lives by balancing high blood sugar.

...mportant supplements used to restore internal biochemical balance. You may not need these supplements. (g=gram, mg=milligram)

	Vitamins & Supplements	Recommended per Day	PRINCIPAL ACTION
PROTECTIVE ANTIOXIDANTS	Alpha Lipoic Acid	30-200 mg	Recycles other antioxidants
	Vitamin C	0.5 to 1 gram	General antioxidant
	Coenzyme Q-10	30-200 mg	•
	Vitamin E family (all isomers)	400 mg	•
	Tocotrienols family	35-75 mg	•
	Lutein	20 mg	•
	Lycopene	5 mg	•
	Grape Seed Extract	50 mg	•
	Vegetable Extracts	1000-2000 mg	Mixture of antioxidants
	Melatonin	1-3 mg at bedtime	Helps sleep, protects brain
ESSENTIAL OILS	Omega-3 Oils	1-5 grams Salmon Oil Flaxseed Oil	See chapter text
	Omega-6 Oil Gamma Linolenic Acid	1-3 grams Borage Oil / Primrose Oil	Anti-inflammatory Omega-6 fat helps skin integrity, joint lubrication
BRAIN AND NERVES	Ginkgo Biloba	60 mg	Improves brain function
	N-acetyl-carnitine	0.5 to 1 gram	
	Choline / Inositol	1-2 grams	
MINERALS	Calcium	1-2 grams	For bone health and biochemical reactions
	Magnesium	500 mg	
	Zinc	7-15 mg	
	Copper	2-4 mg	
HAIR	Saw Palmetto Oil	80-160 mg	Reduces DHT
	Soy Flavonoids	30-300 mg	Estrogen effects
Elements of Collagen and Extracellular Matrix Proteins	MSM	0.5 to 1 gram	For joints and hair
	Vitamin C	500-1000 mg	For collagen
	Glucosamine	0.5 to 1.5 grams	For skin extracellular matrix and joints
	Chondroitin Sulfate	0.4 to 1.2 grams	For skin extracellular matrix and joints
Nitric Oxide Releasers	Arginine / Ornithine / Citrulline	1-6 grams	Vasodilator
OTHER	Extra Soluble Fiber	5-20 grams	Intestinal motility
	Red Wine	5-15 oz	Increases happiness, reduces illness
	Folic Acid	400 mg	Reduces illness
	DHEA	25-100 mg	Increases sexual and metabolic hormones and blocks cortisone damage

Also supplements such as methylsulfonylmethane (MSM) has long been used to speed hair growth in horses while vitamin C helps synthesize collagen needed for contraction and tightening skin. Omega-3 fish oils, and flaxseed and borage oil help smooth the skin.

RDA (Recommended Daily Allowance) is Not Adequate for Older Humans

The Recommended Daily Allowance (RDA) listed on the labels of processed foods and vitamin products provide the percentage of each of 19 essential nutrients you get per serving or dose. However most people do not realize that the RDA was originally developed as the minimum nutrients required for young rats to successfully breed. The labeling fails to consider the changing nutritional needs of seniors and those with special diseases such as diabetes and heart disease.

While slight adjustments in the RDA have been introduced to reduce birth defects and heart disease, these underestimate your needs as you grow older. Many vital biochemicals, such as DHEA and alpha lipoic acid, decline dramatically with age. Also, our antioxidant defenses greatly weaken and cells are more easily damaged by various types of molecules that cause oxidative damage to cells and tissues. As a result, the biochemical balances that produced a youthful body weaken and this accelerates aging.

The chart on the previous page provides supplements recommended by experts on human aging. Many of these nutrients can reduce the risk of age-related disease and some can even rejuvenate the body. However, take note, that we are all unique with individual dietary requirements.

Depending on your health, you may only need a few of these supplements. For example, a person with cardiovascular disease may benefit more from omega-3 fats than the average person. Above all, please keep in mind that supplements do not substitute for high quality foods that contain a wide range of helpful nutrients, some of which science has not yet discovered.

For example, fruits and vegetables contain synergistic blend of many vitamins, antioxidants and phytonutrients. Our bodies are complex and so are the nutrients in foods we consume. It's all a balancing act to find what works best for ourselves.

Dosages and Driving Reactions - A Little Chemistry

Although few will dispute that daily supplements provide health benefits, many disagree about the recommended dosages. Nutritionists often advise far higher dosages than commonly used. However, some of these elevated requirements can be viewed as quirks in chemistry; chemists define this as **"Driving a Reaction."**

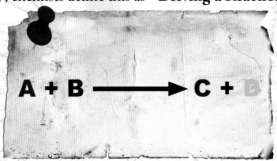

$$A + B \longrightarrow C + D$$

If we want our body to produce more of a needed biochemical, for example **C** or Collagen for fingernail growth, then when we raise the concentration of one of the starting materials (for example compound **A** or MSM) by 10 fold, we speed up the reaction. Now we may not accelerate the reaction ten times, but the production might easily double. In the case of MSM, as an example, the result of a higher concentration may react in faster fingernail growth. Studies on MSM supplementation found that about 2 grams daily will increase nail growth. This is a high, but safe and effective dosage. The great majority of dietary supplements are non-toxic. Excess amounts are excreted from the body.

Food Wars—Veggies vs Paleolithic Diets

Vegetarians argue that a meatless or nearly meatless diet is the most healthy. At the other end of the spectrum is the Paleo Diet that emphasizes a version of the ancient diet of wild plants and some meats from animals that the human species consumed during the Paleolithic era—a period of about 2.5 million years that ended around 10,000 years ago with the development of agriculture. The Paleo diet's intellectual argument is that the human genome adjusted to such a diet during the 2.5 million year Paleolithic period but has not yet adjusted to more modern foods such as grains. The recommended Paleolithic diet consists mainly of grass-fed pasture raised meats, fish, vegetables, fruits, roots, and nuts, and excludes grains, legumes, dairy products, salt, refined sugar, and processed oils.

NOTE: Some supplements can affect the action of pharmaceutical drugs, so always inform your health care provider of your supplements.

As for which is best, there is little evidence. A 21-year follow-up study from the German Cancer Research Center (Heidelberg, Germany) of 1,225 vegetarians and 679 health-conscious non-vegetarians found no difference in overall mortality, although both groups had 41% lower death rates than the general German population. Meat eaters had twice the rates of smoking of the vegetarians. In both groups, smoking increased mortality while moderate to high physical exercise reduced mortality (Chang-Claude et al 2005).

It may be that just being careful about one's diet is the most important. An 80-year study from University of California Riverside of 1,500 people found that the best predictor of longevity was conscientiousness, forethought, planning, and perseverance in one's professional and personal life (Friedman & Martin 2011). Other studies have found the similar longevity benefits of conscientiousness (Hill et al 2011). The fact that you are reading this book means you are already high on the conscientiousness score.

So what can we do about our dietary choices? Well, a lot! By examining our evolutionary past and the changes that occur as we grow older, since we are not young rats, we can make intelligent choices about our nutrition today and in the future.

HEALTHY FATS We are often barraged with differing views for what makes up good vs bad fats. To decipher the confusion, we only need take a peak into fats consumed by our ancestors. Today's diet now differs from that of our predecessors who hunted wild game, fished and gathered their food. They consumed a diet low in saturated fat and high in essential fatty acids (EFAs). The foods of early humans contained omega-6s and omega-3s in a ratio of about 2:1 which contained significant amounts of CLAs (conjugated linoleic acid omega-6 fats) from hunted animals. Today, people eat about 14 times more omega-6 fats (mostly from vegetable oils) than omega-3 EFAs. This imbalanced ratio makes our skin more prone to inflammation.

Flaxseed oil, an omega-3 fat called AHA, offers health and beauty benefits while maintaining the recommended ratio between omega-6 GLA fats and omega-3 fats.

A study at Heinrich-Heine-University Dusseldorf in Germany found that daily supplements of 2.2 grams of borage oil or flaxseed oil for 12 weeks improved skin quality in women. Skin hydration increased and the skin was less prone to irritations. A surface evaluation of living skin revealed that roughness and scaling of the skin were significantly decreased. (De Spirt et al 2009)

Cold water fish (salmon, sardines, herring and mackerel) provide excellent sources of omega-3 fatty acids that are found mostly in fish and seafoods. You need about 300 to 600 mgs daily of the omega-3s which are composed of DHA (docosahexaenoic acid), and EPA (eicosapentaenoic acid). Seafood, grass fed animals, and alpha-linolenic fat found in many vegetable oils, provide excellent sources of these beneficial fats. As for CLAs, in grass-fed beef, the fat contains about 1.1% omega-3s, 3.3% omega-6s, and 0.9% CLAs.

Both inflammatory omega-6 and anti-inflammatory omega-3 fats contribute to our health in ways that balance each other. Omega-6 fats fight infections, heal wounds, stimulate skin and hair growth, maintain bone health, regulate metabolism, and maintain the reproductive system. Omega-3 fats curb inflammation, improve cognitive function, reduce heart disease, possibly stroke, some cancers, inflammatory bowel disease, and other autoimmune diseases such as lupus and rheumatoid arthritis. The CLA fats possess anti-diabetic, anti-cancer and weight management properties. Some researchers recommend getting at least 3% of daily calories from EFAs and CLAs.

Although we should limit our intake of omega-6 fats, GLA (gamma linolenic acid) may provide the exception when taken in moderation. GLA is found in vegetable oils such as primrose oil, borage oil, flaxseed oil, and canola oil. GLA confers health and beauty benefits. It is an anti-inflammatory that improves skin health, lubricates joints, and treats PMS.

Excellent sources of GLA such as borage oil, flaxseed oil, primrose oil and blackcurrant seed oil help keep your skin healthy and dazzling. They can drench your skin in beautifying moisture and treat inflammatory skin disorders such as eczema. You can take 2 to 3 grams daily to alleviate skin conditions. However, once the condition clears up, some researchers recommend a basic maintenance dosage of no more than 7 milligrams a day.

FRUITS AND VEGETABLES We should emphasize diets rich in fruits and vegetables. This gourmet garden of delicacies provides our bodies with many vitamins, valuable phytonutrients and antioxidants. A fundamental change in the human diet over the centuries has been the diminished intake of low-calorie plant foods. The colorful fruits and vegetables sold at your neighborhood grocery store provide a wide variety of more than 600 phytonutrients that benefit 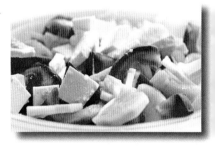 our health, including terpenes, organosulfides, isothiocyanates, indoles, dithiolthiones, polyphenols, flavones, tannins, and protease inhibitors. Fruits and vegetables also contain carotenoids, a rich source of vitamin A and antioxidants.

The carotenoids lutein (abundant in spinach and other green leafy vegetables) and lycopene (found in tomatoes) possess particularly strong antioxidant activity. Another powerful group of antioxidants are proantocyanidins that are present in blueberries, red grapes, and many other deep colored fruits and berries. This is important because as we age, our antioxidant defenses decline and must be enhanced to reduce free radical damage.

Fruits and Vegetables are Powerful Antioxidants

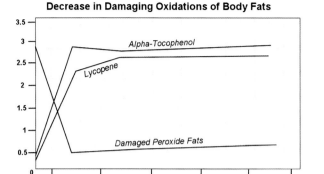

Decrease in Damaging Oxidations of Body Fats

Alpha-Tocophenol

Lycopene

Damaged Peroxide Fats

Days on Supplementation with Dehydrated Fruit and Vegetable Powders

Decrease in Damaging Oxidations of Body Fats (Based on: Wise et al)[2]

FRESH versus
Processed Juice

Many of us enjoy a daily jolt of juice: What a tasty way to imbibe on fruits and veggies! But some juices may be better for us than others. While processed juice contains health benefits, many nutritionists say that freshly squeezed or extracted juice is far more nutritious. Fresh raw juice provides a concentrated dose of antioxidants and enzymes that aid digestion. Fresh juice also contains a significant level of hydrogen peroxide, which some scientists say serves as a natural stimulant to the immune system. Human mothers milk also contains a significant level of hydrogen peroxide. Unfortunately, the amount of hydrogen peroxide in juice drops rapidly during storage. For the highest quality juice, a twin gear press juicer or single auger machine is the machine for you. This type is more efficient (especially for juicing leafy greens) than the other juicers. Since this type operates at a low RPM, the oxidation that occurs while juicing is minimized maximizing the nutritional value in the juice. Beware that many processed fruit juices contain a high amount of added sugar. Try to buy only juices **with no sugar added** or better yet, juice your own fruit. My slogan? A glass of freshly squeezed apple juice a day keeps high fructose corn syrup away!

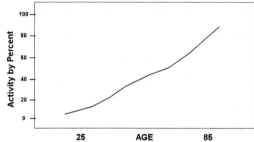

Level of Oxidative Damage with Age

Activity by Percent

AGE

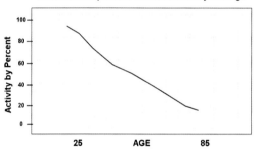

Antioxidant Superoxide Dismutase Activity with Age

Activity by Percent

AGE

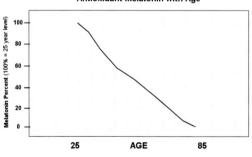

Antioxidant Melatonin with Age

Melatonin Percent (100% = 25 year level)

AGE

Charts Based on: Linnane A.W. et al

Extracts of fruits and vegetables can reduce damaging lipid peroxidation products in the blood by as much as **75%** within one week.

Antioxidants Need Not Be Expensive

Wise and colleagues reported that the daily supplement of 1.5 grams of dried extracts of fruits and vegetables reduced damaging lipid peroxidation products in the blood by 75 percent within one week. Lipid peroxidation products provide an excellent measure of the rate of damaging oxidations within the body. Conversely, protective antioxidants such as alpha-tocopherol and lycopene sharply rose. The fruit and vegetable supplements consisted of dried fruit and vegetable powders obtained by drying juices from apples, oranges, pineapples, papaya, cranberries, peaches, carrots, parsley, beets, broccoli, kale, cabbage, spinach, and tomatoes (see figure on previous page) (Wise et al 1996).

Sugars and Carbohydrates

Say no to simple sugars found in a myriad of processed foods. Be aware that FDA regulations only label sucrose as sugar. However there are many other types of sugar molecules not identified as sugar on packages of white bread and other non-sweet foods. These other sugars are labeled fructose, glucose, high fructose corn syrup and maltose, fruit juice concentrates, honey, dextrose, lactose, maltose, and molasses, all of which are sugars that are no better than sucrose.

Excess sugar damages the skin by increasing 'AGE' (advanced glycosylation end-products). These substances form a harmful waste that can prematurely age skin. They attach to your collagen and break it down which increases wrinkles. Whole fruits, vegetables and unprocessed grains provide essential sugars from complex carbohydrates without affecting blood sugar levels and increasing the need for insulin. But processed carbohydrates such as white bread, cake, potatoes and pasta are quickly broken down and raise blood sugar levels (Bruce et al 2000). When you overproduce insulin after eating too much sugar, your blood sugar falls and your energy level plummets. As a result, you crave more processed carbs and the cycle begins anew. Thus the more sugar you eat, the more you crave as you ride the blood sugar roller coaster.

Dietary Fiber

Are you ready for yet another reason to indulge in succulent plant foods? Plants contain an abundance of healthy fiber. One advantage of fiber is that it makes you feel full and does not raise your blood sugar. Most Americans do not eat enough fiber; some nutritionists recommend that we consume 40 to 50 grams a day, but the average American gets only 12 grams. Dietary fiber comes in two forms which provide different benefits: soluble, the type in oatmeal 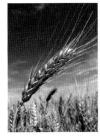 that gets sticky when wet, and insoluble, the sponge-like version in bran, fruit and vegetables that absorbs water and helps to prevent constipation. Insoluble fiber improves digestion and is predominant in plant skins, husks, and the tough part of plants. Soluble fiber helps reduce blood cholesterol and the risk of heart disease and is found in pectin, guar, barley, and oat bran. You can increase your intake of both insoluble and soluble fiber by eating more whole-grain foods, cereal products, fruits, and vegetables.

Current culture is filled with conflicting ideas of quasi-religious advice on health. This has produced a public boredom and also disbelief in most advice.

Not Vitamins, but Vitamin Families

Vitamins are natural substances necessary in small amounts in the diet for the normal growth and maintenance of our bodies. Each of the six main vitamins (A, B, C, D, E and K) has its own vitamin family. For example, the vitamin C family consists of at least seven forms of vitamin C, while vitamin E has four forms plus its closely associated tocotrienol cousins. Vitamin A and beta-carotene are part of a family of at least 400 members. According to recent research, mixtures of vitamins may provide more health benefits than the use of a pure vitamin.

The Mediterranean Diet: A High Fat Diet

How would you like to be lion hearted—or shall I say lyon hearted? If you want a healthy heart, take heed of the Lyon Heart Diet Study. This small, but influential study was based on the Mediterranean Diet. This diet is based on Cretan diets where men had exceptionally low death rates from heart disease despite moderate to high intake of fat. The primary foods include high consumption of olive oil, legumes (such as peas, beans, lentils), unrefined cereals and bread, *no day without* fruit, plus root and green vegetables, moderate to high consumption of fish, moderate consumption of dairy products (mostly as cheese and yogurt), moderate portions of poultry, less beef, lamb and pork, and butter and cream replaced with margarine high in α-linolenic acid. The Mediterranean diet is high in salt from foods such as olives, salt-cured cheeses, anchovies, capers, salted fish roe, and salads dressed with olive oil.

The trial consisted of more than 600 patients who had recovered from a first heart attack. They were randomly selected to either continue their present diet or eat a Mediterranean-style diet. Although the Lyon Heart Diet did not reduce blood lipids, the diet did lower cardiac deaths and coronary events by 70 percent within one year (rising to 76 percent reduction after two years). These results correlated with the combination of monosaturates and omega-3 content of the diet. Blood samples found that the diet increased blood antioxidants (vitamins E and C) and omega-3 fats while reducing omega-6 fats. Surprisingly, those on the Lyon Heart Diet experienced no change in blood pressure or cholesterol as compared to the control (normal diet) patients. The diet also reduced cancer by 61 percent after four years perhaps due to not only the anti-cancer actions in olive oil but to the variety of fruits, vegetables and omega-3 fats (de Lorgeril et al 1998).

It must be emphasized that regional diets in other parts of the world, such as Okinawa, the mountains of Peru, and the Hunza Valley of Pakistan, have been studied as nutritional models that can provide a template for healthier lives since their populations have longer than average lifespans.

Can Food Fight Wrinkles?

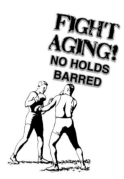

A healthy diet can not only benefit your internal health, it may also protect your skin from wrinkles as well! A study from Monash University of Australians over age 70 (177 Greek-born persons living in Australia, 69 Greeks living in rural Greece, 48 Anglo-Celtic Australians elderly living in Australia and 159 Swedes living in Sweden) found a decreased level of actinic sun damage with a diet high in vegetables (best), olive oil (second best), fish, legumes and fruit and low in butter, margarine, sugar, and whole milk products.

DO YOU REALIZE THAT: Beyond breeding and chronological survival, we still do not know what dietary elements counter the actions of aging and keep a person happy, mentally functional and serene, sleeping-well, filled with high energy and productive.

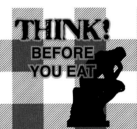

Ethnic Greek skin remained younger on a high intake of green leafy vegetables, broad beans, cheese, mousaka, eggplant dip, garlic, low fat yogurt, polyunsaturated oil and a low intake of milk, coffee, meat, pudding, butter and dessert. Swedes did best with a high intake of egg, skimmed milk, yogurt, lima bean and spinach pie and a low intake of roast beef, meat soup, fried potato, cantaloupe, grapes, canned fruit, ice cream, cakes and pastries, jam and soft drinks.

Anglo-Celtic Australians did best on a high intake of sardines, cheese, asparagus, celery, vegetable juice, cherries, grapes, melon, apple, fruit salad, jam, multigrain bread, prunes and tea (Purba et al B 2001). This study also found those with the least skin wrinkling had the highest blood levels of DHEA (dehydroepiandrosterone) (Purba et al A 2001).

Limit Calories

If we want to extend a healthy maximum lifespan, many researchers on human aging, recommend CR (calorie restriction). Our hunter-gatherer ancestors ate when the hunting was ripe and had to fast for long periods when game was scarce. Studies show that calorie restriction can not only increase longevity, it may offer protection against heart disease, strokes, Alzheimer's and Parkinson's disease.

In order to benefit from CR today, you need not go hungry. In fact the good news is you can actually increase the volume of food. You simply replace the low volume processed bread, cake and cookies with higher volume low calorie fruits and vegetables. Fruits and vegetables have low calorie density. Direct fasting reduces calorie intake and was an ancient method used to improve health. Some people choose to reduce calories by skipping a meal or fasting for one or more days. Others, who don't wish to fast, just consume smaller densely nutritious foods several times a day.

CAN YOUR DIET SUPPLY EVERYTHING THAT YOU NEED?

Yes, when you are young. But as you grow older, there comes a day when the best diet alone cannot retard the progression of age-related dysfunction. Remember, the human body is a finely tuned machine programmed to raise children from birth to adulthood after which the body, like a computer ending its session, shuts itself off. By the age of 18, our levels of growth hormones drop drastically. Sexual hormones peak around age 18, then slowly decline with time. The anti-oxidant defenses rapidly decline after age 45.

Every scientist that we have met, who has seriously researched aging in a laboratory and published original discoveries, has told us they believe diets alone cannot retard or reverse aging and that dietary supplements are necessary to counter the deleterious changes of aging. The unanswered question is what supplements to use and what dosage to take. The great Linus Pauling, who created modern chemistry and stopped nuclear testing in the atmosphere, was heavily criticized by many for his advice on antioxidants but worked actively and published research articles throughout his entire life. He lived to the age of 92.

The Sunshine Vitamin—Vitamin D

Make no bones about it: Vitamin D strengthens bones. But there's more to vitamin D than building 'dem bones.' This sunshine vitamin boasts many health claims–some may even sound contradictory. You've probably heard that sunlight may prevent cancer. How can that be when we also hear sun exposure causes cancer?

The answer may lie with the power of vitamin D. A small amount of sun exposure, which produces vitamin D in the body, can reduce the risk of certain cancers while keeping bones strong. And a slew of new studies suggest that the vitamin offers a lot of other benefits: Diets high in D may ward off diabetes, gum disease, multiple sclerosis and auto-immune diseases. Vitamin D is a powerful weapon aiding the immune system to defend cells, the brain, liver, nerves, intestines, kidneys, pancreas, and skin keratinocytes.

Virtually all great dietary "breakthroughs" vanish when subjected to controlled, double-blinded studies.

So what is the best way to enjoy the sunshine vitamin? The best source is full body exposure to sunlight for 15-20 minutes a day which produces about 10,000 units of the vitamins. Many researchers recommend taking 5,000 units of supplemental vitamin D daily.

Drinking Alcohol May Improve Brain Function As We Age

The general recommendation? Imbibe in two drinks per day. Now that's just what the doctor ordered! But so many opinions and emotions swirl around drinking ethyl alcohol that one never knows what is healthful. The two best, long-term studies have provided some unexpected and strange results about drinking.

The Framingham Study in Massachusetts found in 1,053 women and 733 men of ages 55-88, the highest cognitive ability (verbal memory, learning, visual organization and memory, attention, abstract reasoning, and concept formation) occurred in men who drank four to eight drinks daily and women who had two to four (Elias et al 1999).

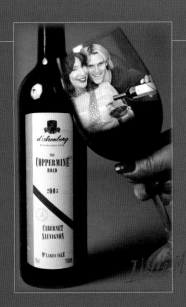

Healthy Selection Menu
COPPER IN MY GARDEN

FLOW COPPER MINE WINE, DIVINE WITH LUSTFUL MIXTURES TO NOURISH LOVE AND NURTURE SKIN WITH LUSCIOUS FRUIT ELIXIRS.

LIKE ROSE BOUQUETS OF GHK, SNIFF COPPER GRAPES. COME ON...LET'S PLAY. LET'S LAUGH THE DAY AWAY.

INCENSE INSIDE MY GARDEN

NOW TAKE A WHIFF. SWISH SUN SWEPT KISS, ACIDIC HINTS OF CITRUS. DO I DETECT LacSal TO PEEL AWAY MY YEARS WITH LIVELY HINTS OF LEMON ZEAL TART AS MY MAN PAL?

KISS SCENTS INSIDE MY GARDEN WITH LIPS SO FINE, TURN BACK TIME. FLOW GHK BOUQUETS TO BLOSSOM CUPID'S VINE.....

Use Moderation to Avoid Excessive Ethyl Alcohol

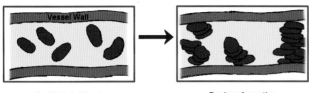

Red Cells in Blood

Rouleau formation
blocks small vessels

The Whitehall II study of British Civil Servants found in 4,272 men and 1,761 women of ages 46-68, the highest cognitive ability (five standard tests of short term memory, verbal and mathematical reasoning, inductive reasoning, and verbal fluency) were found in those drinking at the highest weekly levels (men > 241 grams of alcohol, women >161 grams). In men, this corresponded to over 30 drinks weekly (Britton et al 2004).

We do not recommend you chug down such exorbitant amounts, but as you grow older you may have to choose whether you desire a functioning mind or a functioning body. Now isn't that something? The choices we have to make may persuade us to drown away our sorrows with alcoholic beverages! But alas, here's the dark side of too much fine wine! Excessive alcohol also increases accidents, causes the body to generate high levels of free radicals that overwhelm the liver's antioxidant defenses and thus damages our health in many ways.

When we rapidly chug down alcohol, blood can sludge in the smaller vessels due to rouleau formation as red blood cells bind to each other and form stacks of cells. This stops oxygen and nutrients from flowing to the affected tissues and can produce a rupture of the blood vessels.

Probably the best advice is to spread drinks out—avoid binging. And drink some water before and while imbibing. If you are thirsty, it is very easy to drink much, too fast. Sipping drinks intermingled with a glass of water or two slows alcohol absorption.

Now let me personally make a toast to your healthy skin, heart, body, mind and senses. Enjoy healthy foods and pour yourself a glass of wine or two. Eat and be well. Bon Appetite!

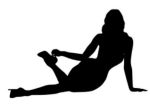

*Perhaps we should also keep in mind the diet habits of **Hugh Hefner**, the still-active 85-year-old owner of **Playboy** who is still famous for his many beautiful girlfriends. He grew up on an Illinois dairy farm and still favors corn-on-the-cob, potatoes and gravy, fried chicken and country-fried steak. He also likes burgers and fries, and oatmeal cookies prepared with extra butter that yields flatter, crispier cookie. Maybe it's his "conscientiousness" that protects him from his diet.*

But perhaps any advice on diet and health is no better than that from Luigi Cornaro (1467–1566) who was a Venetian nobleman near death at the age of 35 as a result of his dissolute way of life.

He modified his eating habits and wrote *The Sure and Certain Method of Attaining a Long and Healthful Life*, which went through numerous editions; this was followed by three volumes on the same subject, composed at the ages of eighty-six, ninety-one and ninety-five respectively. He died in Padua at the age of 98:

"I further reminded them of the two proverbs, which say: he who has a mind to eat a great deal, must eat but little; eating little makes life long, and, living long, he must eat much; and the other proverb was: that, what we leave after making a hearty meal, does us more good than what we have eaten.

But my arguments and proverbs were not able to prevent them teasing me upon the subject; therefore, not to appear obstinate, or affecting to know more than the physicians themselves, but above all, to please my family, I consented to the increase before mentioned; so that, whereas previous, what with bread, meat, the yolk of an egg, and soup, I ate as much as twelve ounces, neither more nor less, I now increased it to fourteen; and whereas before I drank but fourteen ounces of wine, I now increased it to sixteen."

Excerpt from: *Luigi Cornaro*

(18)

THE SCIENCE BEHIND SRCPs
My Quest for the Molecular Fountain of Youth

SRCPs, the miraculous molecules that inspired this book, arose from my passion to reverse aging. In the process, I uncovered this exquisite copper elixir which ancients proclaimed holds the power to heal. As the name Skin Remodeling Copper Peptides implies, SRCPs remodel the skin. However, this molecular gem ignites a powerhouse of other activities that promise to promote health and reverse aging. In addition to skin, SRCPs activate the repair and remodeling of other tissues in the body, including hair follicles, stomach lining, intestinal tract, bones, and liver. Recent studies revealed even more beneficial actions of SRCPs such as their ability to re-charge skin's stem cells and prevent malignant tumors from developing.

I embarked upon this biochemical journey over four decades ago. However, my passion for science began even earlier—when I was a young boy. The path that led me to pursue a career in medical research began in the Minnesota heartland where I grew up. I still recall that we often fished for dinner from Minnesota's rivers and lakes.

BEYOND INTELLECT: THE MAGIC MOLECULES When I was young my grandparents, aunts, and uncles would talk about the health fears of their generation. They would say if a person had an infection and red streaks appeared on the skin, the person would always die. They also talked about young people they knew who had died lingering and painful deaths from juvenile diabetes.

I was a healthy nature lover until I caught a severe and very painful throat infection at the tender age of 10 years old. I was bedridden for over two weeks. Fortunately, I was nursed back to health when my doctor injected me with penicillin. One shot was all it took! I was up and around within 2 hours.

215

As the years went by, I never forgot how penicillin rescued me. The idea that the discovery of penicillin could have such a powerful impact on health care left a lasting impression on me.

Previously, I had been fascinated by electronics and physics. They are logical and pleasant pursuits. But molecules like penicillin and insulin were to me a magical realm of science. To be ill yourself or know desperately ill people who are suddenly restored to their happy life by simple molecules is more magic than intellect.

Experiments on Aging Reversal

After graduating from the *University of Minnesota* armed with a degree in chemistry and math, I began my work at the *Sansum Foundation*, a gerontological aging research laboratory in Santa Barbara. It was here, in lovely Southern California, that my work started which ultimately led to the discovery of the human copper peptide complex GHK-Cu. Initially I researched ways to reverse the detrimental changes that occur during human aging. I aspired to suppress the synthesis of the blood fibrinogen, a blood protein that rises with age. The level of this protein can accurately predict our mortality. Elevated fibrinogen levels increase blood coagulation and decrease tissue nutrition by increasing the thickness of blood in the capillaries.

To understand these changes, I compared the synthesis of fibrinogen in liver biopsy samples from young patients in their 20's with those of patients between 60 to 80 years of age. As expected, the liver tissue from the older group produced more fibrinogen. However, if tissue from the older patients was incubated in the blood from the younger group, it functioned in nearly the same way as the younger liver tissue. Conversely, incubation of the younger liver tissue with blood from the older patients changed the synthesis pattern to that of older tissue. I came to the natural conclusion that a factor in young blood caused the older tissue to act like younger tissue.

I isolated this factor while completing my PhD thesis in biochemistry at the *University of California*. I attended this northern California campus during the heyday of the 60's when many students were protesting the Vietnamese war. I was busy protesting a different war—the war on aging. The factor in young blood that

After high school, I spent three satisfying years in the U.S. Army working at Fort Huachuca with scientists and engineers on experimental computers long before user-friendly computers became household items. As much as I enjoyed the complex workings of computers, I was much more fascinated with the inner workings of the human body, being the humanist that I am. I subsequently enrolled at the University of Minnesota with the intent of making a career of medical research. I decided to concentrate on a relatively new field: human aging. This was the 1960's, when medical researchers believed they would find a cure for cancer and heart disease in the next 10 years. I concluded that by concentrating on human aging, I would always have a job and perhaps live to a ripe old age as I pursued the molecular fountain of youth.

caused older tissue to behave like young tissue turned out to contain a small peptide called glycyl-histidyl-lysine, or GHK, plus another unknown factor (Pickart 1973, Pickart & Thaler 1973).

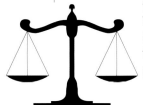

Note on word usage: Studies of GHK use either the copper-free peptide or GHK chelated to copper 2+. Because GHK has a very high affinity for ionic copper 2+ and can obtain copper from the biological milieu, it is difficult to know what form is active.

GHK? or GHK-Cu?

While both forms may have biological actions, in every case where both forms were tested, the copper chelate was the most active form. However, aged skin is often copper deficient; this is why it is prudent to use GHK-Cu in anti-aging cosmetics.

The chemical structure of GHK looked like a copper-binding site, and an analysis by Merle Millard (*Department of Agriculture Labs, Albany California*) found copper in the extracts, so we knew that the active material was a copper peptide complex (Pickart et al 1979).

In 1974, Boris Weinstein of the *University of Washington Chemistry Department* contacted me. He proposed that he, being an organic chemist, and his colleague Norman Rose, an inorganic chemist, could collaborate to determine what role GHK played in the human body. I decided to join forces with them and focus my efforts on GHK's actions on cells and tissues while Weinstein's group established the chemical properties of the molecule (Pickart et al 1980).

During the throes of passionate research, GHK's properties and actions came to light. Proof of GHK's structure was established by David Schlesinger (*Harvard University Chemistry Department*) (Schlesinger et al 1977). Groups at the *University of Washington*, the *Hospital for Sick Children at University of Toronto*, and the *Albert Einstein Medical School* defined the detailed interactions of GHK with the copper 2+ ion.

In the body, both GHK and GHK-Cu co-exist, so both structures may have biological actions. On the basis of the available data, we proposed that GHK-Cu can facilitate copper intake into the cell (Pickart et al 1980, Lau & Sarkar 1981, Laussac et al 1983).

In 1980, I moved to the beautiful Emerald city of Seattle to continue my work at the *Benaroya Research Institute*. To this day, I make my home in the Seattle area. By 1983, I had discovered that GHK accelerates wound healing and contraction, improves the take of transplanted skin, and also possesses anti-inflammatory actions. Since then numerous other laboratories (see below) have confirmed the wound-healing actions of GHK (Downey et al 1985, Pickart et al 1986, Pickart Patent 1987 Pickart 1987, Pickart & Lovejoy 1987).

In 1985, Barbara Weinstein and I started a company called Procyte to develop the GHK findings into useful products. Mrs. Weinstein was the widow of my colleague, Boris Weinstein, one of the most decent and cultured men whom I have ever met. He tragically passed away during the prime of his life.

I feel blessed to have had friends like Barbara and Boris Weinstein. It is much easier to start a small company when you have a network of colleagues. John Majnarich, offered me free lab space, to start both Procyte in the 80s and Skin Biology in the 90s. John is a brilliant biochemist who invented the standard fish vaccines used for salmon farms.

Between 1986 and 1990, I discovered a potential breakthrough in the application of GHK for skin care. I found that when GHK creams are applied to human skin, the dermis and epidermis thickens, skin elasticity increases, wrinkles diminish, skin imperfections such as blotchiness and sun damage marks are reduced and subcutaneous fat cells increase. However, these were small studies and were not further pursued at that time (Pickart Patent A 1992 and Pickart Patent 1994).

Around the same period, H. Paul Ehrlich of *Shriner's Burn Center in Boston* noted with puzzlement that GHK simultaneously increased both collagen synthesis and collagen breakdown during the healing of wounds (Ehrlich 1991).

Remodeling and a Cat Named Collagen

QUOTABLE QUOTES: *There's more than one way to skin a cat.*

The major breakthrough on SRCPs and skin remodeling came from the biochemistry group at the *University of Reims in France*. In 1985, my wife and I attended a scientific conference in Rome where we met Jacque-Paul Borel and his wife Nadine. My observations on GHK and wound healing sparked Borel's interest, whose research focused on collagen metabolism, to such a degree that he named his family cat Collagen.

So you see, there is more than one way to skin a cat... especially when the skin is thick with collagen. Over the next 14 years, Borel's research group (later headed by François Maquart) unraveled many key actions of GHK on cells critical to skin repair.

In 1988, Borel's group discovered that GHK at very low concentrations strongly stimulated collagen synthesis in fibroblasts. They also noted that the GHK sequence is present in the alpha 2(I) chain of type I collagen and suggested that in the organism GHK might be liberated by proteases at the site of a wound healing. At this time they coined a word "matrikines" to describe a class of regulatory molecules that are liberated from the extracellular matrix by proteolytic enzymes after wounding. They proposed that these molecules serve as a first emergency response, recruiting and activating other molecular forces needed for swift repair (Maquart et al 1988, 1990, 1993, 1999, 2005).

REMOVE DAMAGE - REBUILD NEW EXTRACELLULAR MATRIX

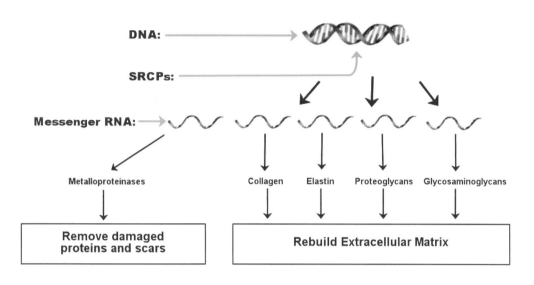

GHK also accelerated wound healing in rats and increased an accumulation of collagen and water-binding glycosaminoglycans in wounds (Wegrowski et al 1992).

Eventually, Borel-Maquart's group discovered that GHK activates and controls the skin's remodeling process, which was evident from its ability to trigger synthesis of messenger RNAs for both metalloproteinases (the family of enzymes that dissolves skin proteins), and anti-proteases (the inhibitors of skin's proteins breakdown) (Simeon et al 1999, 2000A, 2000B).

The ability of GHK to modulate an activity of metalloproteinases and their

SKIN REMODELING: MESSAGES FROM THE MOLECULE

Skin remodeling was once thought of as simply the removal of scar tissue associated with the early stages of healing and the replacement of normal skin. But experiments on GHK reveal remodeling as a far more complex and coordinated process. GHK possesses a diverse multiplicity of actions connected with skin remodeling.

inhibitors becomes especially important in light of recent studies that revealed a new function of these proteins in wound healing and the skin remodeling process. It turns out that metalloproteinases are involved in regulating all phases of the wound healing process.

For example, they can loosen cell-to-cell contacts, allowing skin cells to migrate and cover the wound. They can liberate different matrikines from the extracellular matrix, creating an influx of molecular regulators. They can digest or cleave growth factors and cytokines, altering their activity and, finally, they can alter cell response to cytokines, digesting some receptors for growth factors (Gill 2008).

Therefore, the ability of GHK to modulate both metalloproteinases and their inhibitors places it right at the steering wheel of the skin healing and remodeling process.

The best direct evidence supporting this remodeling role came from a series of placebo-controlled facial studies in women that gave evidence of skin remodeling. GHK products, applied to uninjured skin were found to increase skin collagen, reduce skin irritation and redness, tighten loose skin, improve elasticity, thicken older skin, improve firmness, reduce fine lines and depth of wrinkles, smooth rough skin, improve overall appearance and reduce age spots, photodamage, and hyperpigmentation (the studies are reviewed in detail later in this chapter).

Anti-inflammatory Action

Inflammation is one of the hallmarks of skin aging and one of its key mechanisms. It is now evident that chronically inflamed skin constantly produces free-radical molecules that damage skin's proteins and deplete its antioxidant storage. Chronic inflammation also over-activates metalloproteases—enzymes that break down skin's water binding gel (glycosaminoglycans) and destroy its essential proteins such as collagen and elastin, causing wrinkles and skin sagging (Thornfeldt 2008).

The good news is that the GHK system possesses an array of actions that suppress the "acute-phase" inflammatory and scar-forming events after wounding. The acute phase is a localized and systemic response to tissue injury that serves to stop bleeding, destroy invading bacteria, and quickly cover the wound surface with a protective layer. If this phase is not suppressed and remodeling is not complete, as often occurs after radiation burns, then scars and inflammation may persist for months or years.

In 1984, I observed that GHK possesses an antioxidant activity similar to the enzyme superoxide dismutase, which manifests itself as a calming of red and

Actions of the Human TriPeptide Gly-His-Lys

GHK (Gly-His-Lys) was discovered during studies on human aging. Blood serum from young humans supports cultured cells and tissues better than serum from old humans. GHK was isolated as a serum molecule that maintained the viability of cells and tissues. GHK declines from a serum level of about 0.59 micromolar at age 20-25 to 0.24 micromolar at age 60-70.

GHK has a very high affinity for copper 2+ and can obtain copper 2+ from the copper-binding site on human albumin.

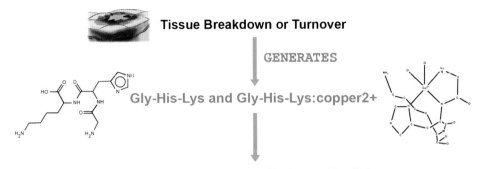

Tissue Breakdown or Turnover

GENERATES

Gly-His-Lys and Gly-His-Lys:copper2+

GHK Acts on Community 15 "Controlling" Genes
435 Genes (268 up / 167 down)

GHK Modulates Expression of About 3,900 Genes

PROTEINS

INCREASES
Vascular Endothelial Growth Factor
Integrins
Fibroblast Growth Factor 2
Protein P63
Erythropoietin
Neurotropins 3 & 4
Nerve Growth Factor
Superoxide Dismuatase
Decorin
Proteoglycans
Metalloproteinases
Anti-proteases
Collagen
Elastin

DECREASES
Interleukin-1
Transforming Growth Factor beta-1
Tumor Necrosis Factor alpha
Release of oxidizing iron
Free radical damage
Protein glycation

CELL EFFECTS

Increases stem cells and activates quiescent stem cells

Repairs DNA damaged by X-rays

Increases fibroblasts, keratinocytes, and chondrocytes

Angiogenesis

Nerve Outgrowth

Attracts healing cells (macrophages, mast cells, and capillary cells)

Protects keratinocytes from ultraviolet damage

Helps break Hayflick Limit

ORGAN EFFECTS

Improves aged intact skin (increases elasticity and firmness, tightens skin, reduces fine lines, wrinkles, photodamage and hyperpigmentation)

Increases hair follicle size and hair transplant success

Speeds healing of wounds (surgical, burns, wound chambers)

Heals stomach & intestinal ulcers

Heals bone tissue

Protects hepatic tissue from tetrachloromethane poisoning

Increases resistance to bacterial infection

Vasodilator – lowers blood pressure
Binds to angiotensin AT 1 receptor

Based on publications from over 80 laboratories

irritated skin. *Steve Aust's lab at Utah State University* discovered that GHK blocks the damage-induced release of oxidizing iron molecules from ferritin. Aust also said SRCPs did a great job of healing wounds in his horses (Pickart et al 1986, Pickart Patent B 1988, Pickart Patent 1990, Miller et al 1990).

Further discoveries followed. In 1995, Vinci et al (*University of Catalina, Italy*) reported that GHK blocks tissue damage by interleukin-1. Soon after, *Robert Koch's lab* (*Stanford University*) reported that GHK shuts down the production, by normal and keloid fibroblasts, of the scar-forming protein transforming growth factor-beta-1 or TGF-ß-1. Interestingly, they also found that retinoic acid, which is thought to trigger remodeling, actually increases this scar-forming factor (McCormack et al 2001).

Canapp et al (*University of Florida*) found GHK suppresses the tissue damaging cytokine TNF-alpha (tumor necrosis factor-alpha) and shifts the balance of proteases, that dissolve proteins, and anti-proteases toward more anti-protease activity (Canapp et al 2003). Arul et al (*Central Leather Research Institute in Chennai, India*) found that in wound healing models, biotinylated GHK increases the production of anti-inflammatory proteins such as copper, zinc-superoxide dismutase that detoxifies oxygen radicals (Arul et al 2005, 2007).

GHK also acts by removing some toxic products of free radical reactions. For example, GHK binds alpha,beta-4-hydroxy-trans-2-nonenal—a toxic product of fatty acids lipid peroxidation that plays an important role in the pathogenesis of several age related conditions such as Alzheimer's disease, neuropathy, retinopathy, atherosclerosis and diabetes. GHK binds and removes acrolein—another toxic product of lipid peroxidation involved in the development of many age related degenerative disorders. It was proposed that GHK may be used for prevention of some age related pathologies. Since lipid peroxidation plays an important role in skin aging and UV-induced skin damage, the ability of GHK to remove toxic by-products of lipid peroxidation has protective effect against skin aging and photo-damage (Beretta et al 2007, 2008).

GHK also inhibits the damaging glycation of copper, zinc-superoxide dismutase caused by fructose and is more active than carnosine in this respect (Cebrian et al 2005, *Lipotec S.A. Barcelona Bioinorganic Institute, University of Milan*; Beretta et al 2007 and 2008, *University of Milan*).

Re-establishment of Blood Flow and Blood Pressure Control

The re-establishment of blood flow into the damaged area is a crucial factor determining the rate and outcome of wound healing. Insufficient circulation leads to slow healing and ulcer formation.

Express VEGF, FGF-
Angiogenesis
Anti-Coagulation, Vasodilatio
Increase Erythropoietin
Nerve and Blood Vessels Growth
Reinnervation
Express NGF, NT-3, N
(+) Enlarge Hair Follicles

One of the characteristics of aging skin is reduced blood flow—that is why older people usually do not have the rosy glow of the youth. GHK helps re-establish blood flow into damaged tissues and aged skin through a mixture of three actions: angiogenesis (new blood-vessel formation), anti-coagulation, and vasodilation. GHK increases the expression of basic fibroblast growth factor and vascular endothelial growth factor, both of which aid blood vessel formation (Pollard et al 2005, *Stanford University*).

GHK induced angiogenesis was documented by Pietro Guillu's lab at the *National Cancer Institute in Bethesda* (Raju et al 1982, 1984). Rabenstein et al (*University of California Riverside*) demonstrated that GHK formed strong complexes with heparin (Rabenstein et al 1995). Both GHK and heparin stimulate angiogenesis.

In Seattle, Helen Sage (*University of Washington*) observed that endothelial cells at the site of an injury express a protein called SPARC that contains the GHK sequence. SPARC protein itself inhibits blood vessel growth, but after the tissue is damaged, it breaks down, releasing an array of GHK and GHK-containing copper-binding peptides, which stimulate new vessel growth. Apart from revealing GHK's ability to regulate blood vessel development, Helen Sage's study confirmed the idea from Maquart's research group that GHK is present in connective tissue proteins and released after an injury (Lane et al 1994, Sage & Vernon 1994).

In safety studies, GHK lowered blood pressure in goats and in isolated perfused rabbit hearts (Pickart 1993). Leslie Manot of the *University of Reims* confirmed the ability of GHK to increase blood flow and dilate blood vessels (Manot 1997). GHK tightly binds to the blood-pressure-controlling angiotensin II AT1 receptor and this is likely to be the causative (Garcia-Sainz & Olivarez-Reyes 1995, *Universidad Nacional Autónoma de México, México D.F.*).

GHK also increases erythropoietin in rats which increases blood cell production (Naughton et al 1982, *New York University*).

Chemoattraction, Repair, and Skin Contraction

GHK is a powerful attractant for capillary cells that build new blood vessels, an action that was discovered by my lab (Pickart et al 1986). At Harvard University, Bruce Zetter's lab found similar actions of GHK on macrophages and mast cells. Macrophages remove damaged cellular debris and secrete a cornucopia of 20 or more proteins (fibroblast growth factor, epidermal growth factor, and so on) important for healing in the area of tissue damage. Mast cells stimulate skin contraction (Poole & Zetter 1983, Zetter et al 1985). In wound-healing experiments, I observed GHK to both heal wounds and induce a powerful skin contraction around the wound.

Promotion of Nerve Outgrowth

When wound healing is inadequate, the healed area is often devoid of sensory abilities. In cell cultures, both Monique Sensenbrenner's lab (*University of Strasbourg, France*) and Gertrude Lindler's lab (*Karl Marx University, Berlin Germany*) found that GHK stimulates nerve outgrowth, an essential attribute of skin repair (Sensenbrenner et al 1975; Lindner et al 1979).

Ahmed and colleagues at the *Neurochemistry Lab in Chennai, India* wrote that when severed nerves are placed in a collagen tube impregnated with GHK, there is an increased production of nerve growth factor and the neurotrophins NT-3 and NT-4 (Ahmed et al 2005).

GHK Repairs DNA Damage in Cells

Wound healing and normal skin renewal require well coordinated and balanced activity of many cells such as fibroblasts, immune cells etc. The outcome of skin renewal and remodeling depends on how well this repair team functions. And one of the problems that often arises during wound healing is that the cells that are supposed to conduct repair are themselves damaged or impaired due to advanced age of the patient, underlying health conditions or external factors such as radiation. For example, the main skin repair cell (the fibroblast) that produces a multitude of important growth factors, is a very sensitive cell that is often damaged by radiation or toxins. One of the fascinating effects of GHK-Cu is an ability to restore damaged fibroblasts.

In specimens obtained from patients who had undergone radiation therapy for head and neck cancer, GHK restored normal fibroblast replication after X-ray damage and increased basic fibroblast growth factor and vascular endothelial growth factor production (Pollard et al 2005, *Stanford University*).

GHK and LED Lights Stimulate Fibroblasts

Huang et al evaluated the effect of GHK alone or in combination with LED irradiation (light emitting diode irradiation, 625-635 nm) on human fibroblasts. Combined GHK and LED treatment resulted in 12.5-fold increase in cell viability, 230% increase in basic fibroblast growth factor (bFGF) production, and 70% increase in collagen I mRNA production compared with the LED irradiation alone (Huang et al 2007, *Industrial Technology Research Center, Hsinchu Taiwan*).

Since fibroblasts are the key cells in skin reparative and renewal processes, the ability of GHK to support these cells, increasing their functional activity greatly contributes into its wound healing and skin rejuvenating activity.

Also, GHK was found to attract skin repair immune cells (macrophages and mast cells) plus capillary cells to the site of injury, which is another explanation of its wound healing promoting activity (Poole & Zetter 1983; Zetter et al 1985; Pickart et al 1986).

Suppression of Sebum Production

In 2007, Schagen (*University of Basel*) found that GHK reduced sebum production but did not affect other cell lipids (Schagen et al 2007).

Remodeling of Aged Skin

My early observations, which showed GHK reverses skin damage (accumulated during aging), gathered dust for a decade. Finally, starting in 1998, more extensive human studies started to validate my observations. At present, GHK undoubtedly has more scientific support data than any peptide used in today's cosmetic practice. Its efficacy was confirmed in several placebo-controlled independent trials:

♦ Abdulghani at the *Robert Wood Johnson Medical School* compared the effect on the skin's production of collagen after using creams containing copper-peptides, vitamin C, or retinoic acid. Volunteers applied the various creams to their thighs daily for one month. The study found that after one month, copper-peptides stimulated more new collagen production than retinoic acid or vitamin C (Abdulghani et al 1998).

♦ A GHK eye cream, tested on 41 women for twelve weeks with mild to advanced photodamage, was compared to a placebo control and an eye cream containing vitamin K. The GHK cream performed better than both controls in terms of reducing lines and wrinkles, improving overall appearance, and increasing skin density and thickness (Leyden et al C 2002, *University of Pennsylvania*).

♦ In another 12 week facial study of 67 women between 50-59 years with mild to advanced photodamage, a GHK cream was applied twice daily and improved skin laxity, clarity, firmness and appearance, reduced fine lines, coarse wrinkles and mottled hyperpigmentation, and increased skin density and thickness. The result was assessed visually by a trained technician (wrinkles, pigmentation, laxity, roughness, overall appearance) as well as using ballistometer (firmness of the skin) and ultrasound (skin density). The GHK cream also strongly stimulated dermal keratinocyte proliferation as determined by histological analysis of biopsies. At the same time, GHK-containing cream proved to be very safe. GHK complex at 20 times the use level was proved to be non-allergenic. It also did not produce eye irritation (Leyden et al A 2002; Leyden et al B 2002; Finkey et al 2005, *University of Pennsylvania, University of California at San Francisco*).

♦ GHK containing liquid foundation and cream concealer was tested in an 8 week study. It improved skin appearance and increased skin elasticity and epidermal thickness (Appa et al 2002, *Neutrogena Corporation*).

♦ GHK in a SPF 20 skin cream containing Octinoxate (7.5%), Octisalate (5%), Zinc Oxide (1.9%) improved skin tone and texture in an 8 week study (Stephens et al 2003, *Dallas Research Center Texas*).

♦ After laser resurfacing, a 2% GHK cream improved cosmetic outcome as measured by greater patient satisfaction (Miller et al 2006, *Facial Aesthetic Concepts San Clemente California*).

Today peptide based cosmetic products continue gaining popularity. However, peptides that are used in today's cosmetic products have very little or no scientific data confirming their efficacy. Also the main problem with peptide-based cosmetics is that most peptides cannot pass through the stratum corneum and therefore cannot reach viable layers of epidermis. Since peptides are used for their cell regulatory activity, inability to permeate the stratum corneum is a serious handicap.

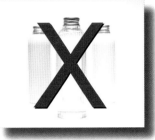

OTHER "PEPTIDE" PRODUCTS
DO NOT REMODEL SKIN

GHK is able to pass with ease through the lipid barrier of the stratum corneum in order to reach epidermal cells (Mazurowska & Mojski 2007 and 2008, *Warsaw University of Technology, Poland*; Hostynek et al 2010 and 2011, *University of California, San Francisco*).

WOUND HEALING In rats and mice, GHK stimulated wound closure of surgical and burn wounds and the establishment of skin grafts (Downey et al 1985, *Virginia Mason Hospital in Seattle, Washington*; Pickart et al 1986, Pickart 1987, Pickart & Lovejoy 1987).

GHK has systemic effects on healing in rats, mice, and pigs. For example, if GHK is injected into thigh muscles it activates healing through the animals, even at sites distant from the administration point (Ehrlich 1991, *Shriners Burn Center, Boston Massachusetts*; Pickart Patent B 1992). It markedly increases collagen production, angiogenesis, and wound closure. This healing effect also restores healing in immune depressed animals. The level of GHK used in pigs corresponds to a dosage of 5 to 50 mg in humans, and would be very safe.

Mice / Rats / Pigs:
Inject GHK-Copper into thigh muscle ⟶
Result: Activates systemic healing

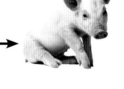

Comparable Human Dosage:
Introduce 5 to 50 mg GHK-Copper ⟶
by injection or dermal patch

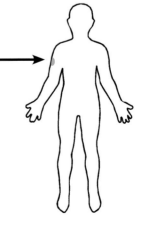

Enhancement of systemic tissue repair would be especially helpful after internal surgeries and after procedures such as implanted artificial joints in elderly patients.

GHK Healed Dog "Paw" Wounds and Surgical Wounds

In dog paw wounds closure, contraction and production of granulation tissue all increased (Swaim et al 1993; Swaim et al 1996, *Auburn University*). Tensile strength of linear incision wounds increased by 74% and neovascularity by 69% (Schmidt et al 1994, *University of Akron*).

Pig Wounds

In pigs, punch biopsies were used to create localized wounds. The defects were filled with graded amounts of GHK in a cream or control substances. In a dose dependent manner, GHK stimulated wound healing and collagen synthesis. The effect was highly localized to the immediate skin area that was treated (Counts et al 1992).

GHK improved healing of ischemic open wounds in rats. Wounds displayed faster healing, decreased concentration of metalloproteinases 2 and 9 as well as of TNF-alpha (a major inflammatory cytokine) compared with vehicle alone or with untreated wounds (Canapp et al 2003, *University of Florida*).

Wound Healing in Rabbits

Healing using GHK with copper and zinc oxide was compared. Median time for the coverage of the wound bed with granulation tissue was significantly shorter with GHK. Neovascularization was best observed in the GHK-Cu group. The authors suggest that GHK-Cu is a better choice in the treatment of open wounds than zinc oxide.

Also GHK alone and in combination with high dose helium neon laser stimulated granulation, increased the formation of new blood vessels and elevated the level of antioxidant enzymes in the dermal wounds in rabbits (Cangul et al 2006; Gul et al 2008, *Uludag University, Turkey*).

Human Wound Healing Trials

During early open clinical trials at the *University of Reims*, Bernard Kalis (dermatology) and Marc Leutenegger (diabetology) treated 60 patients and found that GHK creams accelerated healing of skin ulcers (Aupaix et al 1990).

Unfortunately these special creams that I developed, which showed great promise to cure skin ulcers, were never tested in larger FDA clinical trials. A later controlled clinical trial on venous stasis ulcers failed to reach clinical significance. Another open study in one hospital used a GHK gel on 120 diabetic patients, after their skin ulcers were surgically excised of dead or infected tissue to reduce bacterial contamination. The percentage of closure of plantar ulcers was three times faster than with standard care. The incidence of ulcer infections significantly lessened (7% incidence compared with 34% for vehicle) (Mulder et al 1994, *Wound Healing Institute, Aurora Colorado*).

However, a later trial in numerous hospitals of 530 patients treated with a GHK gel with standard care, failed to demonstrate efficacy.

While GHK failed to prove effects in some studies, all other growth factors and cytokines tested for wound repair have similarly failed. The problem with using growth factors may result from the previously unknown influence of bacteria biofilms that colonize skin ulcers. These feisty bacteria are resistant to anti-microbial agents, and secrete proteases that can degrade GHK, and other growth factors, in minutes.

Fishing for Second-Generation SRCPs on a Boat called Regenerate

As I was stewing over these problems, I was struck with a sudden blood clot while traveling by airplane. A slow recovery from heart surgery forced me to leave Procyte. However, this gave me more time to think about new and better approaches to copper-based tissue repair.

What better way to solve problems than to go fishing? Having time to fish and regenerate the soul can offer a wellspring for new ideas. So I bought a boat and named it ***Regenerate*** for that very purpose. I needed time to rethink mixed results with GHK clinical trials. I also had to regenerate from heart surgery. So I went fishing.

I theorized that after skin damage, the body's breakdown processes generate a blizzard of small peptides, including GHK, in the damaged area. Since GHK has a robust affinity to bind copper (II) ions and can obtain copper ion from tissue fluids, it occurred to me that other small peptides might act as SRCPs if pre-loaded with copper ions.

Therefore, in 1994 my wife Charlene and I started our company, Skin Biology to develop stronger second-generation skin regenerative/remodeling copper peptides with enhanced potency, breakdown resistance, and high adherence to skin.

My goal was to use breakdown-resistant copper peptides with regenerative actions. To accomplish this, I isolated peptide fragments from soy enzymatic digests that possessed the desired qualities when chelated to copper (II).

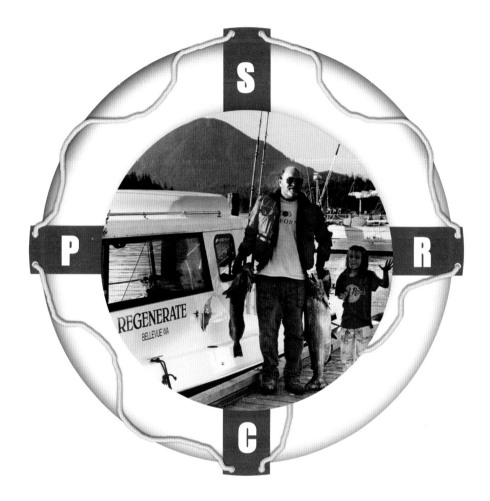

These peptide fragments are very resistant to further breakdown by bacteria. Such peptides have a long history of safe use in cosmetic products. In human and veterinary studies, creams made from these new copper complexes showed superior healing actions in all of my standard tests. They accelerated wound closure, produced greatly enlarged hair follicles, possessed anti-inflammatory actions as good as cortisone, increased the synthesis of collagen and elastin, and produced rapid and scar-free healing in dogs after spaying operations and in young horses after leg straightening operations.

Howard Maibach's group (*University of California, San Francisco*) tested the second-generation copper peptides in four small placebo-controlled human studies.

They found that creams made from the new copper complexes produced significantly faster skin healing and reduced redness and inflammation after mild skin injuries brought on by tape stripping, acetone burns (removal of skin lipids), 24-hour detergent irritation, and nickel allergy inflammation (Zhai et al 1998 A, B, C; Zhai et al 1999).

While the second-generation SRCPs were originally developed to help prevent skin damage in nursing homes and hospitals, somewhat accidentally, women and men began using them on their skin. They were thrilled with the results. Excitingly, the breakdown-resistant SRCPs can be used with hydroxy acids and retinoic acid to enhance skin remodeling and the removal of many types of blemishes and scars.

Other Uses of GHK and Other SRCPs

While the proceeding discussion focused on skin actions, research has determined that SRCPs have many other positive effects on the hair and other parts of the body, as follows.

Improved Hair Growth and Condition

In 1985 I observed that, after treating skin wounds with GHK, hair follicles at the wound edge enlarged profoundly. Further work with radioisotopes indicated that SRCPs stayed present at the site of injection for only about 30 seconds before they cleared from the area.

This meant that a very brief exposure of the hair follicle to SRCPs was sufficient to produce an increase in follicle volume. Such an exposure increased hair growth in mice four- to eight-fold within 12 days, as the following photos demonstrate (Pickart Patent 1987, Pickart Patent 1993, Pickart Patent A 1996, Pickart Patent B 1996).

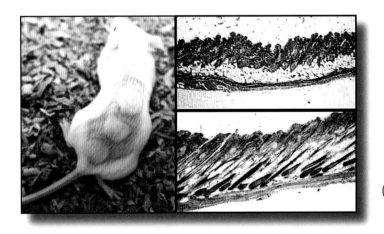

NORMAL
HAIR FOLLICLES

ENLARGED
HAIR FOLLICLES:
(After injection of SRCPs)

A 25 day-old mouse was shaved and injected intradermally in three spots with a SRCP. Twelve days later, hair growth was stimulated at the injection sites.

Effect of GHK in Mammals

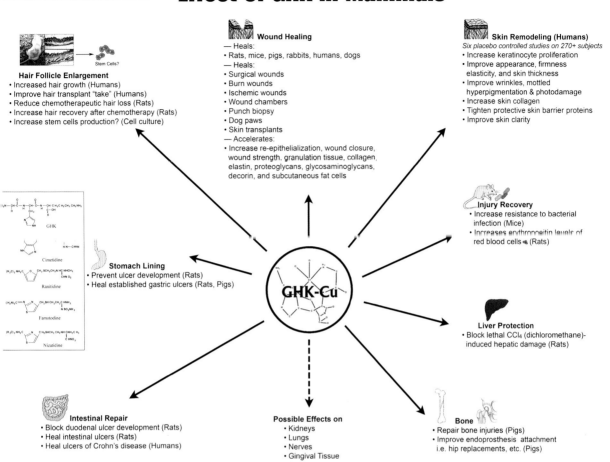

Hair Follicle Enlargement
- Increased hair growth (Humans)
- Improve hair transplant "take" (Humans)
- Reduce chemotherapeutic hair loss (Rats)
- Increase hair recovery after chemotherapy (Rats)
- Increase stem cells production? (Cell culture)

Wound Healing
— Heals:
- Rats, mice, pigs, rabbits, humans, dogs
— Heals:
- Surgical wounds
- Burn wounds
- Ischemic wounds
- Wound chambers
- Punch biopsy
- Dog paws
- Skin transplants
— Accelerates:
- Increase re-epithelialization, wound closure, wound strength, granulation tissue, collagen, elastin, proteoglycans, glycosaminoglycans, decorin, and subcutaneous fat cells

Skin Remodeling (Humans)
Six placebo controlled studies on 270+ subjects
- Increase keratinocyte proliferation
- Improve appearance, firmness elasticity, and skin thickness
- Improve wrinkles, mottled hyperpigmentation & photodamage
- Increase skin collagen
- Tighten protective skin barrier proteins
- Improve skin clarity

Injury Recovery
- Increase resistance to bacterial infection (Mice)
- Increases erythropoietin levels of red blood cells (Rats)

Stomach Lining
- Prevent ulcer development (Rats)
- Heal established gastric ulcers (Rats, Pigs)

GHK-Cu

Liver Protection
- Block lethal CCl_4 (dichloromethane)-induced hepatic damage (Rats)

Intestinal Repair
- Block duodenal ulcer development (Rats)
- Heal intestinal ulcers (Rats)
- Heal ulcers of Crohn's disease (Humans)

Possible Effects on
- Kidneys
- Lungs
- Nerves
- Gingival Tissue

Bone
- Repair bone injuries (Pigs)
- Improve endoprosthesis attachment i.e. hip replacements, etc. (Pigs)

GHK, Cimetidine, Ranitidine, Famotodine, Nizatidine

When I attached fat-like molecules, such as fatty acids or hydrophobic amino acid residues to GHK, hair follicles enlarged dramatically and stimulated hair growth in undamaged mouse skin. Hideo Uno extended these studies (*University of Wisconsin*). Uno had written The UpJohn Company's textbook for physicians when Rogaine® (minoxidil) was first marketed.

Bernard Kalis (*University of Reims*) was the first researcher to demonstrate that SRCPs have positive actions in humans. His studies found SRCPs caused a greater proportion of human follicles to switch from the dormant telogen state into the hair-growing anagen state.

Uno's laboratory found that in fuzzy rats a copper binding peptide PC1031, a structural analog of GHK (GHKVFV-copper complex) affected hair growth with its effect comparable to that of minoxidil. Both 5% minoxidil and 5% PC1031 almost doubled follicle size after 3-4 months of treatment, and caused 80% increase in the number of anagen hair follicles. An increased DNA synthesis and cell proliferation was confirmed in the enlarged hair follicles (Trachy et al 1991, Uno & Kurata 1993, Timpe et al 1996, Trachy et al A 1996, Trachy et al B 1996).

Only the surface of what the GHK molecule can truly do for human tissues has been scratched...

231

Human Study of AHG Copper vs Minoxidil

Compared GHK-Cu analog in Tricomin® with 2% minoxidil. Tricomin® 2.5% increased hair count by 97 non-vellus hairs per unit area while 2% minoxidil increased count by 73 non-vellus hairs after 3 months (Procyte Corp. Press Release 1997). The mechanism of GHK-Cu induced hair growth was investigated in experiments with GHK-Cu analog—AHK (L-alanyl-L-histidyl-L-lysine-Cu2+). It was found that AHK-Cu stimulated dermal papilla cells (DPCs)—specialized fibroblasts important in the morphogenesis and growth of hair follicles. AHK caused elongation of hair follicles, and stimulated proliferation of DPCs while decreasing programmed cell death (apoptosis) (Pyo et al 2007, *Seoul National University, Korea*).

Improved Hair Transplantation

In addition to stimulating hair growth, SRCPs have been shown to improve human hair transplantation. When used in the post-operative regimen, GraftCyte®, a SRCP product sold by ProCyte, results in faster healing of transplants and earlier regrowth of the hair shafts. Perez-Meza (*Mexico City, Mexico*) et al found the GraftCyte® system provided enhanced healing of the transplanted follicles and more immediate hair growth. In their study, patients saw new hair growth in six weeks, versus the normal 10 to 14 weeks. In most cases, skin crusting after transplantation is reduced from 10 to 14 days to five days (Perez-Meza et al 1998).

A second study of GraftCyte® by Gary Hitzig (*New York City, New York*), involving 30 hair transplant patients, found that GraftCyte® reduced the shedding of transplanted hair from 30 percent with saline to 10 percent with GraftCyte®. The healing time of the transplanted grafts was cut in half. Regrowth of new hair from the transplants occurred in six to eight weeks with saline and four to six weeks with GraftCyte®. Patient satisfaction after transplantation rose from 80 percent to 95 percent (Hitzig 2000).

Accelerated Hair Regrowth after Chemotherapy

Awa and Nogimori (*Kaken Pharmaceuticals, Japan*) found that mice pre-treated with SRCPs blocked the hair loss induced by the cancer chemotherapy drugs cytosine arabinoside and doxorubicin. If the mice were first treated with chemotherapeutic drugs to induce hair loss, subsequent treatment with SRCPs accelerated the recovery of lost hair (Awa et al 1995). At Skin Biology, the second-generation SRCPs also strongly stimulated hair growth in mice. To enhance the uptake of SRCPs into the hair follicles, natural penetrating agents, such as emu oil and squalane from olives, pushed more SRCPs into the follicle area.

Restoration of Damaged Liver
Liver Protection

GHK improves liver organ cultures. It also increases repair of liver damage in rats (Pickart & Thaler 1973, *University of California, San Francisco*; Fouad et al 1981, *Max Planck Institute, Germany*; Globa et al 1996, *Russian Academy of Sciences,*

Moscow; Kawase et al 1999 A, B) (*Kagama University, Japan*). Researchers at *Kursk Medical University in Russia* found that in rats, GHK increased the replication of hepatocytes (liver cells) while decreasing hepatic immune reactivity (delayed hypersensitivity reaction). Pretreatment with GHK prevented acute lethal damage to the liver caused by tetrachloromethane (carbontetrachloride), and restored normal liver functions and immune responsiveness (Smakhtin et al 2002, Smakhtin et al 2003).

Reduction of Stomach Ulcers and Intestinal Damage

 Stomach Lining

Intestinal and Stomach Healing—GHK has potent effects on the healing of stomach ulcers and intestinal inflammations. It reduces stomach acidity and increases the production of gastric mucous. GHK healed experimental stomach ulcers and intestinal damage in rats (Pickart Patent A 1988, Pickart Patent B 1991, Pickart Patent C 1992). GHK protected intestinal mucosal tissue from lipid peroxidation by oxygen-derived free radicals (Alberghina et al 1992, *University of Cantania, Italy*).

Sixteen patients with refractory inflammatory bowel disease were treated with rectally administered solutions of GHK. After the 12 week treatment, there was a 60% reduction in severity as measured by endoscopy, histopathology, and symptoms (Levine et al 1995, *University of Washington*). Recently GHK loaded Zn-pectinate microparticles in a form of coated tablets were proposed as a possible treatment for inflammation in inflammatory bowel disease (Ugurlu 2011, *Marmara University*).

Accelerated Bone Healing

Bone

GHK accelerates the healing of bones by increasing the formation of healing granulation tissue in damaged bones. GHK has also been shown to increase collagen synthesis by bone chondrocytes from chickens and pigs, increase the growth of human marrow stromal cells, and promote the attachment of human osteoblastic cells.

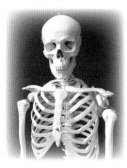

Milan Adam's group at the *Medical University in Prague* developed a GHK gel that was shown to promote the filling of bone defects in femurs and bone attachment to cementless endoprostheses. The GHK gel, when used with cementless endoprotheses, produced vivid osteogenic activity at the interface of bone and metal stem. Such gels may aid in the establishment and retention of artificial joints (Pickart Patent A 1991, Pesakova et al 1995, Adam et al A 1995, Adam et al B 1995, Pohunkova et al 1996, Adam et al 1997).

Suppression of Infections

A testing lab (*Panlabs*) found that GHK suppresses infections (Staphylococcus aureus, Streptococcus, and Pseudomonas aeruginosa) in mice during unpublished safety studies at Procyte in 1989. Later, a group at *Aristotle University* rediscovered these anti-infection actions (Liakopoulou-Kyriakides et al 1997).

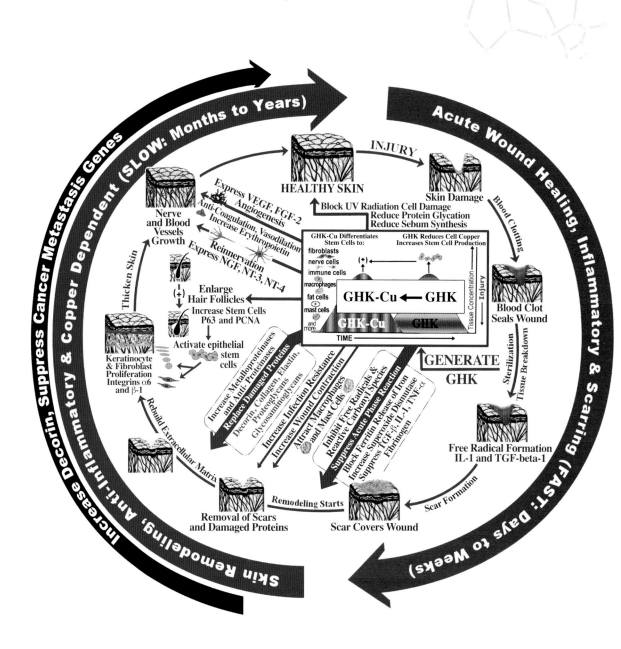

This diagram of the mechanism of Skin Remodeling and GHK-Cu's role in human skin health and repair has taken nearly a decade to develop.

Hair Follicles to Stem Cells

During World War II, physicians discovered that after burns to the skin, when hair follicles appeared at the edge of the healing wound, scar-free healing followed. If no follicles were observed, healing was incomplete and the scar remained. Likewise, when I studied the morphology of experimental wounds treated with GHK, the wound edge was always filled with enlarged hair follicles possessing greatly enlarged sebaceous glands. Yet there was no logical connection between hair follicles and skin repair. Then in 2000, a research group in Paris broadened our understanding of healing skin when they found that stem cells for skin are secreted from enlarged sebaceous glands protruding from the enlarged hair follicles.

Skin's stem cells are its "gold reserve"— a resource for renewal and rejuvenation. When skin is damaged (either by accident or by cosmetic procedures such as lasers or chemical peels), it recruits and activates these hidden reserves, prompting stem cells to multiply and differentiate into cells needed for repair. It was long believed that in aged skin stem cells undergo senescence, losing their ability to repair skin.

However, today there is accumulating evidence that stem cells in aged skin resemble Sleeping Beauty—even though they appear dormant and inactive, they remain eternally young and can be activated with the right stimulus. Just as Sleeping Beauty needed a kiss from Prince Charming to rise from her slumber, GHK is that Prince Charming, awakening the skin's stem cells.

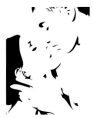

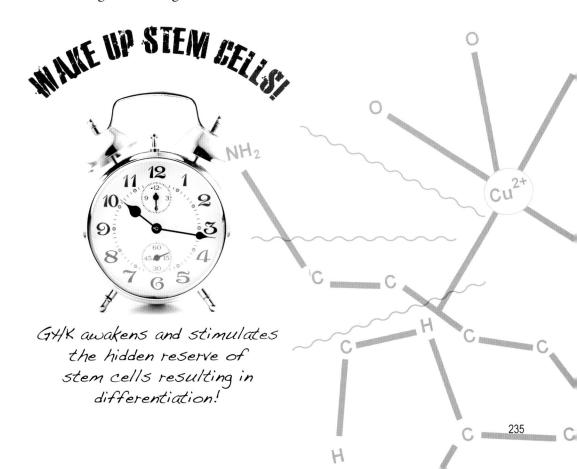

GHK awakens and stimulates the hidden reserve of stem cells resulting in differentiation!

235

In 1995, Godet and Marie (*Lariboisiére Hospital, Paris France*) found GHK increases replication of human mesenchymal stem cells (A.K.A. Marrow Stromal Cells) (Godet & Marie 1995). Later, Tony Peled et al (*Gamida Cell in Jerusalem, Israel*) reported that GHK (without copper) stabilized undifferentiated hematopoietic stem cells from human donors or from neonatal umbilical cord blood. In contrast, GHK-Cu increased stem cell differentiation (Peled et al 2002, 2005, Patent 2005).

In 2009, a group of researchers from the *Seoul National University* (*Republic of Korea*) demonstrated that GHK is able to "re-charge" skin stem cells. In particular, after GHK addition, skin stem cells produced more p63 protein, which is considered to be an "anti-senescence protein". They also acquired a shape that is typical for stem cells in younger skin and restored their ability to proliferate in response to skin damage (Kang et al 2009).

These recently discovered GHK effects on skin's stem cells may explain the dramatic, almost miraculous results that GHK based cosmetics produce in aged and photo-damaged skin.

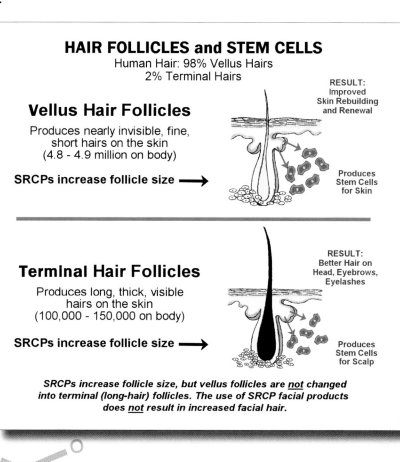

HAIR FOLLICLES and STEM CELLS
Human Hair: 98% Vellus Hairs
2% Terminal Hairs

Vellus Hair Follicles

Produces nearly invisible, fine, short hairs on the skin
(4.8 - 4.9 million on body)

SRCPs increase follicle size ⟶

RESULT:
Improved
Skin Rebuilding
and Renewal

Produces Stem Cells for Skin

Terminal Hair Follicles

Produces long, thick, visible hairs on the skin
(100,000 - 150,000 on body)

SRCPs increase follicle size ⟶

RESULT:
Better Hair on
Head, Eyebrows,
Eyelashes

Produces Stem Cells for Scalp

SRCPs increase follicle size, but vellus follicles are not changed into terminal (long-hair) follicles. The use of SRCP facial products does not result in increased facial hair.

GHK Suppresses
Human Cancer Metastasis Genes

There is no effective treatment for aggressive, metastatic cancer. Two skin remodeling molecules, GHK at 1 micromolar and the plant alkaloid, securinine at 14 micromolar, inhibit cancer metastasis genes. Only these compounds, of 1,309 bioactives tested, suppressed messenger RNA production in 70% of 54 human genes overexpressed in patients with aggressive metastasis of colon cancer (Hong et al 2010).

GHK may inhibit cancer genes by its increasing production of decorin, a proteoglycan. Decorin's regenerative and anti-inflammatory actions (regenerating nerves, muscles, and suppressing scar formation) mimic those of GHK. Numerous studies have found decorin to inhibit tumor growth and metastasis (breast, prostate, osteosarcoma) in animal models.

These observations and results suggest that metastatic cancer cells may activate the same migration-inducing genes utilized in the early stage of wound healing which requires rapid migration of repair cells into the wounded region. Since the later remodeling stage shuts down this migration, substances that promote skin remodeling may act by downregulating the migration/metastasis genes (Pickart & Pickart 2011).

Proposed Mechanism of GHK Effects on Cell Migration

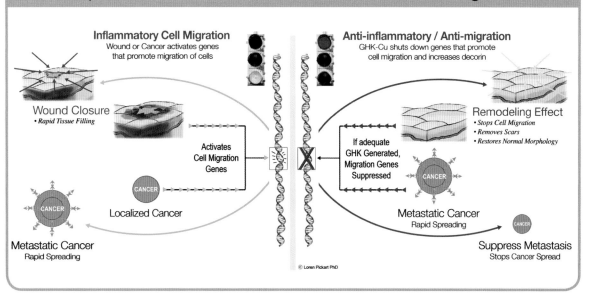

© Loren Pickart PhD

237

A Possible Mechanism Whereby
Skin Remodeling May Suppress Cancer Metastasis Genes

Loren Pickart and Francoise Pickart

Skin Biology
4122 Factoria Boulevard — Suite #200
Bellevue, Washington 98006
Email: lorenpickart@skinbiology.com

Two skin remodeling molecules, the human peptide GHK (Gly-His-Lys) and the plant alkaloid, securinine, inhibit cancer metastasis genes. Only these compounds, of 1,309 bioactives tested, suppressed RNA production in 70% of 54 human genes overexpressed in patients with aggressive metastasis of colon cancer. (Hong, et al., Clin Exp Metastasis. 2010;27:83-90).

Both GHK (which has regenerative and anti-inflammatory actions) and securinine, (a component of traditional African and Chinese medicines for skin injuries and rashes) promote wound healing, extracellular matrix remodeling, and activate macrophages. They suppressed the cancer genes at low and non-toxic concentrations: GHK at 1×10^{-6} M and securinine at 18×10^{-6} M.

GHK has been extensively studied. (Pickart, J Biomater Sci Polym Ed. 2008:19:969-88, Pickart and Margolina, SOFW Journal 2010;136:10-20). Because of GHK's extraordinary copper binding properties, it likely exerts effects as GHK-Cu, its copper complex. GHK-Cu, at 0.1-10 micromolar, activates quiescent adult epithelial stem cells by increasing protein P63 and integrins. (Kang, et al., Arch Dermatol Res. 2009;301:301-6). GHK possesses many regenerative and anti-inflammatory activities. The Broad Institute's Connectivity Map of human gene activity found that GHK, at 1 micromolar, alters RNA production by 50% or more in approximately 2,199 to 3,949 genes in various cell lines (Average change: 74% increased, 26% decreased).

GHK may inhibit cancer genes by increasing production of decorin, a proteoglycan. Decorin's regenerative and anti-inflammatory actions (regenerating nerves, muscles, and suppressing scar formation) mimic those of GHK. Numerous studies have found decorin to inhibit tumor growth and metastasis (breast, prostate, osteosarcoma) in animal models.

These observations and results suggest that metastatic cancer cells may activate the same migration-inducing genes utilized in the early stage of wound healing which requires rapid migration of repair cells into the wounded region. Since the later remodeling stage shuts down this migration, substances that promote skin remodeling may act by downregulating the migration/metastasis genes.

Society for the Advancement of Wound Care and the Wound Healing Society
April 14-17th, 2011
Dallas, Texas

Copper Peptides Suppress Cancer in Mice

So does the above mean that copper peptides could actually suppress cancers in humans? Experiments in mice suggest they would.

In 1983, Linus Pauling's Group reported that the combination of Gly-Gly-His:copper 2+ and ascorbic acid slowed cancer growth and "cured" Ehrlich ascites cancer in 40% of mice (Kimoto et al 1983). I repeated this type of experiment in 1985, using the same dosages but with GHK-copper 2+ and ascorbic acid. This caused a strong inhibition of the growth of a fibrosarcoma in mice (Pickart et al 1983, Pickart 1985). Unfortunately, I could not obtain funding to pursue this work.

Possible Non-Toxic Cancer Therapy Methods

The combination of GHK-copper 2+ and ascorbic acid used on the above mouse cancer is very non-toxic. This could possibly be combined with other molecules which suppress cancer at low and non-toxic concentrations such a retinoic acid and arsenic trioxide (Park & Tallman 2011). The general idea is that such molecules do not kill cancer cells but cause them to revert to "normal" differentiated cells.

While non-toxic methods appear very promising, don't expect much interest in such ideas. The cancer treatment establishment is wedded to very toxic therapies for human cancers (which are also very profitable).

GHK & Cimetidine

Both components have anti-ulcer properties. The drug cimetidine has a chemical structure similar to GHK and avidly binds copper 2+. Cimetidine possesses many anti cancer actions and is used as a treatment for horse melanoma

GHK

Cimetidine

Understanding the Biochemistry of Cancer

The cancer establishment uses therapies based on a very simplistic idea which is that cancer cells are "bad" and must be destroyed. But the GHK work suggests that cancer is just part of a spectrum of regenerative states.

Healthy regeneration (Regenerative Homeostasis) is controlled perhaps by GHK and decorin. Skin problems such as long-lasting scars, skin tags and moles are the result of less control. Metastatic cancer is the most extreme version of the effect.

DEFINING REGENERATIVE HOMEOSTASIS IN HUMANS

Regenerative homeostasis in humans can be viewed as a spectrum ranging from a healthy, normal regenerative response to increasingly unhealthy results. In this sense, metastatic cancer is the most extreme example of an unhealthy response.

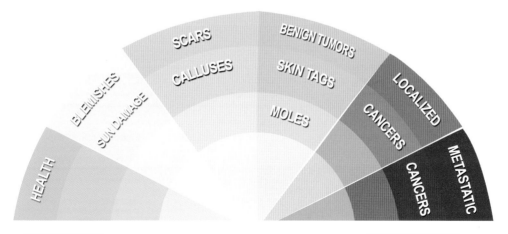

ADEQUATE GHK
Strong Tissue Remodeling
Results in healthy normal tissue

INSUFFICIENT GHK
Weak Tissue Remodeling
Results in aberrant tissue growth

The Broad Institute: GHK Data

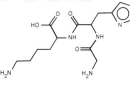

The Broad Institute in Boston (Harvard and MIT) tests bioactive molecules for their effects on human genes and biochemical reactions. Their tests generate huge amounts of information. This information is freely available to other scientists.

GHK was recently tested in their systems. *The actions of GHK on suppressing metastatic cancer genes arose from Broad Institute data.* There is now at least 10 times more information than was collected since 1973 when GHK was discovered. We are *slowly* analyzing the mountains of GHK data to fully understand GHK's role in the human body.

From the Broad Institute Connectivity Map we now know that GHK controls (or influences) about 3,000 of the 20,500 human genes. As we dig out the data in the next year, this will allow us to know what genes GHK "turns on" and which it "turns off".

GHK Modulates Expression of About 3,900 Genes

CONNECTIVITY MAP 02

instances   query   results   admin   downloads   help

instance query

selected instances:

batch	cmap name	dose	cell	instance_id	
1040	Gly-His-Lys	1 µM	PC3	6570	remove instance

up threshold: 0.4   3176 probes found   down threshold: −0.4   773 probes found
(0.67 is equivalent to 2-fold, 0.4 is equivalent to 1.5-fold)

check tags   execute query

The Broad's Connectivity Map also compares the similarity of actions between GHK and other biological compounds and pharmaceutical drugs.

Similarity of Actions of GHK, Decorin, and 6-Bromoindirubin-3'-Oxime

ACTION	GHK	Decorin	(BIO) 6-bromoindirubin-3'-oxime
Stimulates Regeneration	Increases stem cell activity or "stemness" Wound Healing Gastrointestinal Track Nerves Anti-scarring	Wound Healing Nerves Anti-scarring	Increases stem cell activity or "stemness"
Anti-Cancer	Increases Decorin Suppresses many genes overexpressed in aggressive metastatic human colon cancer Anti-scarring	Suppresses metastasis of breast, prostate, and osteosarcomas in animal models	Suppresses human multiple myeloma, leukemia, hepatomas in human or animal models
Human Gene Activity	Affects mRNA production of 2,000 to 3,900 genes	Not tested	Second most-similar to GHK in gene effects of 1,308 molecules tested
Action on Telomerase	Binds telomerase	Unknown	Suppresses telomerase synthesis

detailed results

Gly-His-Lys [45005] (17-FEB-11)

total instances: 6100, *signature:* Gly-His-Lys, *export:* Excel
permuted results | isolate shaded

Similarity of Gene m-RNA Synthesis between GHK and 1,308 other bioactives

rank	batch	cmap name	dose	cell	score	function	Activity of GHK
1	1036	Gly-His-Lys	1 µM	PC3	1		
2	1036	STOCK1N-35874	14 µM	PC3	.877	anti-glaucoma	(MAYBE) GHK reduces blood pressure
3	1036	6-bromoindirubin-3'-oxime	500 nM	PC3	.683	Maintains stem cell "stemness" Suppresses telomerase & cancer growth	YES
4	762	tiletamine	15 µM	PC3	.506	anesthetic	PROBABLY YES many copper complexes are anesthetics
5	653	cefalexin	11 µM	MCF7	.496	antibiotic	YES
6	610	minoxidil	19 µM	PC3	.488	hair growth	YES
7	706	Prestwick-857	12 µM	MCF7	.485	unknown	UNKNOWN
8	711	citiolone	25 µM	MCF7	.466	liver therapy	YES
9	692	nystatin	4 µM	PC3	.466	antibiotic	YES
10	748	bambuterol	10 µM	MCF7	.465	asthma drug	PROBABLY YES
11	642	prilocaine	16 µM	MCF7	.465	local anesthetic	PROBABLY YES
12	734	quipazine	9 µM	PC3	.456	seratonin receptor	UNKNOWN
13	628	epirizole	17 µM	PC3	.455	anti-inflammatory	YES
14	702	flunisolide	9 µM	PC3	.454	anti-inflammatory	YES
15	628	heptaminol	22 µM	PC3	.450	vasodilator	YES
16	628	isoflupredone	10 µM	PC3	.449	anti-inflammatory	YES
17	761	enalapril	8 µM	PC3	.447	vasodilator	YES
18	680	monensin	6 µM	PC3	.447	antibiotic	YES

PLUS 1,290 MORE COMPOUNDS COMPARED TO GHK

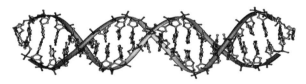

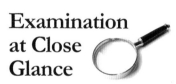

Examination at Close Glance

GHK inhibits human telomerase which could be an anti-cancer action. On the other hand, it also functions to help maintain healthy thyroid cells in culture for over 200 generations. So suppression of telomerase in cancer cells is not necessarily connected to longevity.

ACTION	GHK	Decorin	(BIO) 6-bromoindirubin-3'-oxime
Anti-Cancer	Increases Decorin Suppresses many genes overexpressed in aggressive metastatic human colon cancer Anti-scarring	Suppresses metastasis of breast, prostate, and osteosarcomas in animal models	Suppresses human multiple myeloma, leukemia, hepatomas in human or animal models
Action on Telomerase	Binds telomerase	Unknown	Suppresses telomerase synthesis

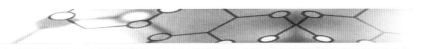

CHEMBANK

Gly- His- Lys

Names: 379527 *(NSC)*, Gly- His- Lys *(common)*, glycyl- histidyl- lysine *(MeSH, chemical)*, glycyl- L- histidyl- L- lysine *(IUPAC)*

Another important source of information is The Broad's ChemBank where GHK has been tested on about 790 proteins, enzymes, and cellular systems. GHK's highest activity in the Broad Institute ChemBank is inhibiting human histone deacetylase or HDAC. GHK inhibits HDAC based on its very strong binding to HDAC and its gene actions. Such inhibitors seem to kill cancer cells but not normal cells. They also kill cells with latent HIV and have anti-Alzheimer actions.

Some such inhibitors cause cell senescence while others do the opposite. Since GHK has been used as an ingredient in the long term cell culture (over 200 generations or 5-times the Hayflick Limit) of normal rat adult thyroid cells to "Break the Hayflick Limit", it is obviously not a senescence factor. During aging, many genes are silenced and stop producing proteins. Young DNA is rather open so that proteins can be made. During aging, HDACs cause a tightening of the DNA strands by removing acetyl groups from DNA which silences the DNA. Inhibitors of HDAC increase acetyl groups on the DNA thus producing more proteins like younger DNA.

HDAC inhibitors such as Vorinostat and Trichostatin suppress many types of cancers. Such inhibitors have in vivo effects against latently HIV infected T-cells. This means it might be possible to remove the virus from infected cells. A brief look at other effects are based on the first 8 tests of about 370. It appears that GHK strongly inhibits proteins causing aging itself plus the problems of cancer, arthritis, HIV, HIV nerve damage, psychiatric disease, malaria, immune suppression for transplantations, and Alzheimers. Every one of the proteins that GHK affects is the object of intense research by drug companies.

It also inhibits the Wnt pathway, a signaling system involved in embryogenesis and in many other processes in living cells, it has been implicated in many cancers. And we have just touched the surface of this data.

Project Name	Assay Name	Assay Type	Plate	Well	Z-score	Composite Z-Score	Standard Hit
Commercial HDACs	ManualSNR(1122.0012)	small-molecule microarray	1122.0012.2099.C	N17	3.16456309043623	5.734	0.0
DihydroorotateDehydrogenase	Calc(E1-E2)(1021.0020)	HTS (homogeneous)	1021.0020.2099.B	N17	3.95	5.5321	0.0
PETLigandSMM	ManualSNR(1153.0015)	small-molecule microarray	1153.0015.2099.C	N17	3.4293	4.6602	0.0
S836	AutoSNR(1146.0006)	small-molecule microarray	1146.0006.2099.C	N17	1.1908	4.5127	0.0
NeuroSMM	ManualSNR(1069.0005)	small-molecule microarray	1069.0005.2099.C	N17	3.30983550471318	4.3427	0.0
PDI Slides	ManualSNR(1129.0009)	small-molecule microarray	1129.0009.2099.C	N17	2.85540370902437	4.0791	0.0
Commercial HDACs	ManualSNR(1122.0007)	small-molecule microarray	1122.0007.2099.C	N17	2.05202405573315	3.9861	0.0
NeuroSMM	ManualSNR(1069.0003)	small-molecule microarray	1069.0003.2099.C	N17	2.16829671489896	3.947	
HumanTelomeraseRNASMM	AutoSNR(1114.0001)	small-molecule microarray	1114.0001.2099.C	N17	2.89676057956012	3.7393	

Possible Mechanism of GHK-Cu Action

It is now well established that the biological significance of GHK-Cu primarily results from its unique relationship with copper. GHK has a strong affinity for copper and it can obtain copper from plasma albumin to deliver into tissues. Since copper ions are used by many enzymes involved in different biological processes in the cell, supplying the tissues with copper can improve many aspects of tissue metabolism including antioxidant defense, tissue repair, oxygenation etc.

Although copper is vital for the human organism, free ionic copper needs to be tightly controlled because of its high chemical reactivity. While GHK can deliver copper to cells, the plasma protein albumin dominates this function.

GHK appears to function in cellular signaling and activate specific cellular receptors that maintain Regenerative Homeostasis, that is healthy tissue regeneration. The molecule can also act directly on biochemical reactions such as suppressing free radical formation.

As for signaling, low tissue copper prompts proliferation of stem cells, while sufficient tissue copper is required for stem cell differentiation into cells needed for tissue repair. An inadequate level of copper can prevent stem cells from differentiation and hamper tissue repair.

Since copper has signaling function, it should be delivered precisely when and where needed—both dosage and timing are important. By modulating copper levels, GHK-Cu may act as a "switch" that curbs inflammation and prompts skin healing and the remodeling process. Small size and mobility allow GHK-Cu easy access to molecular receptors and speedy travel in the extracellular space.

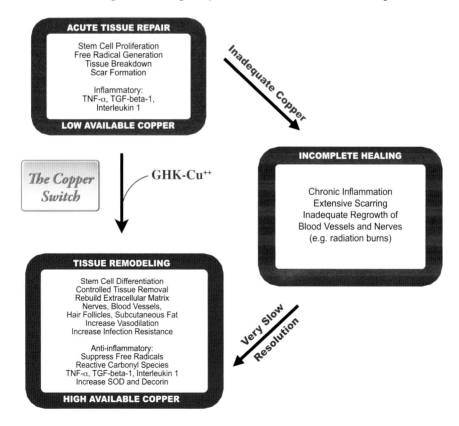

CAN COPPER PEPTIDES REVERSE HUMAN AGING OR IMPROVE THE HEALTH OF OLDER PERSONS?

Causes of Human Aging—The major causes of human aging are:

PRINCIPAL CAUSES OF AGING	ANTI-AGING ACTIONS OF GHK
Older humans and other mammals have numbers of tissue stem cells similar to younger animals. But in the older group, the adult stem cells are not producing needed differentiated cells.	GHK increases stem cell replication and progression to differentiated cells.
Lack of organ repair and renewal.	GHK increases and activates stem cells. It increases regeneration of skin, hair follicles, bone tissue, gastric lining, and intestinal lining.
Increased Inflammations (heart disease, kidney disease, etc.)	GHK increases anti-oxidant proteins while suppressing inflammatory cytokines. It protects tissues from damage by oxygen radicals and reactive carbonyl species. It blocks the release of oxidizing iron from ferritin.
Increased infections	GHK suppresses bacterial infections in mice.
Increased cancer	GHK plus ascorbic acid suppresses two cancer lines in mice. GHK topped the list of 1,309 compounds tested at the Broad Institute for the suppression of genes overexpressed in aggressive, metastatic human colon cancer.
DNA produces less healthy types of proteins in older humans	Data so far (analysis of gene effects is just beginning) indicates that GHK induces the production of healthier proteins such as decorin (cancer suppressing), collagen, water-holding glycosaminoglycans and proteoglycans, superoxide dismutase, tissue remodeling metalloproteinases and anti-proteases. GHK suppresses inflammatory proteins (TGF-beta, interleukin-1, TNF-alpha), Alzheimer associated genes, and suppresses about 37 genes overexpressed in aggressive, metastatic colon cancer.

Regulation of Genes?

What does it mean when we say that GHK is able to influence (up- or downregulate) certain genes? Scientists long believed that DNA, a repository of genetic information, remains unchanged through the life of an individual unless its structure is somehow damaged. According to a modern concept, DNA resembles

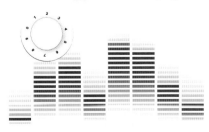

an extremely complex and sophisticated control panel, where different knobs (genes) are switched on and off, turned up or down by molecular regulators. In human aging and diseases "youth and health" genes are being turned down or even completely switched off, while genes that favor inflammation, cancerous and metastatic growth are turned up. In light of recent scientific data, GHK emerges as one of the most important molecular regulators that help maintain DNA in the most productive and youthful state.

GHK from an Evolutionary Perspective

The cornucopia of positive findings raises questions, namely: Why does this molecule have so many reparative actions? It may be that GHK originated from an ancient marine signaling system dependent on levels of copper ion, that was swept into mammals on the tides of evolution, and predates more modern growth factors and cytokines. Free ionic copper proves highly toxic to primitive marine invertebrates such as mollusks, crustaceans, worms, corals, sponges, barnacles and jellyfish. GHK detoxifies the free copper by binding it and aids the growth of several primitive life forms. It is a potent attractor of barnacle larvae, causing them to metamorphosize and colonize surfaces to form barnacles (Rittschof & Cohen 2004). Barnacles date back at least 400 million years. Copper plates and copper-containing paints were used in the past to protect vessels from barnacle larvae that settled on the hulls. Copper is toxic to roundworms, very primitive animals, but GHK adds to their growth (Stromberg et al 1977). GHK also acts as a "pumping pheromone" for spiny lobsters, another early sea creature, and causes them to release internal eggs and larvae (Ziegler & Forward 2007).

Probable Evolution of GHK

GHK system may be very old, dating back to primitive organisms

Humans and Other Mammals:

↑
- Anti-Inflammatory
  (May have started as a protective system)
- Tissue Repair
  (May be more recent)

Reptiles

↑

Primitive Parasitic Worms:

↑
GHK induces differentiation and promotes growth
- Ascaris
- Litomosoides

GHK and similar marine peptide-like pheromones:

↑
- Spiny Lobsters — Act as "pumping pheromone" for egg release
- Barnacles — Act as chemoattractors and induce settling on surface
  (Copper used to repel barnacles)
  GHK strongly competes for receptor binding with pheromones inducing settlement

GHK-like molecules de-toxify copper:

↑
- Act as anti-inflammatory

 Worms Algae Sponges

↑

Early ocean's free copper toxic to primitive organisms

Healthy Living for 350 Years? Breaking the "Hayflick Limit" and Protein p63

The Hayflick Limit asserts that normal human cells can replicate for only about 40 generations before they become senescent or cancerous. GHK is one of six growth factors (GHK, insulin, thyrotropin, transferrin, hydrocortisone, somatostatin) used to culture normal adult thyroid cells. In this system, the cells have been cultured over 200 generations without becoming senescent or cancerous (Ambesi-Impiombato et al 1980).

GHK increases the anti-senescence protein p63 which maintains the proliferative capacity in stratified epithelial stem cells (Kang et al 2009, Senoo et al 2007). This promotes stem cell maintenance and genomic stability, thereby suppressing senescence and preventing premature tissue aging (Keyes & Mills 2006, Beaudry & Attardi 2009, Su et al 2009).

So if the Hayflick Limit does control longevity, then the above thyroid cells exceeded this by five-fold. This would imply that a 70 year old (whose cells remained healthy for 200 generations) might hypothetically live for 5 x 70 years = 350 years.

What If?

What if turning back the clock was as simple as administering GHK?

Elderly Woman takes her supplement of GHK daily...

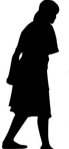

GHK begins to affect genetic aging...

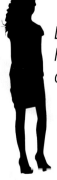

Life span increases and health improves to that of a young woman!

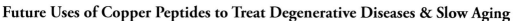

Future Uses of Copper Peptides to Treat Degenerative Diseases & Slow Aging

With GHK-Cu, it is possible to produce systemic wound healing in mice, rats, and pigs. For example, if GHK is injected into the thighs of pigs, wounds heal more rapidly throughout the body such as the upper back or the ears. If wound healing can be accelerated this way, it is very likely that all other GHK actions could be activated (Pickart Patent B 1992).

> GHK is the human body's regulator of protective and regenerative mechanisms for the health and beauty of our skin. There is nothing like it. When using GHK based cosmetics, you are tapping into your skin's own regenerative and age reversal power—something that presently cannot be achieved by any other ingredient!

By incorporating GHK-Cu into the proper type of liposomes, they could be taken as an oral supplement which would pass through the stomach, be released in the intestines, and absorbed into the bloodstream. The GHK could be used as a nutritional supplement or used for various medical treatments (e.g. cancer, kidney failure, general aging and senescence). GHK-Cu is very non-toxic but drastically drops blood pressure when overused. However, the effective therapeutic dosage for tissue regeneration is about 300 times lower than the level that causes dangerous side-effects. GHK could also be used in combination with other aging-reversal methods such as stem cell infusion and pharmaceutical telomerase activators.

IN CONCLUSION My idealistic dream to find a cure for aging led me to the discovery of a fascinating molecule—the copper binding tripeptide GHK. Now more than 49 years after starting this search, science finally started to unveil at least some of its secrets. Scientific data from over 80 research laboratories all over the world confirm that GHK is a central regulator of reparative and renewal processes in the skin, and quite possibly the entire human body. It maintains stem cell reserves, regulates proliferation of many skin cells such as fibroblasts and keratinocytes, stimulates production of reparative growth factors (while suppressing the scar forming and inflammatory ones); regulates skin remodeling by balancing skin protein breakdown and synthesis; stimulates synthesis of glycosaminoglycans (improves the water-holding capacity of the skin) and increases skin collagen.

The amazing GHK prevents chronic inflammation and scarring, increases antioxidant defense and speeds up wound healing. It also improves aged skin, wrinkles, mottled pigmentation, skin tonus and elasticity. Hair growth is enhanced as well. By balancing the cycle of skin remodeling, it helps to eliminate buried skin defects.

Now adding the recently discovered anti-cancer and gene regulating actions, you get a perfect skin wellness and rejuvenation molecule! The most exciting part is that this fascinating molecule has been transformed into a beauty elixir that works together with the natural healing and restorative mechanisms in your body creating healthier, younger looking and radiantly beautiful skin.

REVERSE SKIN AGING ALLOWED WITH COPPER PEPTIDES

19

THE ESSENTIALS OF COPPER
YOUR BODY'S PROTECTIVE AND ANTI-AGING METAL

At the dawn of the copper age, (5500 to 3000 B.C.), ancients had a love affair with this lustrous metal. Copper, an excellent conductor of heat, was thought to stimulate a warm flow of healing energy. Used throughout, Egypt, Greece, Rome and Asia, ancients created copper crowns, ceremonial vessels, bejeweled tools and ornate décor. As one of the oldest metals used and cherished by humans, many referred to copper as the metal of healing and the metal of love.

Our ancestors had keen insight. As the adage states, 'they were right on the money' or perhaps we might say 'right on the copper coin'. In Greek mythology, copper is the metal of Venus and the Goddess of Love. Throughout this book, we have explored how copper turns back the clock to a beautiful complexion and healthy body. When we look and feel our best, Aphrodite may indeed be just around the corner making it easy to attract love.

COPPER MISCONCEPTIONS Quite often, modern scientists toil for decades only to discover something that our ancestors knew all along from observation and keen intuition. Even after the essential discovery is made, it may take years before the official health guidelines catch up with the scientific research. It is because of this that copper, an absolutely essential element for human health, has only recently started to attract the attention of nutrition gurus. Still today, not many people know that they are at risk of copper deficiency which may put them in danger of many illnesses, not to mention accelerated aging of skin and hair.

The slow process of recognizing the importance of copper was best highlighted by Dr. Leslie Klevay in his paper published in 1996 ["Deliberations and evaluations of the approaches, endpoints and paradigms for dietary recommendations about copper", Klevay & Medeiros 1996]. He reviewed the last 10 editions of the Recommended Daily Allowances (RDAs) guidelines and observed that in the 1943 edition the recommended daily amount of copper was estimated at 1-2 mg/day, and in a 1958 edition (15 years later), it was stated that "2 mg/day will maintain adults in balance".

In the same 1958 edition, he found a statement that mentioned "a typical diet" usually supplies 2-5 mg of copper a day, and that the deficiency of this metal is very rare. However, in the 1989 edition, we see a reference to the National Food Consumption survey conducted in 1987-1988, according to which an average intake of copper was 1.2 mg/day for males and only 0.9 mg/day for females—a statistic well below the recommended 2mg/day. In this same edition it was also stated that copper intake as high as 3 mg/day may be necessary to maintain good health. The current RDI (Recommended Dietary Intake established by the U.S. Food and Drug Administration) for copper is 2 mg/day.

Another reference that should be considered is the estimated safe and adequate daily dietary intakes or ESADDI (Natural Research Council, 1989) which recommends a daily intake of 1.5-3 mg of copper. Recently, U.S. dietary guidelines underwent another major revision and RDAs were replaced by The Dietary Reference Intakes (DRI) established by the Food and Nutrition Board of the Institute of Medicine, 1997-2001. The World Health Organization gives 10 mg/day as the tolerable upper limit of copper intake.

Copper Deficient Skin

Impaired collagen synthesis:
Lax skin / wrinkles

Disruption of anti-oxidant defense:
Accelerated aging

Increased glycation of proteins:
Brittle collagen / wrinkles

Delayed
wound healing

Impaired pigment synthesis:
Graying of hairs

Increased
inflammation

Out of the blue, the recommended intake of copper was set up as 0.9 mg/day —a number that is clearly not enough to assure adequate copper intake! For example, a paper published in 2010 by Chambers et al studied the effects of copper deficiency and excess. This study came to the conclusion that to prevent copper deficiency optimum intake for copper should be 2.6 mg/day (which is well below the level where any adverse effects can be seen).

The sudden drop in the recommended intake of copper is more interesting when you take into consideration that estimated daily loss of copper is about 1.3 mg/day. This is one of the reasons why it is so dangerous to lower copper consumption below 2 mg/day (Williams 1983). Active males should also be aware that additional daily loss of copper due to sweating may be as high as 0.34 mg/day (Jacob 1981).

But is copper really that important and worth such an in depth discussion? Absolutely! In fact, copper deficiency may be a leading cause of many so-called "diseases of civilizations" that currently plague the population in the United States. Furthermore it may also be the main reason why our skin and hair lose their health and vitality as we age.

Since SRCPs contain copper, our clients often ask about the function of copper within the body. As they learn about how copper works and experience its benefits, they also want to know about its safety.

Copper is an essential metal necessary for many processes in the human body. A deficiency in copper can contribute to a host of health problems, including a higher rate of: cellular oxidation, cancer, cardiovascular disease, atherosclerosis, LDL "bad cholesterol", lipid oxidation, aortic aneurysms, osteoarthritis, rheumatoid arthritis, osteoporosis, chronic conditions involving bone and connective tissue, brain defects in newborns, obesity, graying of hair, sensitivity to pain, Alzheimer's disease, reproductive problems, depression, and fatigue; as well as lowering HDL "good cholesterol", reduction in the pleasure producing brain enkephalins, and impaired brain function.

Copper—There is Nothing Like It

The first evidence for the essential role copper plays in the human body was obtained in 1928. When rats were kept on an iron-free milk diet, they developed severe anemia. Surprisingly, iron supplementation alone couldn't reverse this condition. It turned out that not only iron, but also copper deficiency, contributed to the observed symptoms of anemia. Since then copper/iron supplements have been used to correct anemia in malnourished infants (Hart et al 2002).

In Australia, farmers were long puzzled by an array of problems that sheep and cattle (brought from the mainland) had been experiencing after grazing on indigenous soil. Poor wool quality in sheep, neurological problems (swayback) in newborn lambs and aorta ruptures in cattle drove farmers crazy until it was discovered that the indigenous soil had very little copper. As soon as livestock began taking copper supplements, the mysterious diseases became a thing of the past (Harris 2003).

Today, we know that copper is absolutely essential for life. No other metal can replace it. Fortunately, severe deficiency of this metal is rare and is observed mostly in experiments of animals kept on copper-free diets. We are lucky that most of our foods contain at least some copper. However, even marginal copper deficiency can be dangerous and have long term consequences.

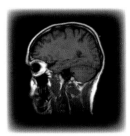

For example, when pregnant rats were kept on a marginally copper-deficient diet, their copper indexes were often within norm, and yet their offspring were born with marked differences in their immune status. What's more, those rats developed copper deficiency in the brain (which could not be reversed by copper supplementation). Young rats with copper deficient brains exhibited altered behavior and neurological characteristics (Prohaska & Hoffman 1996).

So why does our body need copper? To answer this question we need to talk about an important kind of biological molecule called enzymes.

Copper and The Chemical Balance in Our Body

Our bodies are constantly transforming chemical substances into other substances, using and releasing energy, breaking down and building biological compounds over and over again. Our well-being completely depends on the delicate chemical balance within our cells. The same principle holds true for our beauty.

For example, production of the most important proteins in our skin (collagen and elastin) occurs through a series of precisely balanced chemical reactions. The majority of chemical reactions in our cells cannot occur spontaneously under normal physiological conditions. If this wasn't the case there would be no order, no organization, no harmony. So in order to maintain this balance and order within the cells, our body uses special molecules that carefully guide every substance through its precise chemical transformation process. Such molecular organizers are called **enzymes**.

There is a special enzyme for each and every biological reaction. Many of them are not active by themselves but require metal ions in order to function. More than a dozen important enzymes (cuproenzymes) require copper (Camakaris et al 1999). Some of them are listed in the table on the following page.

> **Did You Know?** Most of the body's copper binds into proteins where it plays an important role in biological activities such as antioxidant effects, energy generation, and tissue regeneration. In fact, over a dozen important enzymes in the human body require **copper**. Our brain contains more copper than any other organ except the liver, where copper stores are tapped on as needed. This fact suggests that copper plays a role in brain functions.

A New *Ethereal* Understanding of GHK and Copper

Controls or influences about 17% of human genes

Increases anti-inflammatory proteins
Increases anti-oxidant proteins

Suppresses inflammatory proteins

Protects tissues from oxygen radicals and reactive carbonyl species

Blocks the release of oxidizing iron

Suppresses bacterial infections

Suppresses many genes overexpressed in aggressive, metastatic cancer

Produces biologically younger skin

Accelerates healing of wounds, bones, stomach, intestine healing, and hair growth

Improves hair transplants

Breaks "Hayflick Limit" on maximum cell generations

Increases anti-senescence protein p63

Blocks proteins that shut down DNA during aging

Repairs cellular DNA damage

Understanding of Copper Before GHK

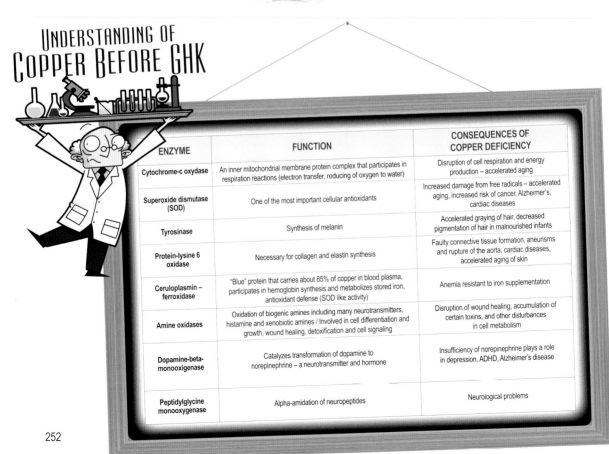

ENZYME	FUNCTION	CONSEQUENCES OF COPPER DEFICIENCY
Cytochrome-c oxydase	An inner mitochondrial membrane protein complex that participates in respiration reactions (electron transfer, reducing of oxygen to water)	Disruption of cell respiration and energy production – accelerated aging
Superoxide dismutase (SOD)	One of the most important cellular antioxidants	Increased damage from free radicals – accelerated aging, increased risk of cancer, Alzheimer's, cardiac diseases
Tyrosinase	Synthesis of melanin	Accelerated graying of hair, decreased pigmentation of hair in malnourished infants
Protein-lysine 6 oxidase	Necessary for collagen and elastin synthesis	Faulty connective tissue formation, aneurisms and rupture of the aorta, cardiac diseases, accelerated aging of skin
Ceruloplasmin – ferroxidase	"Blue" protein that carries about 85% of copper in blood plasma, participates in hemoglobin synthesis and metabolizes stored iron, antioxidant defense (SOD like activity)	Anemia resistant to iron supplementation
Amine oxidases	Oxidation of biogenic amines including many neurotransmitters, histamine and xenobiotic amines / Involved in cell differentiation and growth, wound healing, detoxification and cell signaling	Disruption of wound healing, accumulation of certain toxins, and other disturbances in cell metabolism
Dopamine-beta-monooxigenase	Catalyzes transformation of dopamine to norepinephrine – a neurotransmitter and hormone	Insufficiency of norepinephrine plays a role in depression, ADHD, Alzheimer's disease
Peptidylglycine monooxygenase	Alpha-amidation of neuropeptides	Neurological problems

Later in this chapter we will discuss copper's role in skin health. But for now it should be clear that copper deficiency (even if it is slight) can have serious consequences for our organisms. Should we really be concerned about this? Yes, we should.

Are You At Risk?

Copper—this precious metal essential for maintaining the chemical balance within our cells, enters our bodies with food and water. The richest sources of copper are red wine, chocolate, cocoa, legumes, nuts (especially Brazilian nuts), seaweed, oysters and other shellfish, fish, liver and organ meats, well water in certain regions (depending on copper content in soil) or soft, acidic water that has passed through copper pipes.

At the same time, some dietary and lifestyle factors can prevent our organism from obtaining enough copper either by increasing its excretion or by lowering its absorption. Some of those factors can also exacerbate symptoms of copper deficiency. Sadly, all of these factors are present in the typical American diet.

First of all, copper levels may be lower in people who routinely consume too much zinc (this is due to zinc interfering with copper absorption) (Klevay 2001). The most dramatic example of copper deficiency in primates caused by excessive zinc is the "white monkey syndrome" that develops in infant monkeys kept in galvanized cages. It manifests itself by elevated zinc, low copper, loss of pigment in skin and hair (hence the name "white monkey syndrome"), immune deficiency, alopecia, severe dermatitis and other problems (Frost et al 2004). Since monkeys are our closest animal relatives, we should pay close attention to this example.

Most people are aware of the importance of zinc. Of course, commercial food manufacturers use this knowledge to increase sales—almost all processed food products in the United States are generously fortified with zinc and iron. In addition, all vitamin/mineral complexes contain zinc and iron. As a result, people who consume large amounts of processed foods and regularly take vitamin/mineral supplements may actually get too much iron and zinc, thereby putting themselves at risk of copper deficiency.

Many Americans prefer meat over all other protein sources. However, meats (with the exception of organ meats) are rich in zinc but low in copper. So those who consume muscle meat as opposed to organ meat and who do not consume enough legumes and seafood, may also develop copper deficiency. In one experiment, rats were fed a red meat based diet and had 23% lower bone density compared to the control animals. It is a known fact that osteoporosis is one of the common consequences of low copper (Klevay & Wildman 2002).

Another factor that can lower copper is the high consumption of fructose, sucrose and other refined sugars (Klevay 2010). If you have a sweet tooth or regularly consume soda that is usually high on sugar, you may need more copper in your diet!

Finally, many Americans today drink bottled water or soda instead of natural well or spring water, thus cutting themselves from another source of dietary copper. The long-lived people who reside high in mountain valleys about 2000 meters above sea level enjoy copper-rich water from natural glaciers. They are living testaments to the health benefits of copper. Cultures in the Hunza region of the Hindu Kush, the Vilcabamba valley of Ecuador, the Caucasus mountains of Georgia, Northwest Tibet, and Lake Titicaca of the Peruvian Andes all have diverse diets but drink the same hard water from 'icy blue' glaciers, which contains an exceptionally high mineral content. In all of these regions, the lifespan and health of the elderly is extraordinary with many centenarians. In contrast, regions with soft water that is low in minerals experience high rates of cancer and heart disease. In the past, physicians would send their patients to sanatoriums where they drank mineral water and also bathed in it.

The popularity of bariatric surgery as a fast means to eliminate obesity also puts many people at risk of copper deficiency, since it lowers copper absorption in the intestine (Ernst et al 2009).

Does Your Diet Contain Adequate Copper?

Vegetarians have higher levels of copper in their diets than non-vegetarians. In a controlled study using females (USDA Nutrition Center in Grand Forks, North Dakota), it was found that lacto-ovo vegetarians took in 1.45 milligrams of copper daily of which 33% was taken into the body (0.48 milligrams). In contrast, the non-vegetarians took in 0.94 milligrams of copper daily of which 42% was taken into the body for an intake of 0.39 milligrams daily (Hunt & Vanderpool 2001).

So ask yourself the following questions:

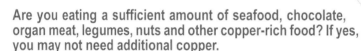

Are you eating a sufficient amount of seafood, chocolate, organ meat, legumes, nuts and other copper-rich food? If yes, you may not need additional copper.

Are you a vegan/vegetarian, consuming a diverse diet? If yes, you may not need additional copper.

Do you regularly consume sweets, soda and other sugar and fructose enriched foods? If yes, you may be in need of copper.

Do you regularly consume processed foods and take vitamin/mineral supplements? If yes, you may still be in need of copper if your vitamin/mineral complex doesn't contain it.

In addition, you should worry about copper deficiency if you have had gastric bypass, malabsorption syndrome, celiac disease or if you are pregnant or lactating.

COPPER DEFICIENCY The majority of the data on the symptoms of severe copper deficiency came from animal studies, studies in malnourished children or studies on the rare genetic abnormality of Menkel syndrome. Recently, scientists began to pay attention to signs and consequences of marginal copper deficiency as well.

The main sign of severe copper deficiency in animals and humans is anemia that is unresponsive to iron therapy and is accompanied by severe abnormalities in bone marrow. Other symptoms include low white cell count in blood, increased incidence of infections, impaired growth and low weight in infants, bone abnormalities (fractures of long bones and ribs, osteoporosis, spur formation, formation of bone tissue outside of bones), impaired collagen synthesis, impaired melanin synthesis, hypotonia, and heart problems (including heart failure) (Elsherif et al 2003, Cartwright & Wintrobe 1964). These symptoms coincide with low levels of copper in plasma and are reversed by copper supplementation (Uauy et al 1998).

Fortunately, such prominent symptoms are rare. However, many people can have a borderline copper deficiency. Today, insufficient copper is thought to contribute to an increased risk of cardiovascular diseases, elevated level of total cholesterol and in particular "bad cholesterol", neuro-degenerative conditions such as Alzheimer's and Parkinson diseases, accelerated skin and hair aging, low immune status, impaired antioxidant defense, diabetes and osteoporosis.

Copper Deficiency Can Harm Your Skin

Collagen, as you all well know, is a protein that maintains the suppleness, firmness and resilience of your skin. Faulty collagen leads to wrinkles, sagging and loose skin. There is no other way to remove wrinkles and tighten skin except through the stimulation and restoration of collagen synthesis.

In order to do this, we need special enzymes that build collagen. One of those enzymes is lysyl oxidase—an enzyme that absolutely depends on copper. Animals deficient in copper show multiple connective tissue abnormalities, including rupture and aneurism of major blood vessels due to defective collagen.

But could the copper in lysyl oxidase be replaced with another similar mineral? It turns out that nothing can replace copper. Researchers have tried to supplement lysyl oxidase with ions of cadmium, iron, zinc, magnesium and cobalt, but failed to restore enzyme activity. Therefore, if your diet does not contain enough copper, you need to deliver it to your skin.

Without adequate copper no other means of stimulating collagen synthesis (no expensive cosmetic procedure or advanced topical product) can restore your collagen (Gacheru et al 1990).

Another risk factor that results from copper deficiency is skin aging due to glycation of skin proteins, a reaction that we've discussed earlier in this book.

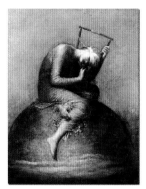

Furthermore, it is known that copper deficiency results in hyperglycemia, which leads to enhanced glycosylation of proteins. Increased peroxidation and glycation are the most likely causes of general damage associated with copper deficiency. It has been demonstrated that some effects of severe copper deficiency in rats, such as cardiac enlargement and anemia, can be reduced by treatment with anti-glycosylation agents. On the contrary, consumption of a sucrose rich diet with starch exacerbates the symptoms of copper deficiency. Food restriction that reduces peroxidation and glycation also reduces symptoms of copper deficiency (Saari et al 1995).

Another reason why insufficient copper can speed up skin aging is decreased function of SOD—a major antioxidant enzyme that requires copper in order to be active. It has now been established that copper is required not only for this enzyme to be functionally active, but also for activation of the genes necessary for SOD synthesis (Itoh et al 2009).

Faulty collagen and increased protein damage due to glycation and peroxidation would be enough to make a significant impact on your complexion, but there is much more! Copper deficiency has such a widespread deleterious influence on our bodies that our beauty may suffer painful punches from numerous directions.

For example, how would you feel about a disruption of your immune functions and increase of inflammation? It can affect your joints and heart while it also impacts your skin. Cardiac problems are strongly associated with copper deficiency and decreased circulation is not good for your skin nor for your whole body. In addition, low copper can lead to numerous neurological problems affecting nerve growth and production of important neuromediators.

So what should this mean to you personally? Well, if you do not consume enough copper rich foods and do not take copper supplements and indulge in sweets and soda, your skin may be at risk of accelerated aging associated with protein glycation. Glycation can make your skin protein stiff and brittle, contributing to wrinkles and other signs of aging. As you restore your internal copper supply, it is very important to use copper peptide products on your skin.

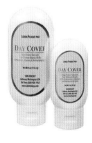
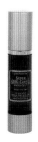
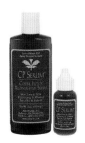
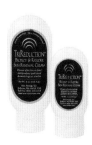

THE TWO FORMS OF COPPER   Have you ever wondered why copper peptide cosmetics look blue while copper in metal appears bronze? In the human body, copper moves between the cuprous (copper (I) or Cu 1+) form and the cupric (copper (II) or Cu 2+) form. Copper (II) is the form of copper that induces tissue regeneration and skin repair. It gives a blue color in water and a blue-to-green color when formulated into creams, lotions, and solutions. Copper (I) has no tissue regenerative or skin-repair activity and is colorless in water.

HOW MUCH COPPER DO YOU NEED?   Most nutritionists recommend a daily copper dosage that ranges from 1 to 3 mg, but there is no certainty to this number. Many scientists who study copper and its health benefits take 4 mg daily. Studies in humans have found that daily supplemental copper, ranging from 4 to 7 mg, promotes positive actions, such as reducing damaging cellular oxidation, lowering LDL levels, and increasing HDL levels. Such high intakes may reduce the risk of some degenerative diseases, but nutritionists also recommend not exceeding 10 mg of copper daily.

Copper deficiency diseases follow the pattern of major degenerative diseases in the U.S. Thus, copper provides preventative benefits for all conditions with only one exception: copper should not be taken if one has Wilson's disease, a rare genetic condition that affects 1,600 people in the U.S.

Something to consider is that copper works synergistically with other minerals and nutrients. Copper needs to be taken in the proper ratio with zinc and other minerals like iron in order to maximize absorption. Since copper and zinc compete for uptake in the body, a high copper intake reduces zinc absorption, and, conversely, a high zinc intake reduces copper absorption. Thus, a balance should be maintained between these two metals. The best guess is to take a ratio of seven parts zinc to one part copper. In addition to supplements, you can boost your daily intake of copper by eating tasty copper-rich foods. These include seafood, shellfish, nuts, seeds, beans, whole-grain breads, cocoa, and chocolate.

Uptake of Copper from SRCP Products

Very little copper from SRCP products penetrates the skin. Charged molecules, including copper and peptides, do not readily permeate the skin barrier. Numerous safety studies of SRCP products have failed to find a rise in blood copper or any other negative action.

So do not worry about factoring the copper from copper peptide products into your daily copper intake. If you were to use two grams of copper peptide product daily that contained 2 mg of copper, assuming the skin uptake was at 0.1 percent penetration, this would introduce only about 0.002 mg of copper into your body.

How much copper can we expect to actually penetrate our skin? This question was recently answered by renowned professor of dermatology Howard Maibach at the *University of California San Francisco School of Medicine*. According to the findings of his study, if a 0.68% aqueous solution of GHK-copper stays on the skin for 48 hours, then about 0.13 mg of copper will pass through the skin (Hostynek 2010 and 2011).

The amount of copper that can penetrate the skin from cosmetics is even less and is just enough to restore balance in the skin's copper metabolism, without incurring any risk of upsetting it.

It has been shown that GHK-Cu exhibits its beneficial actions at a very low concentration (as low as 10^{-9}-10^{-10} M). That explains why our topical products containing copper peptides are so efficient in restoring the skin's health and beauty.

Copper vs. GHK-Cu

If copper has so many beneficial actions on its own, why do we need GHK? Copper is a very active element and as such it has to be handled carefully.

Think about fire. When it burns on a stovetop or in the fireplace, it brings warmth and life. But this same fire burning freely in a house brings destruction. Now think of electricity. When it is safely contained within electrical wires, it can work for us, lighting our houses and powering our appliances. But this same electricity in a form of a lightning bolt can be deadly. Even oxygen, this indispensable element of life, can be dangerous and toxic.

Copper is similar. Even though copper salts are often used to supplement copper without any side effects, it is still better to have it enter the body in the form of "bio-copper" or "innocuous copper", which is copper (II) bound to a protein/peptide. This is the form of copper that you will typically find in foods and the type of copper that Skin Biology products contain.

In the human organism there is very little free ionic copper (estimated 10^{-18} molar), approximately one copper ion per cell. Nearly 95% of copper in plasma is bound to ceruloplasmin, however this copper is not readily available.

Of more importance is the portion of copper that is bound to albumin, because it constitutes labile, metabolically active copper. A very small amount of metabolically active copper is exchanged between plasma and tissues in form of

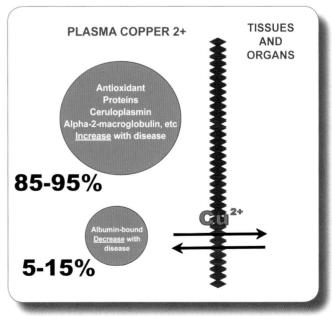

low molecular weight copper complexes. A complex network of copper "chaperones" (carriers and receptors) ensures the safe exchange of copper between plasma and tissues as well as copper delivery into the cells. Any extra copper entering the body is instantly interiorized, packaged, and safely distributed. The same proteins that ensure targeted and safe copper delivery detoxify excess copper (Cabrera et al 2008, Boal & Rosenzweig 2009).

Today our knowledge about this wonderfully complex system of copper delivery and regulation is still very limited. But from clinical observations and animal experiments, we can conclude that copper (either in foods that naturally contain copper or in the form of GHK-Cu) is the most safe, beneficial and smart way to deliver copper to your skin.

Should I Worry About Copper Excess?

One of the fascinating things about copper is the precision with which this essential mineral is regulated in the body. In one study of copper transport in the blood, scientists tried to create an elevated level of copper in plasma, injecting dogs and healthy human volunteers with high doses of copper. To their amazement, all excess copper magically disappeared from the blood shortly after injection!

For example, 50 mg of copper injected in healthy human volunteers (which amounts to 25 times the recommended 2 mg of copper a day) completely cleared from the blood in just 4 hours (Gubler et al 1953).

In experimental settings, researchers gave healthy volunteers 4-8 mg of copper a day for 1 to 3 months without any adverse effects. Due to the efficient mechanism of copper homeostasis, even this high dosage didn't change the plasma concentration (Harvey et al 2003, Turnlund et al 2005).

In a multicenter European study performed in 2000, researchers investigated the effect of extra copper on oxidative processes in the blood cells of middle aged people. Again, they were amazed that even 7 mg/day of copper taken during the 6 week period did not produce any increase in oxidative damage. On the contrary, it improved anti-oxidant defense (Rock et al 2000).

The only dietary source of copper that a person should worry about is in contaminated water, since it supplies inorganic copper not bio-complexes of copper. If you drink water that contains 4-8 mg of copper per liter as your only water source for several weeks, you may experience nausea and other gastric symptoms. However, such problems occur only in Third World countries, where water quality is low. In the United States drinking water does not contribute much to copper intake (Araya et al 2001).

As you can see, our bodies are well equipped with a system of copper balancing proteins and peptides that regulate copper absorption and elimination, swiftly correcting copper excess. Even though copper toxicity may occur (if we ingest too much copper salts or drink copper-loaded water or work in the copper industry), for the majority of us, the issue of copper deficiency is much more worrisome than that of copper excess.

More Support for a Copper-Rich Diet

The copper-containing protein copper-zinc superoxide dismutase (CuZnSOD) provides the primary antioxidant defense in the human body. Animals with higher levels of CuZnSOD have longer lifespans. However because humans usually have a short supply of copper (II), CuZnSOD has only about 50 percent of the copper it needs (zinc supplies are usually adequate). This shortage markedly reduces CuZnSOD's antioxidant powers and presents yet another reason why a higher level of dietary copper benefits our health.

While CuZnSOD requires two metals, copper and zinc, only copper seems to regulate the antioxidant activity. Restricting dietary copper quickly impairs the catalytic function of CuZnSOD in numerous tissues. However, when we supplement our diets with copper, our CuZnSOD activity is quickly restored (Harris 1992).

Animal studies have found that a reduced copper intake increases cellular oxidation which promotes a wide variety of the types of degenerative diseases associated with aging. On the other hand, higher dietary copper reduces cellular oxidation.

Confusion Over Copper and Disease

Of all the copper in our blood serum, only a small fraction is metabolically active. We can find ninety-five percent of active copper in the antioxidant protein ceruloplasmin. During stress or illness, the body increases ceruloplasmin levels as a protective antioxidant mechanism. Because metabolically active copper is technically difficult to measure, most copper and disease studies report only the level of copper in the blood serum. This often leads to false conclusions as to the role copper plays in disease states (Sorenson 1985, Sorenson 1987, Sorenson 1989, Frieden 1986, Sorenson et al 1989).

For example, total blood plasma copper elevates during diseases such as cancer, heart disease, and arthritis, but this increase is due to increased ceruloplasmin in the blood. Some misinformed individuals have interpreted this increase in blood copper as an indication that a high level of copper causes disease.

But when copper supplements are given to animals and humans, the additional dietary copper has been found to lower carcinogenesis and tumor growth, inhibit the development of cardiovascular problems, and reverse many arthritic effects. So let us now take a closer look at how copper impacts various health conditions.

Copper and Cancer

The Center for Disease Control states that copper has not been shown to cause cancer in people or animals. In fact, evidence mounts daily revealing copper's ability to help fight cancer.

As an example, let us consider colon cancer, the second most deadly form of cancer in the U.S. APC, a gene known to suppress the formation of tumors, mutates during the development of colon cancer. Individuals possessing these mutations develop numerous intestinal polyps (precancerous lesions). A species of mice that has a mutation similar to APC was studied. As with APC, the mutation causes intestinal polyps and colon cancer. Nutritionist Cindy D. Davis of the Human Nutrition Research Center in North Dakota found that when these mice were fed a copper-deficient diet (20 percent lower than normal), they developed a significantly higher incidence of small intestine tumors and mass than mice fed adequate dietary copper. Davis says these results have important implications because 80 percent of the population in the United States does not ingest adequate amounts of copper (Davis & Johnson 2002).

Copper complexes cause some types of cancer cells to revert to non-cancerous growth patterns. John R. J. Sorenson of University of Arkansas for Medical Sciences and colleagues treated rats which had solid tumors with various copper complexes (such as copper salicylate) and found that this treatment decreased tumor growth and increased survival rates. While these copper complexes did not kill cancer cells, they often caused them to revert to the growth patterns of normal (differentiated) cells.

In another study, Sorenson found that numerous copper complexes with superoxide dismutase activity retarded the spontaneous development of cancers in mice (Oberley et al 1984). Copper stimulates the production of the tumor-suppressor protein p53, which inhibits the growth of tumors in the body (Greene et al 1987, Narayanan et al 2001). Also see Chapter 18.

Copper and Cardiovascular Disease

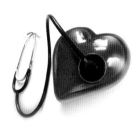

If we want a healthy heart, we need to control our good and bad cholesterol. That's where copper comes to the rescue. Human and animal studies demonstrate that copper deficiency increases plasma cholesterol, "bad" LDL cholesterol, and blood pressure while decreasing "good" HDL cholesterol, thus increasing the risk of cardiovascular disease (Klevay 1987; Klevay & Halas 1991; Klevay 1996, 2000A, 2000B, 2002, 2004).

Investigators have found that copper complexes can minimize damage to the aorta and heart muscle following myocardial infarction. Severe copper deficiency results in heart abnormalities and damage (cardiomyopathy) in some animals (Trumbo et al 2001).

A multi-center study found that copper supplementation of 3 to 6 mg daily increased the resistance of red blood cells to damaging oxidation, indicating that relatively high intakes of copper do not increase the susceptibility of LDL or red blood cells to oxidation (Rock et al 2000). Rats on a copper-deficient diet had a decrease in aortic integrity that produced eventual aneurysm (Greene et al 1987).

Copper and Immune System Function

In order to prevent disease, we need to boost our immune system to fight off those pesky germs such as viruses, bacteria and parasites. Copper can help. A medical publication in 1867 reported that, during the Paris cholera epidemics of 1832, 1849, and 1852, workers exposed to copper salts did not develop cholera. Immune impairment can be detected as early as one week after the start of a diet low in copper; conversely, the addition of adequate copper rapidly reverses the immune suppression within one week (Bala & Failla 1992).

The immune system turned out to be so sensitive to copper deficiency that decreased function of immune cells is now considered an accurate indicator of marginal copper deficiency (Bonham et al 2002). Human and animal studies show that copper deficiency lead to low interleukin 2, decreased proliferation of T-cells and reduced number of neutrophils. In addition, even marginal copper deficiency affects neutrophil's ability to ingest and kill microorganisms such as Candida albicans (yeast infection of the skin). Similar changes can be detected in macrophages (Percival 1998).

Animals deficient in copper have an increased susceptibility to bacterial pathogens such as salmonella and listeria (Bala & Failla 1992). A study of 11 infants with copper deficiencies found that the ability of their white blood cells to engulf pathogens increased after one month of copper supplementation (Heresi et al 1985). Adult men on a low-copper diet (0.66 mg of copper a day for 24 days, and then 0.38 mg a day for another 40 days) showed a decreased ability of their mononuclear cells to respond to antigens (Kelley et al 1995). Abnormally low numbers of white blood cells are a clinical indicator of copper deficiency in humans and the functionality of macrophages decreases in even marginally copper-deficient rats (Babu & Failla 1990, Bala & Failla 1992).

Copper and Arthritis

No one likes those achy joints that wake us up from blissful slumber. Copper can help minimize the painful inflammation. John R. J. Sorenson led the scientific groundwork for the use of copper complexes to treat arthritic and other chronic degenerative diseases. He found that copper complexes combined with more than 140 anti-inflammatory agents, such as aspirin and ibuprofen, to be far more active than these compounds without copper. Studies show copper aspirinate to be more effective in the treatment of rheumatoid arthritis than aspirin alone. Studies also reveal that copper prevents or even cures the ulceration of the stomach often associated with aspirin therapy (Sorenson 1982).

In 1885, the French physician, Luton, effectively treated arthritic patients with a salve of hogs lard and 30 percent neutral copper acetate that he applied to the skin over affected joints. He also had his patients take pills containing 10 mg of copper acetate.

Studies of rheumatoid arthritis exemplify the paradox that has so confounded researchers regarding copper and its effects on various diseases. For example, between 1940 and 1970, patients with rheumatoid arthritis were found to have higher than normal serum copper levels. Similar results were discovered for various inflammatory diseases in both humans and animals. Yet, in seeming contradiction, copper complexes were successfully used to treat numerous conditions characterized by arthritic changes and inflammation.

Subsequent research concluded that an increase in serum copper is a physiological response to inflammation, rather than a cause of inflammation. The rise in copper is due to an elevation of the ceruloplasmin in serum, a protein with strong anti-inflammatory activity. Copper deficiency increases the severity of experimentally induced inflammation (Sorenson & Hangarter 1977, Sorenson 1977, Giampaolo et al 1982, Dollwet & Sorenson 1985, Sorenson 1988).

Recent studies found out that patients with severe rheumatoid arthritis are often copper deficient. According to dietary studies, they typically ingest too much fat and not enough fiber, zinc, magnesium and copper. Their consumption of copper was significantly lower than in a typical American diet (Kremer & Bigaouette 1996).

Copper and Mental Health

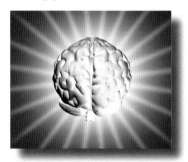

Brain tissue is exceptionally rich in copper and for a good reason. First, brain health and safety depends on the antioxidant enzyme Cu,Zn-SOD. This enzyme protects it against aggressive free radicals of oxygen, which brain cells—highly metabolically active cells—produce in abundance. Faulty SOD due to insufficient copper can have dire consequences, instantly increasing oxidative brain damage. Besides this, copper is essential for a number of other brain enzymes that are involved in the making of important nerve mediators and hormones (Lutsenko et al 2010).

Several neurological conditions have been associated with copper deficiency. Among them is Alzheimer's disease that plagues not only America's seniors, but recently has began to manifest itself at earlier and earlier ages: 40s-50s.

Copper's role in Alzheimer's has long puzzled researchers. In this condition there is focal accumulation of an amyloid beta protein, which traps copper and other metal ions. Only recently has it been discovered that copper deficient brains become prone to beta-amyloid accumulation (Hung et al 2009). Another study demonstrated that copper deficiency increased cell secretion of amyloid-beta. The exact mechanism of this paradox is not yet fully understood, but it is clear that copper deficiency may increase brain's susceptibility to Alzheimer's (Cater et al 2008). Today, there is more and more evidence that copper deficiency in the diet (as well as an excess of zinc) may be the leading cause of Alzheimer's disease (Klevay 2008).

Another neurological symptom of copper deficiency is myelopathy or "human swayback"—a disease similar to that which occurs in sheep grazing on Australian soil lacking copper. Its symptoms include spastic gait or foot dragging and loss of coordination (Kumar 2006).

It is also interesting to note that neurological symptoms often follow bariatric surgery for obesity, which reduces absorption of copper in the intestine. These symptoms may range from neuropathy to encephalopathy and sometimes are irreversible (Kazemi et al 2010).

Copper and Osteoporosis

Dem bones, dem bones, dem dry bones...or so the lyrics go. But who wants to end up with 'dem dry bones' if they can help it? Dry brittle bones or osteoporosis is nothing to sing about. However the good news is that copper contributes to healthy bones and reduces the risk of osteoporosis.

Two hundred years ago, the German physician Rademacher established that copper supplements accelerated healing of broken bones in his patients. Inadequate dietary copper causes osteoporosis in humans and numerous animal species. Copper deficiency is also associated with scoliosis, skeletal abnormalities, and increased susceptibility to fractures. Too little dietary copper lowers bone calcium levels.

A study of elderly subjects found a decreased loss of bone-mineral density from the lumbar spine after copper supplementation of 3 mg daily for two years. Healthy adult males on a low-copper intake (0.7 mgs daily) for six weeks exhibited an increased rate of bone breakdown (Dollwet & Sorenson 1988, Conlan et al 1990, Janas et al 1993, Baker et al 1999).

Ulcer Healing Activities of Copper Complexes

Gastric ulcers are no fun—especially when they give you a stomach ache and kill the pleasure of a hot spicy meal. So next time, add some copper rich oysters and perhaps you'll ward off ulcers.

Studies demonstrate that copper complexes such as copper aspirinate and copper tryptophanate, markedly increased healing rate of gastric ulcers while non-steroidal anti-inflammatory drugs, such as ibuprofen and enefenamic acid, suppress ulcer healing. As a result, these copper complexes promote normal wound healing while at the same time retaining anti-inflammatory activity (Sorenson & Hangartes 1977, Sorenson 1977, Dollwet & Sorenson 1985, Sorenson 1988, Sorenson et al 1982, Alzuet et al 1994, Morgant et al 2000, Lemoine et al 2002, Viossat et al 2005).

Anti-Convulsant Activities of Copper Complexes

 It is important to remember that the brain contains more copper than any other organ with the exception of the liver. This is where copper reserves are tapped into as it is needed by the body. This fact suggests that copper plays a role in brain functions. Since humans and animals are prone to brain seizures when deficient in copper, studies have shown anti-convulsant drugs to more effectively prevent seizures when complexed with copper.

Copper and Pregnancy

In the 1930's, at a sheep station in Western Australia, many newborn lambs lost their coordination, had difficulty standing, and subsequently died. Later it was determined that the pregnant sheep pastured on land that produced grass with a minimal copper content. The grass did not provide sufficient copper for the lambs to develop their normal nervous systems and brains.

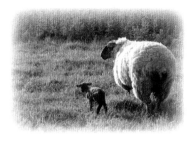

Research at the US Department of Agriculture's Grand Forks Human Nutrition Research Center found that even marginal copper deficiency in pregnant rats produces brain damage and neurological defects in their offspring.

The copper deficient newborn rats have structural abnormalities in the areas of the brain involved in learning and memory and those responsible for coordination and movement. These abnormalities resulted in behavioral changes; for example, the young rats lacked the normal startle reflex as a response to unexpected noises. The copper deficit permanently affected the young rats and could not be corrected by a high-copper diet.

Another study reported that copper deficiency during pregnancy can result in numerous gross structural and biochemical abnormalities, which seem to arise because the copper deficiency reduces free radical defense mechanisms, connective tissue metabolism, and energy production (Ebbs et al 1941, Morten et al 1976, Keen et al 1998, Lonnerdal 1998, Hawk et al 2003, Penland & Prohaska 2004).

Copper Curbs Protein Glycation that AGEs Your Skin

The next time you enjoy a hot smoky steak off the grill, do be aware that you may be aging your skin. Protein glycation, one of the most devastating changes that crops up as we age, occurs when sugar attaches to protein. When you cook meat at high temperatures, a "cross linking" process occurs between the sugar and protein which can lead to stiff brittle skin. As we discussed in an earlier chapter, this process produces a less functional protein. Oxidants can further modify these glycated proteins into "advanced glycation products." These aging products are aptly referred to as AGEs. AGEs not only age our skin, they also cause degenerative diseases such as Diabetes and Alzheimer's. An increased copper intake has been found to reduce protein glycation (Saari et al 1995).

LOW TISSUE COPPER CAUSES:

DO YOU REALIZE THAT: "AGEs" stands for Advanced Glycosylation End-products. These substances that form a harmful waste that can prematurely age skin. Copper has been linked to reducing protein glycation. Low tissue copper has been linked to degenerative diseases.

INCREASED:	DECREASED:
Cardiovascular Disease	Immune System Function
Sensitivity to Pain	Anti-oxidant Activity
Aortic Aneurysms	Energy Production
Diabetes	DHEA
Anemia	HDL
Arthritis	
Blood Pressure	
Cholesterol	
LDL	
Obesity	
Damaging Oxidations	
Tissue Inflammation	
Atherogenic Blood Lipids	
Protein Glycation	
Cancers	
Osteoporosis	
Fatigue	
Psychosis	

The Copper / Stem Cell Paradox

As we seek the key to longevity, stem cells may unlock the doorway to extending lifespan and youthfulness. Could stem cells provide the new wave for organ repair with copper playing catalyst to this process? You bet! One way to repair organ damage that accumulates with age is to introduce stem cells into defective organs. A lack of stem cells causes tissue to deteriorate while increased copper may lead to new stem cells.

Youth — Adequate GHK and Copper 2+

STEM CELLS

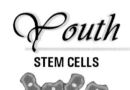

Stem cells are converted to differentiated cells for tissue repair

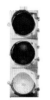

HEALTHY TISSUES

Old Age — Inadequate GHK and Copper 2+

STEM CELLS

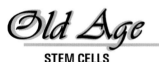

Stem cells fail to differentiate adequate cells for tissue maintenance

DECAYING TISSUES

Scientists concur that low levels of copper stimulate new stem cells. However, a high level of copper causes them to progress into differentiated cells. So on this basis, we would predict that dietary copper that produces low tissue copper would help avoid organ damage. But here's the stem cell paradox: evidence also shows low tissue copper to be associated with degenerative diseases.

How, then, do we resolve this seeming contradiction? Well, it may be that the decline of stem cells results from not having enough available copper to push stem cells into the various types of differentiated cells that organs require. Recent work by Rao,

Hattiangady, and Shetty on the aging of brain tissue in rats found that the stem cells in aging brains are not reduced in number, but there is a reduction in their conversion into neurons (Rao et al 2006). It is possible that additional GHK-Cu would convert more unused stem cells into differentiated cells needed to repair and maintain organs.

Fight Inflammation and Aging

As we learned in Chapter 18, inflammation can wreak havoc on your body and appearance—accelerating disease and aging of your skin. We can fight inflammation with SRCPs. These healing copper molecules can repair skin health and treat the inflammatory diseases of aging. We are often told by clients that SRCPs reduce or sometimes eliminate psoriatic lesions. One theory is that conditions such as psoriasis, psoriatic arthritis, ulcerative colitis, rheumatoid arthritis, ankylosing spondylitis and Crohn's disease are caused by an excess of TNF-alpha, (the tumor necrosis factor involved in inflammation). Since GHK-Cu suppresses TNF-alpha, a low level of GHK (that allows an increased expression of TNF-alpha) may trigger the outbreaks of such conditions and increase inflammatory diseases.

It appears we can use GHK-Cu to biologically repair a variety of issues. As we described earlier in the book, the process of repair begins with a controlled amount of damage. We already know that the molecule helps damage skin, dysfunctional hair follicles, the gastrointestinal tract, the liver, and the bones, but it may also have the ability to repair many other tissues and organs as well. For example, GHK-Cu is very beneficial on kidney and lung organ cultures. Other areas of interest include damaged nerve tissue, inflamed lungs, and knee and hip joints. Some people with gum problems tell me they brush their teeth with SRCPs and have excellent results.

Fibrotic kidney disease may be caused by low GHK levels. The increased incidence of kidney fibrosis that comes with age results from the excessive production of scar-forming TGF-beta-1. TGF beta controls proliferation, differentiation, and other functions in most cell types. Experimental therapies that lower TGF-beta-1 by genetically increasing endogenous levels of anti-inflammatory proteins called decorin or by direct administration of decorin have blocked kidney damage in rat models. GHK-Cu suppresses TGF-beta-1 and increases decorin synthesis. When levels of GHK-Cu drop too low, this may encourage an increase of TGF-beta-1 and diminish levels of decorin, which blocks TGF-beta-1 actions. One day, GHK-Cu might be infused into patients with kidney failure to exert its tissue protective and repair actions.

Does the Copper in Wine Help the French Live Longer?

The French enjoy fine wine, fine dining and live long happy lives. It is indeed a 'French Paradox' that they have healthy hearts while enjoying buttery croissants, Bernaise sauce and mouth watering Duck A L'Orange—all dripping with artery-clogging fats. As we discussed earlier, wine contains reservatrol which can prevent cholesterol plaque from

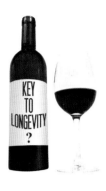

forming. However, here is yet another reason why red wine might contribute to French longevity. Red wine contains an abundance of copper. The copper in wine comes from the skin of the grapes which retain copper from the sulfates used by French vintners. Red wine from France contains about 0.2 mg of copper per liter. So go pour yourself a glass from the wine fountain of youth. Isn't it nice to know you may be sipping your way to a longer life?

Copper and Love

This magic molecule not only provides a door to the future but also offers a window to the past. Ancients believed in copper's power to heal. They wrote that copper was the metal of healing and of love. Throughout this chapter, we have assessed the healing properties of copper—the power of this metal elixir. However according to ancients, copper not only heals, it is also the metal of love. Is this mythology? Maybe not. Today's research has confirmed that copper attracts the molecules that make us feel euphoric pleasure by releasing endorphins. Chemically speaking, love translates into endorphins, serotonin, dopamine, oxytocin, and other brain chemicals. Increased tissue copper has been found to increase brain enkephalins (Bhathena et al 1986). Sorenson determined that copper complexes reduce pain and may activate opioid receptors (Okuyama et al 1987).

Not surprisingly, copper deficiency (even if marginal) can alter the balance of brain chemicals. When healthy males were fed a low copper diet (1 mg/day) for 11 weeks, their plasma opiates level dropped by 80%. As soon as copper was restored (with a diet containing 3 mg/day), it returned to normal (Bhathena et al 1986).

Copper not only contributes to euphoric attraction, it can also play a part in sustaining relationships. During early stages of romantic love, the blood level of NGF (Nerve Growth Factor) nearly doubles. It was also apparent that those who reported the most intense feelings also had the highest NGF levels. But NGF then declines over a years time as passion cools. In wound models, GHK-Cu increases production of NGF.

In addition to feel-good endorphins and NGF levels enhanced by copper, sexual hormones can also boost our sex drives. The hormone DHEA works well with copper to both increase our interest in sex and to lower stress. DHEA converts into the sexual hormones, testosterone and estrogen, which not only promote sex drive but protect against the damaging actions of cortisol. DHEA levels sharply decrease with age while cortisol remains relatively constant. Too much cortisol can result in physical problems and stress related illnesses. The combination of too much stress and decreased sexual hormones can dampen our mood for romance. DHEA is widely used as a dietary supplement to help prevent deleterious changes that occur with age. Klevay and Christopherson found that copper deficiency in rats decreased DHEA in serum by approximately 50 percent. The researchers suggest that eating a higher-copper diet increases the DHEA level in the body (Klevay & Christopherson 2000).

So what about the Metal of Love? While an endorphin-induced sense of euphoric pleasure, coupled with feeling less stress and high personal sexual hormones, may not be love, it is still a good approximation.

ANCIENT IDEAS RISE AGAIN The ancient love affair with copper continues to this day. Modern Spiritualists, like those of thousands of years ago, have reignited their passion for copper's energy into a spiritual evolution. As with most of their beliefs, Spiritualists have taken the true scientific property of a mineral and made it fit their own structure. Because copper conducts electricity and heat, copper is also the conduit of the Spiritualist's belief system.

According to their myths, copper holds the ability to steer spiritual energy back and forth from individuals, crystals, auras, the mind and the spirit world. They also believe in the power of copper to amplify thoughts, to receive and send psychic communication and they use this energy to channel hoaxes throughout the world.

New Age followers carry these metals with their stones and crystals to "straighten" the properties when creating crystal wands to connect with spirits, and for channeling spirits and increasing cosmic awareness. Thus today's Spiritualists find copper to play an essential role in their physical and mental healing rites.

The copper elixir that has ignited our past, will continue to burn far into the future as scientists, Spiritualists, and lovers seek to live a blissful future filled with health, beauty and inner fulfillment.

20

THE MORAL NEED FOR BEAUTY
"MY SKIN IS MY HOBBY" — WHY WE OBSESS OVER SKINCARE

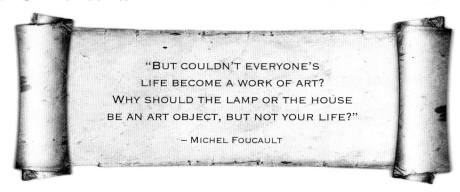

> "BUT COULDN'T EVERYONE'S
> LIFE BECOME A WORK OF ART?
> WHY SHOULD THE LAMP OR THE HOUSE
> BE AN ART OBJECT, BUT NOT YOUR LIFE?"
>
> — MICHEL FOUCAULT

Do you delight in your quest for beauty or do you feel vain? I once knew a woman who lamented with me in jest. As she applied shiny lacquer to plump her lips, she laughed: "I'm vain. I sit here at my vanity table full of vanity items and primp myself in vain." And indeed her vanity table was adorned with exotic bottles of colorful lotions and cosmetic potions (many of which were useless concoctions as we've discussed earlier). However, I assured her that her quest for beautiful skin and hair was not only natural, it was a moral need she inherited from women throughout the ages. It was in her genes. And like many people, she was a bit embarrassed about the price tag of her costly cosmetics. Maybe this was what Shakespeare meant by "unthrifty loveliness" in Sonnet 4. "I feel shallow," she added. However that didn't stop her from applying a lavish coat of mascara. I reassured her that there was nothing shallow about the quest for beauty.

Women decorate their homes and receive praise yet they feel uncomfortable, even a bit embarrassed, about the many hours they spend primping and pruning to look their best. The pursuit of beauty is nothing to be ashamed of. After all, glowing skin and shiny hair have always been linked with good health. So in a sense, the quest for beauty is really the quest for health in all its wonderful aspects.

Good health aside, who can deny the pleasure we receive as we gaze upon men and women who put themselves together well? It's not about looking like a super duper supermodel, but rather about taking the time to enhance your own unique assets, to look and feel your very best. It may take a little time, but aren't you worth it?

COSMETICS, JEWELRY, TECHNOLOGY, ART, AND SYMBOLISM

IT JUST MIGHT BE IN MY GENES!

So OK, maybe your vanity table brims over with a plethora of lipsticks, mascara, blushers, foundation, nail polish, dream creams, perfume, and oh so many products. Dare I say more? It can be a challenge just to sort through this colorful stock pile let alone actually make yourself up. But don't let that turn into unease about your personal vanity. There are those in our society who equate the obsession with self-beauty as some type of moral defect or evil. To deeply care about the beauty of the human body is an essential part of a tight matrix of behaviors that create the best in human nature. The most valued possessions of early humans were cosmetic body paints such as red ochre (a form of iron ore), jewelry such as necklaces made from small seashells or fox teeth, a technology that created finely crafted tools such as arrowheads, spear points, implements for food preparation and sewing, symbolic figurative art objects and geometric forms.

The behavior that creates these objects rises from the deepest recesses of the human psyche. We cannot function properly without them. Red lipstick and computer microprocessors arise from the same deep human drives and needs.

The human body, itself, has been a vessel for artistic expression for hundreds of thousands of years. In all civilizations where art, science, and culture have flourished, women and men found ways to embellish their beauty. And like literature, which reveals inner truth through poetic metaphor, outer beauty can reflect the beauty within. It's our moral right and need to look and feel our best.

It's In Your Genes

Mutual grooming, rubbing, and caressing of skin thrives amongst all social beings. Some birds and primates spend up to 90 percent of their time grooming themselves or others. We humans also love the rub—that special sprucing touch. We share an innate drive for beauty buried deep in our genes. When a masseuse melts your stress away, when you receive an amazing manicure,

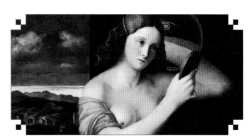

All early human cultures were obsessed with personal beauty.

spend a day adding waves to your hair, pamper yourself with beauty and pleasure, your body increases its level of "happiness hormones." These endorphins enhance your sense of well being. To skyrocket this happiness several notches higher, have someone else groom you. Being pampered by another heightens the pleasure by increasing endorphins even further.

All early human cultures were obsessed with personal beauty. Many presented their bodies as a colorful palette. They painted their skin, pierced various body parts and inserted bones, feathers and shells in the punctured skin. Young and old alike decorated their bodies. Ninety-nine percent of our ancestors lived in small nomadic bands of hunters and gatherers, and our psychological drives still reflect this. In ancient times, physical attributes and body decor attracted partners, contributing to reproduction of our species. Our ancestors were drawn to smooth skin, lush shiny hair and bodies often adorned with body art. These qualities continue to appeal today and guarantee the future of our species.

BODY PAINTING: THE FIRST MAKE-UP

The first make-up, body painting, depicts a fundamental behavior driven by the deep desire for luxury and beauty. Body art is not just the latest fashion. In fact, if the impulse to create art is one of the defining signs of humanity, the body, may well have been the first canvas. Cultures collected red ochre dating back at least 285,000 years. In Africa, people have worn necklaces and painted their bodies for more than 75,000 years. Skeletons sprinkled with red ochre and found in graves, date as far back as the Paleolithic Period, when ice sheets covered Northern Europe and hunters and gatherers roamed the landscape. This ancient burial ritual suggests that body painting already had a long-established practice among the living. Minerals from the earth, chiefly ochre in shades ranging from red to yellow and pyrolosite (manganese) in shades of black and white, were used as pigments. The following examples illustrate the use of body painting recorded throughout the world:

• Archaeological findings suggest Japanese inhabitants were already decorating their bodies in the Neolithic Jomon period (c.10,000-300 B.C.).

• In Egypt, during the time of the pharaohs, upper-class women used face powders and other make-up, perfume, paintbrushes, and polished silver or copper mirrors.

• For thousands of years, Masai warriors applied body decoration and art to express their cultural characteristics.

• In Papua, New Guinea, traditional ceremonial face paint consists of black powdered charcoal. The Huli Wigmen, who live in vibrant valleys, accentuate the nose and mouth with bright colors and apply white clay to emphasize the eye and beard.

• In ancient Athens, noblewomen and courtesans applied white lead carbonate hydroxide foundation with brushes. The Roman poet Ovid wrote that the naked breasts of the Greek women were "rosy buds enhanced with a tincture of gold."

• The ancient Celts wore blue body paint from "woad," a type of mustard plant.

• The American Indian name "Red-Skin" originated from body painting, especially among the prairie Indians.

• In India, extracts of henna plant have been used for centuries as a reddish-yellow hair dye and to decorate the hands and feet.

• In China, during the Chou dynasty of 600 B.C., members of the emperor's family wore gold and silver nail polish. Later, these colors changed to red and black. Well-manicured nails represented the difference between the aristocrats and the working classes.

• In an ancient Peruvian grave, a mummified woman was found perfectly preserved with her light brown hair carefully combed and braided. Her legs, from knee to ankle, were painted red as was the fashion for beauties of Peru in her time. Buried along with her was her "toilet powder" (a fine powder, perhaps scented, for spreading on the body after bathing) for use in the afterlife.

THE ANCIENT ART OF TATTOO The legacy of the tattoo originated over 2000 years ago beginning in Polynesian cultures and spreading throughout the world. The word tattoo stems from the Tahitian word "tatau," meaning to inflict wounds. In the centuries before modern-day tattoo needles, the tattooing process required enduring considerable pain and sometimes took several years to complete. The risk of death by infection loomed as a great concern. Yet, devotees paid this painfully high price for beauty and acceptance. Tribal tattoos marked rites of passage such as puberty, marriage, or a first successful hunt. In Polynesia, tattoo patterns symbolized prosperity and conferred prestige. The following illustrates additional examples of the art of tattoo throughout history:

- In 1000 B.C., Egyptian and Nubian dancers were tattooed on the thigh and pubic areas.

- Japanese aristocrats distinguished themselves with tiny tattoos near the eye. Japanese tattooists followed the lines of the muscle movements, so that when the person moved the pictures would "come alive."

- In 450 A.D., Roman soldiers gave the name "Picts" to Gallic warriors who went to battle naked in order to display their fearsome tattoos.

- The Maoris of New Zealand reserved tattoos for both nobles and free people.

QUOTABLE QUOTES: *Not one great country can be named, from the polar regions in the north to New Zealand in the south, in which the aboriginals do not tattoo themselves. —Charles Darwin, Voyage of the Beagle*

The First Beauty Parlors

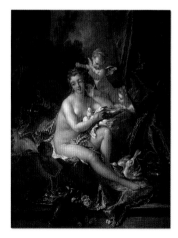

Paleolithic statues show elaborate hair styling and braiding dating back more than 30,000 years. Early cultures worldwide used elaborate top-knots, braids, and other forms of hair styling to attract others. Roman women washed their hair with bleach made from dried nuts and acid, hoping to turn it yellow. When the Roman senate ruled that women with blond hair were to be considered prostitutes, this only increased the popularity of blond hair. In the 1700's, French hairstyles often topped four feet, and the women used wool, paste, glue, and wires to hold their hair in place.

THE POWER OF HUMAN BEAUTY Of all the forms of beauty, it is the allure of the human form that most excites us. The human figure has always been a common object of visual art and chemical attraction. The earliest known depictions of the human body originate from Europe and date between 25,000 and 12,000 years ago. Carved from stone and ivory, these 'Venus' figures represent the female form and may have been associated with fertility. Attraction and fertility are interrelated and fill us with pleasure. When our eyes gaze upon an exceptionally beautiful person, our thought process alters, our breathing changes, our hormones surge, and our brain releases endorphins that fill our body with a sense of bliss. Beauty may even have a positive impact on our health; one Danish/German study found that men who had survived one heart attack, after daily viewing of pictures with nude women, had a 50 percent reduction in new heart attacks.

Studies show that more attractive people are judged by others to have good personalities, be kinder and warmer, have happier marriages, have a more positive outlook on life, be more likely to live longer than average, and be more satisfied with their lives.

QUOTABLE QUOTES: *For the women of my court, hairstyle remains the most important thing, the subject is inexhaustible.*
—Louis XIV

Beyond the way others perceive you, can sprucing up your appearance really make a difference in your life? The answer is yes. The more attractive you look, the more attention you will attract from others—and this in turn builds your sense of self-confidence. The attention you receive in the form of admiring glances and prolonged conversations might even have a positive impact on your health. Researchers have found that when babies are massaged, they gain weight as much as 50 percent faster than un-massaged infants, leading one to conclude that adults also physically thrive from positive attention.

Beauty and Progressive Cultures

Creative ideas and a love of physical beauty are two sides of the same coin. Historically, the areas of the world where the public has been the most attracted to the concept of physical beauty, are the areas where culture, art, science, and basic human freedoms have thrived. Conversely, the areas where physical beauty has been frowned upon or suppressed are the areas where freedom of thought, belief, and other personal liberties have been stifled.

In a sense, an obsession with personal beauty helps ignite the events that raise a society's standard of living, cure disease, and promote freedom. The statues of Athens helped create the logic of Socrates, Plato, and Aristotle. Renaissance Florence found the blend of beauty, art, science, religion, and economic activity that is still our best social model for building a successful and uplifting society.

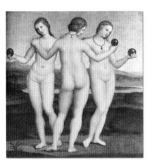

There even appears to be a connection between the number of nude statues and paintings in an area and its economic progress. For example, the most economically vibrant region of the United States is the very tolerant and self-absorbed San Francisco Bay Area. In 2002, the per-capita income of the Bay Area was $67,000. In comparison, the second most prosperous area was Boston at $51,000. The free-living and life-loving culture of the Bay Area attracts and energizes the creative types of people who build a prosperous culture.

QUOTABLE QUOTES: *Fair tresses man's imperial race insnare, and Beauty draws us with a single hair.*
—Alexander Pope

Many of our clients, who love to primp and preen, dress to impress and beguile us with their glowing skin, are highly intelligent, cultured, creative and prosperous. They epitomize the synergy, a special dance that unites their quest for beauty and art, that swirls us around the dance floor of life unfolding nuances of our human nature.

So the next time you reach into that jam-packed drawer of cosmetics, creams, and other concoctions, remember that you are carrying on a tradition that has been passed down through at least 75,000 years and probably much longer: The Universal Quest for Beauty in all its wonderful forms. At the same time, you are also maintaining innate human drives that produce art, science, prosperity, happiness, freedom, and civilized behavior. In revealing how the science of SRCPs is helping men and women turn back the clock, it is my hope that this book will help you reach your personal beauty goals as well.

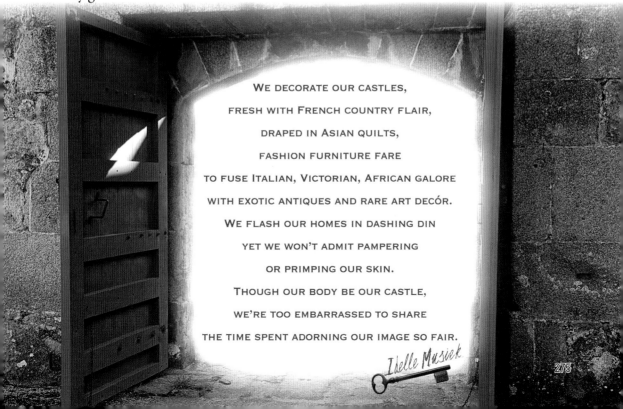

WE DECORATE OUR CASTLES,

FRESH WITH FRENCH COUNTRY FLAIR,

DRAPED IN ASIAN QUILTS,

FASHION FURNITURE FARE

TO FUSE ITALIAN, VICTORIAN, AFRICAN GALORE

WITH EXOTIC ANTIQUES AND RARE ART DECÓR.

WE FLASH OUR HOMES IN DASHING DIN

YET WE WON'T ADMIT PAMPERING

OR PRIMPING OUR SKIN.

THOUGH OUR BODY BE OUR CASTLE,

WE'RE TOO EMBARRASSED TO SHARE

THE TIME SPENT ADORNING OUR IMAGE SO FAIR.

Idelle Musiek

Skin Biology clients often reflect that extraordinary blend of personal beauty and cultural progress. As one of our clients so aptly stated: "My skin is my hobby". Here are a few other comments from clients on how beauty has affected their lives:

My skin is my hobby. My high point of the month is when Vogue Magazine comes out. I love looking at cosmetics in Bloomingdales. I enjoy going to art shows. I study quantum mechanics for entertainment. Every week I meet with my financial adviser." – RG, New York

I am definitely what you would call a beauty 'addict'. I could open a drugstore with all the products I have purchased in the past few years. I also spend a good amount of time in front of a mirror, attempting to fit in all of my exfoliation, moisturizing, buffing, rebuilding, repairing, enhancing etc, etc... The irony of the situation is that my purpose for doing all these things is to eventually <u>decrease</u> the amount of time I have to do them...However, I do seem to find comfort in my beauty rituals, particularly if I see improvement over time. It makes the investment seem worth all the time, money and energy spent." – WN, Wisconsin

I feel totally consumed and obsessed with achieving the most beautiful and flawless skin I know that I have underneath the blemishes and scars. And as long as those imperfections persist, I will never stop the journey – no matter how rocky and tiresome it may become– to skin perfection....I enjoy skin care products, because these products make me feel that I am 'not letting my beauty fade without a fight'...Having clear, beautiful, and flawless skin will allow me to reach my highest potential." – RO, Florida

I love to get a group of us girlfriends together and dedicate the whole day to getting our nails done, or hair done, or a pedicure. Some type of bonding occurs between us and it is unforgettable...There's even something relaxing and enjoyable about doing my own nails. I find myself making designs and playing around with colors all the time." – CM, Washington

Beauty is related to life.

Its opposite, is related to death.
Beauty is like a reflection of light, of sun,
of spring, of happiness, of strength and health.
The Beauty I'm thinking about, is not connected with
an idea of perfection: it's an idea of harmony, of peace.
And, for instance, beautiful and good
skin reflects light." – AM, Italy

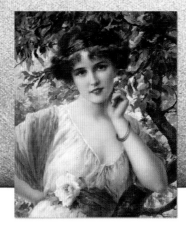

21

RESOURCES

SKIN BIOLOGY PRODUCT GUIDE AND GLOSSARY

Find products at www.skinbiology.com or 1-800-405-1912
Skin Biology – 4122 Factoria Boulevard, Suite #200 • Bellevue, WA 98006 USA

Facial Products

• Protect & Restore Classic Cream
The SRCP complexes contained in this light cream help the skin to regenerate, improving skin firmness and elasticity while helping to increase the skin's natural defense mechanism against oxidative damage.

• Protect & Restore Cream with High Retinol and Oil of Lavender
Helps increase the skin's natural defense mechanism against oxidative damage. Features lipid replenisher retinyl-palmitate which acts as an added moisturizer for very dry skin.

• Protect & Restore Day Cover (with Pure Titanium Dioxide)
Anti-aging copper peptide cream containing pure and safe titanium dioxide that helps reflect UV rays along with high levels of natural absorbers such as squalane and allantoin.

• Regular CP Serum
Light copper peptide serum formula. CP Serum is a skin care serum with SRCPs that helps skin renewal while giving a healthy glow.

• Super CP Serum
Strong copper peptide serum. Best for overall treatment of scars, blemishes, deep wrinkles, and hypo/hyperpigmentation.

• TriReduction Protect & Restore
Specifically designed for clearing blemishes, spots, skin tags, and post-acne scars. This product contains retinyl palmitate added for extra moisturization of dry areas.

• Regular Super Cop Cream
A strong enhancement of our other SRCP serums and creams, still producing the same skin remodeling effects but combines the amazing properties of milder products with the power of a stronger concentration of copper peptide plus hydroxy acid.

• Super Cop Cream 2X - Extra Strength
Strongest copper peptide strength available for skin renewal and damage repair.

• Super GHK-Copper Cream and Serum

Gentle GHK-Copper increases skin elasticity, thickens older skin, improves skin firmness, tightens protective skin barrier proteins, reduces fine lines and wrinkles, while improving skin clarity, "glow" and overall appearance.

• Skin Signals Solution

Triggers two-fold regeneration with a strong copper peptide formula combined with peptides from enzymatically hydrolyzed elastin and collagen to tighten and firm.

• Skin Signals Cream

Technology of both GHK-Copper plus copper peptides produced from hydrolyzed elastin and collagen peptides to help increase new collagen naturally and improve elasticity.

• Sebum Be Gone

A light serum designed to reduce sheen for combination-to-oily skin types. Helps block production of excessive oil.

Specifically for Around the Eye Area

• CP Night Eyes (Premier and Regular)

Specifically developed for the sensitive around-the-eye area to help create a smoother, more elastic, radiant look by helping remove under-eye circles and wrinkles.

Specifically for Hands, Nails & Feet

• TINPEP Hand Cream

Rejuvenate dry hands with the power of tin peptides. Designed to soothe diabetic skin issues and serves as the perfect remedy for chronic dryness.

• Tin Peptide Nail Renewal

Help fingers feel smooth as your nails grow stronger and faster with this tin peptide nail renewal and repair cream.

• Les Pieds Doux Foot Cream

French for "Soft Feet", this luxuriant cream helps regenerate and repair dry, cracked feet with the power of copper peptides.

Hydroxy Acid Exfoliators .... *For stronger acids see: ReverseSkinAging.com/resellers.html*

• Exfol Cream / Exfol Serum

Contains 2% Salicylic Acid to help exfoliate or remove damaged skin proteins and dead skin cells.

• LacSal Cream / LacSal Serum

Mix of Lactic (8.5%) and Salicylic Acid (1.5%) for a total of 10% leave-on hydroxy acid.

• Lactic Power 10

Pure 10% Lactic Acid with added moisturizing ingredients and anti-oxidants to leave the skin smooth, beautiful, and clear.

Beneficial for Tightening Skin

• Two Timing Tightener (DMAE Serum with Pepha-Tight®)
Contains DMAE, a membrane stabilizer that helps give a lift to sagging skin especially around the eye area and neck. Clinical studies show DMAE delves below the skin's surface to prevent facial sagging and helps with collagen synthesis.

SRCP Products for Body Use

• Protect & Restore Body Lotion
Copper peptide body lotion for skin renewal. Aids in the tightening and rejuvenation of body skin.

• Protect & Restore for Breasts, Nipples, and Décolletage
Skin repair cream fortified with protective lipids, retinol and lavender. Helps tighten and improve skin appearance.

• TriReduction Protect & Restore
Specifically designed for clearing blemishes, spots, skin tags, and post-acne scars. This product contains retinyl palmitate added for extra moisturization of dry areas.

Products for At-Risk Skin

• BioHeal
Contains the exceptionally safe skin repair properties of Skin Remodeling Copper Peptides with added camphor and menthol.

• Dr. Pickart's Diabetic Skin Therapy Cream
Gentle and soothing copper peptide cream designed specifically for the treatment of diabetic skin issues.

• Dr. Pickart's Face and Body Cleanser
Originally designed for very sensitive or fragile skin, this cleanser can be used by all skin types. Unlike other soaps, this gentle formula has a pH near neutrality, contains no caustics or free fatty acids, and no chemical foaming agents.

Biological Healing Oils / Moisturizers

• Emu Oil-S Lipid Replenisher for Skin
Biochemically comparable to human skin oil, emu oil has been used for centuries for a variety of skin concerns. Our version is supplemented with anti-oxidants such as lutein, lycopene, tocotrienols and tocopherols to help reduce inflammation.

• Squalane
Squalane from olive oil is a stable moisturizer preferred for skin use. When rubbed on skin, it works to improve skin protection and moisturization. Squalane is absorbed deeply and quickly into the skin and does not leave an oily film.

• Retinol in Squalane
An intensive moisturizer for very dry skin areas. The squalane acts as a penetrating agent to help retinol uptake, while retinyl palmitate is a combination of retinol (pure vitamin A) and palmitic acid to aid skin repair.

• CELES Therapeutic Oil
Specialized mix of Cholesterol Esters, Lanosterol Esters and Squalane designed for the moisturization of extreme dry skin.

• Calypso's Oil
A light, soothing body oil that aids skin moisturizing and healing. Light oils are one of the best protections against dry skin and for promoting skin health in general. Available with essential oils of lavender, jasmine, ylang ylang, nutmeg, asian oud, sandalwood, and patchouli added.

Body Perfumes with Plant Pheromones

- **Body Perfume**
Sensual pheromone fragrance more concentrated than Calypso's Oil. Available with essential oils of lavender, jasmine, ylang ylang, nutmeg, asian oud, sandalwood, patchouli or pheromone only added. Alcohol-free fragrant oil.

Also ask about *Romantic Perfume Oils for Women & Men* and the new *4Sensuous Scents Oil*.

SRCP Products for Post Sun Exposure Skin Care

- **Copper Sun Tanning & Firming Body Lotion**
Tighten skin while helping detoxify oxygen radicals produced by UV rays on the skin's surface with anti-oxidants, UV reflector (pure titanium dioxide), moisturizing agents, and copper peptides.

- **Protect & Restore Body Lotion for Post Tanning Skin Care**
Copper peptide body lotion for skin renewal. Aids in the tightening and rejuvenation of body skin.

SRCP Products for Hair Growth and Condition

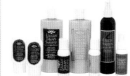

- **Folligen Cream, Lotion, and Spray, Folligen Shampoo / Conditioner**
Copper peptide scalp treatment that helps improve scalp and follicle health and hair vitality.

- **Hair Signals Therapy Solution and Cream**
A synergetic formula using the regenerative power of SRCPs plus Tea Extracts, Saw Palmetto Oil, Pygeum Africanum, and Lavender Oil all of which are effective inhibitors of DHT.

- **Emu Oil-S Lipid Replenisher for Hair**
A biological healing oil supplemented with anti-oxidants (such as CoQ-10, tocotrienols, tocopherols, lutein and lycopene) to help reduce inflammation. Also contains 1% saw palmetto oil (lipidic sterolic extract) to inhibit the formation of DHT.

Skin Cleansers

- **Dr. Pickart's Face and Body Cleanser (Bar and Liquid)**
Originally designed for very sensitive or fragile skin, this cleanser can be used by all skin types. Unlike other soaps, this gentle formula has a pH near neutrality, contains no caustics or free fatty acids, and no chemical foaming agents.

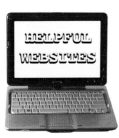

HELPFUL WEBSITES

- www.acne.org
- www.worldhealth.net (American Academy of Anti-Aging Medicine)
- http://dermatology.cdlib.org

Glossary of Terms:

Acne	Acne results due to a disruption in dead skin cell exfoliation in the opening of the oil gland.
Alpha Lipoic Acid	The most important single antioxidant. The best method to raise cellular glutathione which is considered to be the master antioxidant in the body.
Camphor	Produces a cooling effect similar to menthol leaves. Camphor is used in conjunction with menthol as an anti-inflammatory.
Citric Acid	Citric acid is used to adjust the acidity of products. Derived from citrus fruits.
Collagen	Collagen forms the structural network of our skin and is the most abundant protein in the body. As we age, collagen begins to deteriorate and causes the skin to become thinner and eventually sag.
Dermis	The dermis is a thick, supple and sturdy layer of connective tissue (a dense meshwork of collagen and elastin fibers) that makes up about 90 percent of the skin's thickness.
DHT	DHT (dihydrotestosterone) is considered a key contributing factor to the onset and progression of androgenic alopecia and benign prostatic hyperplasia.
DMAE	Dimethylaminoethanol, is an organic compound with strong anti-inflammatory and aging reversal properties. It is a precursor to the chemical that stimulates nerve function and stimulates the muscles to contract and tighten under the skin.
Eczema	Eczema is often associated with dry skin which is also called xerosis, or xerotic eczema (xeros is Greek for "dry").
Elastin	Elastin is a stretchable protein that maintains the skin's elasticity and provides the matrix that holds individual skin cells in place.
Emu Oil	Traditionally used to help alleviate discomfort of arthritis, shingles, eczema, psoriasis and other inflammatory conditions. The fatty acid composition of human skin oil and emu oil are very similar.
Epidermis	The epidermis ("overskin") or top layer of the skin. The epidermis is the thinnest skin layer at a maximum 1 millimeter or as thin as a pencil line.
Free Radicals	Free radicals cause much of the tissue damage responsible for degenerative diseases. The absorption or detoxifying of free radicals would protect our bodies from many of those diseases.
GHK-Cu	GHK-Cu (glycyl-l-histidyl-l-lysine:copper(II)) is a Skin Remodeling Copper-Peptide. The tripeptide, GHK, discovered by Dr. Pickart, is generated by proteolysis after tissue injury. Its high affinity for copper(II) allows it to obtain copper from carrier molecules such as albumin and form GHK-Cu.
Hydrolyzed Soy Protein	Hydrolyzed soy protein (glycine soja) derived from soybeans and broken down by water to form a complex with copper to produce copper peptides.
Lactic Acid	Lactic acid is an alpha hydroxy acid extracted from milk.
Leucine	An essential amino acid. Leucine is used by the body to repair bone, skin and muscle tissue.
Lipids	Lipids and fats in the skin provide the epidermal barrier to transcutaneous (through the skin) water loss.
Lutein	Lutein (from Latin lutea meaning "yellow") is one of over 600 known naturally occurring carotenoids. It is employed by organisms as an antioxidant and for blue light absorption.
Lycopene	Lycopene (solanum lycopersicum) is a tomato extract high in beta carotene, a natural source of vitamin A, which protects and strengthens the skin.
Olive Oil	Olive oil works as an emollient in our skin creams. It is an antioxidant and improves skin moisture. May also protect against UVB damage.
Psoriasis	A chronic skin disease, characterized by itching, scaling and inflammation. Psoriasis develops red patches of thick lesions covered with silvery scales.
Retinoic Acid	The acidic version of vitamin A or retinol. It reduces skin oil by shrinking sebaceous glands and unclogging hair follicles.
Retinyl Palmitate	A combination of retinol (pure vitamin A) and palmitic acid.
Rosacea	Classic rosacea manifests many tiny, visible red blood vessels in the central part of the face. Starts as a tendency to blush easily.
Salicylic Acid	First obtained from the bark of the willow tree, Salix. It is a beta hydroxy acid exfoliator and one of the best known skin renewal methods. Unlike alpha hydroxy acids, it can penetrate into the skin's pores to remove blemishes and reduce acne.
Saw Palmetto	A popular herbal remedy for a type of hair loss and baldness called androgenic alopecia, or male- and female-pattern baldness.
Sebaceous Glands	Clusters of cells that produce an oil called sebum. Two or more sebaceous glands secrete sebum via minuscule tubes in the hair follicle. Sebum helps waterproof the skin and hair.
Squalane	A natural biological oil obtained from olive oil.
SRCPs	Skin Remodeling Copper Peptides that repair and remodel skin. Its actions focus on being able to generate skin remodeling, the skin's renewal process that return it to a younger, healthier state.
Titanium Dioxide	Mineral used as a sunscreen ingredient in cosmetics. Protects skin from UVA and UVB radiation and is considered to have no risk of skin irritation.
Tocopherols	Tocopherols, tocotrienols and tocophersolan are different members of the vitamin E family. Both tocopherols and tocotrienols are fat-soluble antioxidants and have been exhaustively studied.
Ubiquinone (CoQ-10)	Coenzyme Q-10 (Ubiquinone, CoQ10) is a natural part of the body's cell protection function and energy synthesis. Studies have confirmed CoQ10 to be a powerful antioxidant for the skin and effective in reducing wrinkles.

REFERENCES
Scientific Sources for Chapter Information

Abdulghani, AA, A Sherr, S Shirin, G Solodkina, EM Tapia, B Wolf, and AB Gottlieb. "Effects of topical creams containing vitamin C, a copper-binding peptide cream and melatonin compared with tretinoin on the ultrastructure of normal skin - a pilot clinical, histologic, and ultrastructural study " Dis Manag Clin Outcome 1, no. 4 (1998): 136-41.

Adam, M, H Pohunkova, O Cech, and J Vachal. A. "[The effect of collagenous gel on endoprosthesis anchoring]." Acta Chir Orthop Traumatol Cech 62, no. 6 (1995): 336-42.

Adam, M, O Cech, H Pohunkova, J Stehlik, and Z Klezl. B. "[The role of collagen implants containing the tripeptide gly-his-lys in bone healing process]." Acta Chir Orthop Traumatol Cech 62, no. 2 (1995): 76-85.

Adam, M, H Pohunkova, Z Klezl, V Pesakova, and O Cech. "[Use of bioimplants to replace cartilage part II: Application of implants in animal experiments.]." Acta Chir Orthop Traumatol Cech 64, no. 4 (1997): 207-11.

Ahmed, MR, SH Basha, D Gopinath, R Muthusamy, and R Jayakumar. "Initial upregulation of growth factors and inflammatory mediators during nerve regeneration in the presence of cell adhesive peptide-incorporated collagen tubes." J Peripher Nerv Syst 10, no. 1 (2005): 17-30.

Ainsleigh, HG. "Beneficial effects of sun exposure on cancer mortality." Prev Med 22, no. 1 (1993): 132-40.

Alberghina, M, G Lupo, G La Spina, A Mangiameli, M Gulisano, D Sciotto, and E Rizzarelli. "Cytoprotective effect of copper(II) complexes against ethanol-induced damage to rat gastric mucosa." J Inorg Biochem 45, no. 4 (1992): 245-59.

Alzuet, G, S Ferrer, J Borras, and JR Sorenson. "Anticonvulsant properties of copper acetazolamide complexes." J Inorg Biochem 55, no. 2 (1994): 147-51.

Ambesi-Impiombato, FS, LA Parks, and HG Coon. "Culture of hormone-dependent functional epithelial cells from rat thyroids." Proc Natl Acad Sci U S A 77, no. 6 (1980): 3455-59.

Appa, Y, T Stephens, S Barkovic, and MB Finkley. "A clinical evaluation of a copper-peptide containing liquid foundation and cream concealer designed for improving skin condition." Presented at the 60th Annual American Academy of Dermatology Meeting, New Orleans, LA, 2002.

Araya, M, MC McGoldrick, LM Klevay, JJ Strain, P Robson, F Nielsen, M Olivares, F Pizarro, LA Johnson, and KA Poirier. "Determination of an acute no-observed-adverse-effect level (noael) for copper in water." Regul Toxicol Pharmacol 34, no. 2 (2001): 137-45.

Arul, V, D Gopinath, K Gomathi, and R Jayakumar. "Biotinylated GHK peptide incorporated collagenous matrix: A novel biomaterial for dermal wound healing in rats." J Biomed Mater Res B Appl Biomater 73, no. 2 (2005): 383-91.

Arul, V, R Kartha, and R Jayakumar. "A therapeutic approach for diabetic wound healing using biotinylated GHK incorporated collagen matrices." Life Sci 80, no. 4 (2007): 275-84.

Aupaix, F, FX Maquart, L Salagnac, L Pickart, P Gillery, JP Borel, and B Kalis. "Effects of the tripeptide glycyl-histidyl-lysine on healing. Clinical and biochemical correlations." J Invest Dermatol 94 (1990): 390 (abst).

Autier, P, JF Doré, AM Eggermont, and JW Coebergh. "Epidemiological evidence that UVA radiation is involved in the genesis of cutaneous melanoma." Curr Opin Oncol 23, no. 2 (2011): 189-96.

Awa, T, K Nogimori, and RE Trachy. "Hairloss protection by peptide-copper complex in animal models of chemotherapy-induced alopecia." Journal of Dermatological Science 10, no. 1 (1995): 99.

Babu, U, and ML Failla. "Copper status and function of neutrophils are reversibly depressed in marginally and severely copper-deficient rats." J Nutr 120, no. 12 (1990): 1700-9.

Baker, A, L Harvey, G Majask-Newman, S Fairweather-Tait, A Flynn, and K Cashman. "Effect of dietary copper intakes on biochemical markers of bone metabolism in healthy adult males." Eur J Clin Nutr 53, no. 5 (1999): 408-12.

Bala, S, and ML Failla. "Copper deficiency reversibly impairs DNA synthesis in activated T lymphocytes by limiting interleukin 2 activity." Proc Natl Acad Sci U S A 89, no. 15 (1992): 6794-7.

Beaudry, VG, and LD Attardi. "SKP-ing TAp63: Stem cell depletion, senescence, and premature aging." Cell Stem Cell 5, no. 1 (2009): 1-2.

Beresford, SA, KC Johnson, C Ritenbaugh, NL Lasser, LG Snetselaar, HR Black, GL Anderson, AR Assaf, T Bassford, D Bowen, RL Brunner, RG Brzyski, B Caan, RT Chlebowski, M Gass, RC Harrigan, J Hays, D Heber, G Heiss, SL Hendrix, BV Howard, J Hsia, FA Hubbell, RD Jackson, JM Kotchen, LH Kuller, AZ LaCroix, DS Lane, RD Langer, CE Lewis, JE Manson, KL Margolis, Y Mossavar-Rahmani, JK Ockene, LM Parker, MG Perri, L Phillips, RL Prentice, J Robbins, JE Rossouw, GE Sarto, ML Stefanick, L Van Horn, MZ Vitolins, J Wactawski-Wende, RB Wallace, and E Whitlock. "Low-fat dietary pattern and risk of colorectal cancer: The women's health initiative randomized controlled dietary modification trial." JAMA 295, no. 6 (2006): 643-54.

Beretta, G, R Artali, L Regazzoni, M Panigati, and RM Facino. "Glycyl-histidyl-lysine (GHK) is a quencher of alpha,beta-4-hydroxy-trans-2-nonenal: A comparison with carnosine. Insights into the mechanism of reaction by electrospray ionization mass spectrometry, 1h nmr, and computational techniques." Chem Res Toxicol 20, no. 9 (2007): 1309-14.

Beretta, G, E Arlandini, R Artali, JM Anton, and R Maffei Facino. "Acrolein sequestering ability of the endogenous tripeptide glycyl-histidyl-lysine (GHK): Characterization of conjugation products by ESI-MSn and theoretical calculations." J Pharm Biomed Anal 47, no. 3 (2008): 596-602.

Berwick, M. "Counterpoint: Sunscreen use is a safe and effective approach to skin cancer prevention." Cancer Epidemiol Biomarkers Prev 16, no. 10 (2007): 1923-4.

———. "The good, the bad, and the ugly of sunscreens." Clin Pharmacol Ther 89, no. 1 (2011): 31-3.

Bhathena, SJ, L Recant, NR Voyles, KI Timmers, S Reiser, JC Jr Smith, and AS Powell. "Decreased plasma enkephalins in copper deficiency in man." Am J Clin Nutr 43, no. 1 (1986): 42-6.

Boal, AK, and AC Rosenzweig. "Structural biology of copper trafficking." Chem Rev 109, no. 10 (2009): 4760-79.

Bonham, M, JM O'Connor, BM Hannigan, and JJ Strain. "The immune system as a physiological indicator of marginal copper status?" Br J Nutr 87, no. 5 (2002): 393-403.

Britton, A, A Singh-Manoux, and M Marmot. "Alcohol consumption and cognitive function in the Whitehall II study." Am J Epidemiol 160, no. 3 (2004): 240-7.

Bruce, B, GA Spiller, LM Klevay, and SK Gallagher. "A diet high in whole and unrefined foods favorably alters lipids, antioxidant defenses, and colon function." J Am Coll Nutr 19, no. 1 (2000): 61-7.

Cabrera, A, E Alonzo, E Sauble, YL Chu, D Nguyen, MC Linder, DS Sato, and AZ Mason. "Copper binding components of blood plasma and organs, and their responses to influx of large doses of (65)Cu, in the mouse." Biometals 21, no. 5 (2008): 525-43.

Camakaris, J, I Voskoboinik, and JF Mercer. "Molecular mechanisms of copper homeostasis." Biochem Biophys Res Commun 261, no. 2 (1999): 225-32.

Canapp, SO Jr, JP Farese, GS Schultz, S Gowda, AM Ishak, SF Swaim, J Vangilder, L Lee-Ambrose, and FG Martin. "The effect of topical tripeptide-copper complex on healing of ischemic open wounds." Vet Surg 32, no. 6 (2003): 515-23.

Cangul, IT, NY Gul, A Topal, and R Yilmaz. "Evaluation of the effects of topical tripeptide-copper complex and zinc oxide on open-wound healing in rabbits." Vet Dermatol 17, no. 6 (2006): 417-23.

Cartwright, GE, and MM Wintrobe. "The question of copper deficiency in man." Am J Clin Nutr 15 (1964): 94-110.

Cater, MA, KT McInnes, QX Li, I Volitakis, S La Fontaine, JF Mercer, and AI Bush. "Intracellular copper deficiency increases amyloid-beta secretion by diverse mechanisms." Biochem J 412, no. 1 (2008): 141-52.

Cebrian, J, A Messeguer, RM Facino, and JM Garcia Anton. "New anti-RNS and -ROS products for cosmetic treatment." Int J Cosmet Sci 27, no. 5 (2005): 271-8.

Chambers, A, D Krewski, N Birkett, L Plunkett, R Hertzberg, R Danzeisen, PJ Aggett, TB Starr, S Baker, M Dourson, P Jones, CL Keen, B Meek, R Schoeny, and W Slob. "An exposure-response curve for copper excess and deficiency." J Toxicol Environ Health B Crit Rev 13, no. 7-8 (2010): 546-78.

Chang-Claude, J, S Hermann, U Eilber, and K Steindorf. "Lifestyle determinants and mortality in german vegetarians and health-conscious persons: Results of a 21-year follow-up." Cancer Epidemiololgy, Biomarkers, & Prevention 14, no. 4 (2005): 963-68.

Choi, EH, BE Brown, D Crumrine, S Chang, MQ Man, PM Elias, and KR Feingold. "Mechanisms by which psychologic stress alters cutaneous permeability barrier homeostasis and stratum corneum integrity." J Invest Dermatol 124, no. 3 (2005): 587-95.

Coastal, D. "The runner." (1984): 41.

Conlan, D, R Korula, and D Tallentire. "Serum copper levels in elderly patients with femoral-neck fractures." Age Ageing 19, no. 3 (1990): 212-4.

Cornaro, L. Discorsi della vita sobria [Discourses on the sober life]1677.

Counts, D, E Hill, M Turner-Beatty, M Grotewiel, S Fosha-Thomas, and L Pickart. "Effect of lamin on full thickness wound healing." Fed Am Soc Exp Biol (1992): A1636.

Cutler, WB. Love cycles : The science of intimacy. 2 ed. New York: Athena Institute Press, 1996.

Davis, CD, and WT Johnson. "Dietary copper affects azoxymethane-induced intestinal tumor formation and protein kinase C isozyme protein and mRNA expression in colon of rats." J Nutr 132, no. 5 (2002): 1018-25.

De Spirt, S, W Stahl, H Tronnier, H Sies, M Bejot, JM Maurette, and U Heinrich. "Intervention with flaxseed and borage oil supplements modulates skin condition in women." Br J Nutr 101, no. 3 (2009): 440-5.

Dollwet, HH, and JR Sorenson. "Historic uses of copper compounds in medicine." Trace Elements in Medicine 2, no. 2 (1985): 80-87.

———. "Roles of copper in bone maintenance and healing." Biol Trace Elem Res 18 (1988): 39-48.

Downey, D, WF Larrabee, V Voci, and L Pickart. "Acceleration of wound healing using glycyl-histidyl-lysine copper (II)." Surg Forum 25 (1985): 573-75.

Drug and Cosmetic Industry. (1997).

Dwivedi, C, and Y Zhang. "Sandalwood oil prevent skin tumour development in CD1 mice." Eur J Cancer Prev 8, no. 5 (1999): 449-55.

Dwivedi, C, X Guan, WL Harmsen, AL Voss, DE Goetz-Parten, EM Koopman, KM Johnson, HB Valluri, and DP Matthees. "Chemopreventive effects of alpha-santalol on skin tumor development in CD-1 and sencar mice." Cancer Epidemiol Biomarkers Prev 12, no. 2 (2003): 151-6.

Ebbs, JH, FF Tisdall, and WA Scott. "The influence of prenatal diet on the mother and child." J Nutr 22, no. 5 (1941): 515-26.

Ehrlich, HP. "Stimulation of skin healing in immunosuppressed rats." Presented at the Symposium on collagen and skin repair Reims, France, Sept 12-13 1991.

Elias, PK, MF Elias, RB D'Agostino, H Silbershatz, and PA Wolf. "Alcohol consumption and cognitive performance in the Framingham heart study." Am J Epidemiol 150, no. 6 (1999): 580-9.

Ellis, JA, M Stebbing, and SB Harrap. "Genetic analysis of male pattern baldness and the 5alpha-reductase genes." J Invest Dermatol 110, no. 6 (1998): 849-53.

Elsherif, L, RV Ortines, JT Saari, and YJ Kang. "Congestive heart failure in copper-deficient mice." Exp Biol Med (Maywood) 228, no. 7 (2003): 811-7.

Ernst, B, M Thurnheer, and B Schultes. "Copper deficiency after gastric bypass surgery." Obesity (Silver Spring) 17, no. 11 (2009): 1980-1.

Fackelmann, K. "Melanoma madness: The scientific flap over sunscreens and skin cancer " Science News 153, no. 23 (1998): 360.

Farmer, KC, and MF Naylor. "Sun exposure, sunscreens, and skin cancer prevention: A year-round concern." Ann Pharmacother 30, no. 6 (1996): 662-73.

Finkley, MB, Y Appa, and S Bhandarkar. "Copper peptide and skin." In Cosmeceuticals and active cosmetics: Drugs vs. Cosmetics, edited by P Elsner and HI Maibach, 549-63. New York: Marcel Dekker, 2005.

Fouad, FM, M Abd-El-Fattah, R Scherer, and G Ruthenstroth-Bauer. "Effect of glucocorticoids, insulin and a growth promoting tripeptide on the biosynthesis of plasma proteins in serum-free hepatocyte cultures." Z Naturforsch C 36, no. 3-4 (1981): 350-52.

Frieden, E. "Perspectives on copper biochemistry." Clin Physiol Biochem 4, no. 1 (1986): 11-9.

Friedman, HS, and LR Martin. The longevity project: Surprising discoveries for health and long life from the landmark eight-decade study: Hudson Street Press, 2011.

Frost, PA, GB Hubbard, MJ Dammann, CL Snider, CM Moore, VL Hodara, LD Giavedoni, R Rohwer, MC Mahaney, TM Butler, LB Cummins, TJ McDonald, PW Nathanielsz, and NE Schlabritz-Loutsevitch. "White monkey syndrome in infant baboons (papio species)." J Med Primatol 33, no. 4 (2004): 197-213.

Gacheru, SN, PC Trackman, MA Shah, CY O'Gara, P Spacciapoli, FT Greenaway, and HM Kagan. "Structural and catalytic properties of copper in lysyl oxidase " J Biol Chem 265, no. 31 (1990): 19022-7.

Garcia-Sainz, JA, and JA Olivares-Reyes. "Glycyl-histidyl-lysine interacts with the angiotensin II AT1 receptor." Peptides 16, no. 7 (1995): 1203-7.

Garg, A, MM Chren, LP Sands, MS Matsui, KD Marenus, KR Feingold, and PM Elias. "Psychological stress perturbs epidermal permeability barrier homeostasis: Implications for the pathogenesis of stress-associated skin disorders." Arch Dermatol 137, no. 1 (2001): 53-9.

Garland, CF, FC Garland, and ED Gorham. "Could sunscreens increase melanoma risk?" Am J Public Health 82, no. 4 (1992): 614-5.

———. "Rising trends in melanoma. An hypothesis concerning sunscreen effectiveness." Ann Epidemiol 3, no. 1 (1993): 103-10.

———. "Re: Effect of sunscreens on UV radiation-induced enhancement of melanoma growth in mice." J Natl Cancer Inst 86, no. 10 (1994): 798-800.

Gehring, W. "The influence of biotin on nails of reduced quality." Aktuelle Dermatologie (Germany) 22, no. 1-2 (1996): 20-24.

Giampaolo, V, F Luigina, A Conforti, and R Milanino. "Copper and inflammation." In Inflammatory diseases and copper: The metabolic and therapeutic roles of copper and other essential metalloelements in humans, edited by JR Sorenson. Clifton, New Jersey: Humana Press, 1982.

Gilbert, R, G Salanti, M Harden, and S See. "Infant sleeping position and the sudden infant death syndrome: Systematic review of observational studies and historical review of recommendations from 1940 to 2002." Int J Epidemiol 34, no. 4 (2005): 874-87.

Gill, SE, and WC Parks. "Metalloproteinases and their inhibitors: Regulators of wound healing." Int J Biochem Cell Biol 40, no. 6-7 (2008): 1334-47.

Globa, AG, VA Vishnevskiĭ, VS Demidova, Olu Abakumova, and AA Karelin. "[accumulation of ATP in rat and human hepatocyte cell membranes exposed to certain growth factors and phosphatidylcholine]." Biull Eksp Biol Med 121, no. 3 (1996): 271-4.

Godet, D, and PJ Marie. "Effects of the tripeptide glycyl-l-histidyl-l-lysine copper complex on osteoblastic cell spreading, attachment and phenotype." Cell Mol Biol (Noisy-le-grand) 41, no. 8 (1995): 1081-91.

Gonzalez, S, A Wu, MA Pathak, M Sifakis, and DA Goukassian. "Oral administration of lutein modulates cell proliferation induced by acute UV-B radiation in the SHK-1 hairless mouse animal model." The Society for Investigative Dermatology, 63rd Annual Meeting (2002): Abstract 769.

Granstein, R, D Faulhaber, and W Ding. "Lutein inhibits UVB radiation-induced tissue swelling and suppression of the induction of contact hypersensitivity (CHS) in the mouse." 62nd Annual Meeting of the Society for Investigative Dermatology (2001): 497.

Greene, FL, LS Lamb, M Barwick, and NJ Pappas. "Effect of dietary copper on colonic tumor production and aortic integrity in the rat." J Surg Res 42, no. 5 (1987): 503-12.

Gubler, CJ, ME Lahey, GE Cartwright, and MM Wintrobe. "Studies on copper metabolism. IX. The transportation of copper in blood." J Clin Invest 32, no. 5 (1953): 405-14.

Gul, NY, A Topal, IT Cangul, and K Yanik. "The effects of topical tripeptide copper complex and helium-neon laser on wound healing in rabbits." Vet Dermatol 19, no. 1 (2008): 7-14.

Hanson, KM, E Gratton, and CJ Bardeen. "Sunscreen enhancement of UV-induced reactive oxygen species in the skin." Free Radic Biol Med 41, no. 8 (2006): 1205-12.

Harris, ED. "Copper as a cofactor and regulator of copper,zinc superoxide dismutase." J Nutr 122, no. 3 Suppl (1992): 636-40.

———. "Basic and clinical aspects of copper." Crit Rev Clin Lab Sci 40, no. 5 (2003): 547-86.

Hart, EB, H Steenbock, J Waddell, and CA Elvehjem. "Iron in nutrition. VII. Copper as a supplement to iron for hemoglobin building in the rat. 1928." J Biol Chem 277, no. 34 (2002): e22.

Harvey, LJ, G Majsak-Newman, JR Dainty, DJ Lewis, NJ Langford, HM Crews, and SJ Fairweather-Tait. "Adaptive responses in men fed low- and high-copper diets." Br J Nutr 90, no. 1 (2003): 161-8.

Hawk, SN, L Lanoue, CL Keen, CL Kwik-Uribe, RB Rucker, and JY Uriu-Adams. "Copper-deficient rat embryos are characterized by low superoxide dismutase activity and elevated superoxide anions." Biol Reprod 68, no. 3 (2003): 896-903.

Heinrich, U, C Gartner, M Wiebusch, O Eichler, H Sies, H Tronnier, and W Stahl. "Supplementation with beta-carotene or a similar amount of mixed carotenoids protects humans from UV-induced erythema." J Nutr 133, no. 1 (2003): 98-101.

Heresi, G, C Castillo-Durán, C Muñoz, M Arévalo, and L Schlesinger. "Phagocytosis and immunoglobulin levels in hypocupremic infants." Nutrition Research 5, no. 12 (1985): 1327-34.

Hill, PL, NA Turiano, MD Hurd, DK Mroczek, and BW Roberts. "Conscientiousness and longevity: An examination of possible mediators." Health Psychol 30, no. 5 (2011): 536-41.

Hirsch, A. Scentsational sex: The secret to using aroma for arousal: Element Books, 1998.

Hitzig, G. "Enhanced healing and growth in hair transplantation using copper peptides." Cosmetic Dermatol 13 (2000): 18-21.

Hobday, R. The healing sun: Sunlight and health in the 21st century: Findhorn Press, 2000.

Holick, M. "The UV advantage." (2003): 190.

Holstege, G. Presented at the European Society for Human Reproduction and Development, 2005.

Hong, Y, T Downey, KW Eu, PK Koh, and PY Cheah. "A 'metastasis-prone' signature for early-stage mismatch-repair proficient sporadic colorectal cancer patients and its implications for possible therapeutics." Clin Exp Metastasis 27, no. 2 (2010): 83-90.

Hostynek, JJ, F Dreher, and HI Maibach. "Human skin retention and penetration of a copper tripeptide in vitro as function of skin layer towards anti-inflammatory therapy." Inflamm Res 59, no. 11 (2010): 983-8.

———. "Human skin penetration of a copper tripeptide in vitro as a function of skin layer." Inflamm Res 60, no. 1 (2011): 79-86.

Howard, BV, L Van Horn, J Hsia, JE Manson, ML Stefanick, S Wassertheil-Smoller, LH Kuller, AZ LaCroix, RD Langer, NL Lasser, CE Lewis, MC Limacher, KL Margolis, WJ Mysiw, JK Ockene, LM Parker, MG Perri, L Phillips, RL Prentice, J Robbins, JE Rossouw, GE Sarto, IJ Schatz, LG Snetselaar, VJ Stevens, LF Tinker, M Trevisan, MZ Vitolins, GL Anderson, AR Assaf, T Bassford, SA Beresford, HR Black, RL Brunner, RG Brzyski, B Caan, RT Chlebowski, M Gass, I Granek, P Greenland, J Hays, D Heber, G Heiss, SL Hendrix, FA Hubbell, KC Johnson, and JM Kotchen. "Low-fat dietary pattern and risk of cardiovascular disease: The women's health initiative randomized controlled dietary modification trial." JAMA 295, no. 6 (2006): 655-66.

Huang, PJ, YC Huang, MF Su, TY Yang, JR Huang, and CP Jiang. "In vitro observations on the influence of copper peptide aids for the led photoirradiation of fibroblast collagen synthesis." Photomed Laser Surg 25, no. 3 (2007): 183-90.

Hung, YH, EL Robb, I Volitakis, M Ho, G Evin, QX Li, JG Culvenor, CL Masters, RA Cherny, and AI Bush. "Paradoxical condensation of copper with elevated beta-amyloid in lipid rafts under cellular copper deficiency conditions: Implications for Alzheimer disease." J Biol Chem 284, no. 33 (2009): 21899-907.

Hunt, JR, and RA Vanderpool. "Apparent copper absorption from a vegetarian diet." Am J Clin Nutr 74, no. 6 (2001): 803-7.

Itoh, S, K Ozumi, HW Kim, O Nakagawa, RD McKinney, RJ Folz, IN Zelko, M Ushio-Fukai, and T Fukai. "Novel mechanism for regulation of extracellular SOD transcription and activity by copper: Role of antioxidant-1." Free Radic Biol Med 46, no. 1 (2009): 95-104.

Jacob, RA, HH Sandstead, JM Munoz, LM Klevay, and DB Milne. "Whole body surface loss of trace metals in normal males." Am J Clin Nutr 34, no. 7 (1981): 1379-83.

Jonas, J, J Burns, EW Abel, MJ Cresswell, JJ Strain, and CR Paterson. "Impaired mechanical strength of bone in experimental copper deficiency." Ann Nutr Metab 37, no. 5 (1993): 245-52.

Kang, YA, HR Choi, JI Na, CH Huh, MJ Kim, SW Youn, KH Kim, and KC Park. "Copper-GHK increases integrin expression and p63 positivity by keratinocytes." Arch Dermatol Res 301, no. 4 (2009): 301-6.

Kaur, M, C Agarwal, RP Singh, X Guan, C Dwivedi, and R Agarwal. "Skin cancer chemopreventive agent, {alpha}-santalol, induces apoptotic death of human epidermoid carcinoma A431 cells via caspase activation together with dissipation of mitochondrial membrane potential and cytochrome c release." Carcinogenesis 26, no. 2 (2005): 369-80.

Kawase, M, N Kurikawa, S Higashiyama, N Miura, T Shiomi, C Ozawa, T Mizoguchi, and K Yagi. A. "Effectiveness of polyamidoamine dendrimers modified with tripeptide growth factor, glycyl-l-histidyl-l-lysine, for enhancement of function of hepatoma cells." J Biosci Bioeng 88, no. 4 (1999): 433-7.

Kawase, M, N Miura, N Kurikawa, K Masuda, S Higashiyama, K Yagi, and T Mizoguchi. B. "Immobilization of tripeptide growth factor glycyl-l-histidyl-l-lysine on poly(vinylalcohol)-quarternized stilbazole (PVA-SbQ) and its use as a ligand for hepatocyte attachment." Biol Pharm Bull 22, no. 9 (1999): 999-1001.

Kazemi, A, T Frazier, and M Cave. "Micronutrient-related neurologic complications following bariatric surgery." Curr Gastroenterol Rep 12, no. 4 (2010): 288-95.

Keen, CL, JY Uriu-Hare, SN Hawk, MA Jankowski, GP Daston, CL Kwik-Uribe, and RB Rucker. "Effect of copper deficiency on prenatal development and pregnancy outcome." Am J Clin Nutr 67, no. 5 Suppl (1998): 1003S-11.

Kelley, DS, PA Daudu, PC Taylor, BE Mackey, and JR Turnlund. "Effects of low-copper diets on human immune response." Am J Clin Nutr 62, no. 2 (1995): 412-6.

Keyes, WM, and AA Mills. "p63: A new link between senescence and aging." Cell Cycle 5, no. 3 (2006): 260-5.

Kimoto, E, H Tanaka, J Gyotoku, F Morishige, and L Pauling. "Enhancement of antitumor activity of ascorbate against ehrlich ascites tumor cells by the copper:Glycylglycylhistidine complex." Cancer Res 43, no. 2 (1983): 824-28.

Klevay, LM. "Hypertension in rats due to copper deficiency." Nutr Rep Int 35 (1987): 999-1005.

Klevay, LM, and ES Halas. "The effects of dietary copper deficiency and psychological stress on blood pressure in rats." Physiol Behav 49, no. 2 (1991): 309-14.

Klevay, LM, and DM Medeiros. "Deliberations and evaluations of the approaches, endpoints and paradigms for dietary recommendations about copper." J Nutr 126, no. 9 Suppl (1996): 2419S-26S.

Klevay, LM. "Trace elements, atherosclerosis, and abdominal aneurysms." Ann N Y Acad Sci 800 (1996): 239-42.

———. A. "Cardiovascular disease from copper deficiency--a history." J Nutr 130, no. 2S Suppl (2000): 489S-92S.

Klevay, LM, and DM Christopherson. "Copper deficiency halves serum dehydroepiandrosterone in rats." J Trace Elem Med Biol 14, no. 3 (2000): 143-5.

Klevay, LM. B. "Dietary copper and risk of coronary heart disease." Am J Clin Nutr 71, no. 5 (2000): 1213-4.

———. "Iron overload can induce mild copper deficiency." J Trace Elem Med Biol 14, no. 4 (2001): 237-40.

———. "Extra dietary copper inhibits LDL oxidation." Am J Clin Nutr 76, no. 3 (2002): 687-8; author reply 88.

Klevay, LM, and RE Wildman. "Meat diets and fragile bones: Inferences about osteoporosis." J Trace Elem Med Biol 16, no. 3 (2002): 149-54.

Klevay, LM. "Ischemic heart disease as deficiency disease." Cell Mol Biol (Noisy-le-grand) 50, no. 8 (2004): 877-84.

———. "Alzheimer's disease as copper deficiency." Med Hypotheses 70, no. 4 (2008): 802-7.

———. "Metabolic interactions among dietary choletstrol, copper, and fructose." Am J Physiol Endocrinol Metab 298, no. 1 (2010): E138-9.

Kohl, JV, and RT Francoeur. The scent of eros : Mysteries of odor in human sexuality. New York: Continuum Publishing Company, 1995.

Kremer, JM, and J Bigaouette. "Nutrient intake of patients with rheumatoid arthritis is deficient in pyridoxine, zinc, copper, and magnesium." J Rheumatol 23, no. 6 (1996): 990-4.

Kubecova, M, K Kolostova, D Pinterova, G Kacprzak, and V Bobek. "Cimetidine: An anticancer drug?" Eur J Pharm Sci 42, no. 5 (2011): 439-44.

Kumar, N. "Copper deficiency myelopathy (human swayback)." Mayo Clin Proc 81, no. 10 (2006): 1371-84.

Lane, TF, ML Iruela-Arispe, RS Johnson, and EH Sage. "SPARC is a source of copper-binding peptides that stimulate angiogenesis." J Cell Biol 125, no. 4 (1994): 929-43.

Larsen, HR. "Sunscreens: Do they cause skin cancer." Internat J of Alternative & Complementary Med 12 (1994): 17-19.

Lau, SJ, and B Sarkar. "The interaction of copper(II) and glycyl-l-histidyl-l-lysine, a growth-modulating tripeptide from plasma." Biochem J 199, no. 3 (1981): 649-56.

Laussac, JP, R Haran, and B Sarkar. "N.M.R. and E.P.R. Investigation of the interaction of copper(II) and glycyl-l-histidyl-l-lysine, a growth-modulating tripeptide from plasma." Biochem J 209, no. 2 (1983): 533-9.

Lee, A, and R Langer. "Shark cartilage contains inhibitors of tumor angiogenesis." Science 221, no. 4616 (1983): 1185-7.

Lee, J, S Jiang, N Levine, and RR Watson. "Carotenoid supplementation reduces erythema in human skin after simulated solar radiation exposure." Proc Soc Exp Biol Med 223, no. 2 (2000): 170-4.

Lemoine, P, B Viossat, G Morgant, FT Greenaway, A Tomas, NH Dung, and JR Sorenson. "Synthesis, crystal structure, EPR properties, and anti-convulsant activities of binuclear and mononuclear 1,10-phenanthroline and salicylate ternary copper(II) complexes." J Inorg Biochem 89, no. 1-2 (2002): 18-28.

Levine, DD, SB Hanauer, L Patt, and G Koren. "An open study of PC1020 (GHK-Cu) rectal solution in treatment of distal inflammatory bowel disease." Digestive Disease Week Abstract Book (1995).

Leyden, J, G Grove, S Barkovic, and Y Appa. A. "The effect of tripeptide to copper ratio in two copper peptide creams on photoaged facial skin." Presented at the Amer Acad Derm Meeting, 2002: Abstract P67.

Leyden, J, T Stephens, MB Finkey, Y Appa, and S Barkovic. B. "Skin care benefits of copper peptide containing facial cream." Presented at the American Academy Dermatology Meeting, 2002: Abstract P68.

Leyden, J, T Stephens, MB Finkey, and S Barkovic. C. "Skin care benefits of copper peptide containing eye creams." Presented at the American Academy Dermatology Meeting, 2002: Abstract P69.

Liakopoulou-Kyriakides, M, C Pachatouridis, L Ekateriuiadou, and VP Papageorgiou. "A new synthesis of the tripeptide gly-his-lys with antimicrobial activity." Amino Acids 13, no. 2 (1997): 155-61.

Lindner, G, G Grosse, W Halle, and P Henklein. "Uber die wirkung eines synthetischen tripeptids auf in vitro kultiviertes nervengewebe [The effect of a synthetic tripeptide nervous tissue cultured in vitro]." Z Mikrosk Anat Forsch 93, no. 5 (1979): 820-8.

Linnane, AW, C Zhang, N Yarovaya, G Kopsidas, S Kovalenko, P Papakostopoulos, H Eastwood, S Graves, and M Richardson. "Human aging and global function of coenzyme q10." Ann N Y Acad Sci 959 (2002): 396-411; discussion 63-5.

Lipotec S.A., Barcelona, Spain. Brochure "ALDENINE® PBC CODE: P10-PD050." www.reverseskinaging.com/lipotec-aldenine.html.

Lonnerdal, B. "Copper nutrition during infancy and childhood." Am J Clin Nutr 67, no. 5 Suppl (1998): 1046S-53S.

Lopez, A, DE Sims, RF Ablett, RE Skinner, LW Leger, CM Lariviere, LA Jamieson, J Martinez-Burnes, and GG Zawadzka. "Effect of emu oil on auricular inflammation induced with croton oil in mice." Am J Vet Res 60, no. 12 (1999): 1558-61.

Lutsenko, S, A Bhattacharjee, and AL Hubbard. "Copper handling machinery of the brain." Metallomics 2, no. 9 (2010): 596-608.

Manot, L. "Effects du tripeptide GHK-Cu sur le coeur isole de rat." Universite de Reims Champagne-Ardenne, 1997.

Maquart, FX, L Pickart, M Laurent, P Gillery, JC Monboisse, and JP Borel. "Stimulation of collagen synthesis in fibroblast cultures by the tripeptide-copper complex glycyl-l-histidyl-l-lysine-Cu2+." FEBS Lett 238, no. 2 (1988): 343-6.

Maquart, FX, P Gillery, JC Monboisse, L Pickart, M Laurent, and JP Borel. "Glycyl-l-histidyl-l-lysine, a triplet from the a2 (I) chain of human type I collagen, stimulates collagen synthesis by fibroblast cultures." Ann N Y Acad Sci 580 (1990): 573-75.

Maquart, FX, G Bellon, B Chaqour, J Wegrowski, L. M Patt, RE Trachy, JC Monboisse, F Chastang, P Birembaut, P Gillery, and et al. "In vivo stimulation of connective tissue accumulation by the tripeptide-copper complex glycyl-l-histidyl-l-lysine-Cu2+ in rat experimental wounds." J Clin Invest 92, no. 5 (1993): 2368-76.

Maquart, FX, A Simeon, S Pasco, and JC Monboisse. "Regulation de l'activite cellulaire par la matrice extracelulaire: Le concept de matrikines [Regulation of cell activity by the extracellular matrix: The concept of matrikines]." French J Soc Biol 193, no. 4-5 (1999): 423-8.

Maquart, FX, G Bellon, S Pasco, and JC Monboisse. "Matrikines in the regulation of extracellular matrix degradation." Biochimie 87, no. 3-4 (2005): 353-60.

Masuda, A, S Akiyama, M Kuwano, and N Ikekawa. "Potentiation of antifungal effect of amphotericin B by squalene, an intermediate for sterol biosynthesis." J Antibiot (Tokyo) 35, no. 2 (1982): 230-4.

Mazurowska, L, and M Mojski. "ESI-MS study of the mechanism of glycyl-l-histidyl-l-lysine-Cu(II) complex transport through model membrane of stratum corneum." Talanta 72, no. 2 (2007): 650-4.

———. "Biological activities of selected peptides: Skin penetration ability of copper complexes with peptides." J Cosmet Sci 59, no. 1 (2008): 59-69.

McCormack, MC, KC Nowak, and RJ Koch. "The effect of copper tripeptide and tretinoin on growth factor production in a serum-free fibroblast model." Arch Facial Plast Surg 3, no. 1 (2001): 28-32.

Miller, DM, D DeSilva, L Pickart, and SD Aust. "Effects of glycyl-histidyl-lysyl chelated Cu(II) on ferritin dependent lipid peroxidation." Adv Exp Med Biol 264 (1990): 79-84.

Miller, TR, JD Wagner, BR Baack, and KJ Eisbach. "Effects of topical copper tripeptide complex on CO2 laser-resurfaced skin." Arch Facial Plast Surg 8, no. 4 (2006): 252-9.

Moan, J, and A Dahlback. "The relationship between skin cancers, solar radiation and ozone depletion." Br J Cancer 65, no. 6 (1992): 916-21.

Morgant, G, NH Dung, JC Daran, B Viossat, X Labouze, M Roch-Arveiller, FT Greenaway, W Cordes, and JR Sorenson. "Low-temperature crystal structures of tetrakis-mu-3,5-diisopropylsalicylatobis-dimethylformamidodico pper(II) and tetrakis-mu-3,5-diisopropylsalicylatobis-diethyletheratodicopp er(II) and their role in modulating polymorphonuclear leukocyte activity in overcoming seizures." J Inorg Biochem 81, no. 1-2 (2000): 11-22.

Morganti, P, C Bruno, and G Colelli. "[Gelatin-cystine, keratogenesis and structure of the hair]." Boll Soc Ital Biol Sper 59, no. 1 (1983): 20-5.

Morganti, P, C Bruno, F Guarneri, A Cardillo, P Del Ciotto, and F Valenzano. "Role of topical and nutritional supplement to modify the oxidative stress." Int J Cosmet Sci 24, no. 6 (2002): 331-9.

Morton, MS, PC Elwood, and M Abernethy. "Trace elements in water and congenital malformations of the central nervous system in south wales." Br J Prev Soc Med 30, no. 1 (1976): 36-9.

Mulder, GD, L. M Patt, L Sanders, J Rosenstock, MI Altman, ME Hanley, and GW Duncan. "Enhanced healing of ulcers in patients with diabetes by topical treatment with glycyl-l-histidyl-l-lysine copper." Wound Repair Regen 2, no. 4 (1994): 259-69.

Narayanan, VS, CA Fitch, and CW Levenson. "Tumor suppressor protein p53 mRNA and subcellular localization are altered by changes in cellular copper in human Hep G2 cells." J Nutr 131, no. 5 (2001): 1427-32.

Naughton, BA, GK Naughton, P Liu, GB Zuckerman, and AS Gordon. "The influence of pancreatic hormones and diabetogenic procedures on erythropoietin production." J Surg Oncol 21, no. 2 (1982): 97-103.

Oberley, LW, SW Leuthauser, RF Pasternack, TD Oberley, L Schutt, and JR Sorenson. "Anticancer activity of metal compounds with superoxide dismutase activity." Agents Actions 15, no. 5-6 (1984): 535-8.

Okuyama, S, S Hashimoto, H Aihara, WM Willingham, and JR Sorenson. "Copper complexes of non-steroidal antiinflammatory agents: Analgesic activity and possible opioid receptor activation." Agents Actions 21, no. 1-2 (1987): 130-44.

Paffenbarger, RS Jr, AL Wing, and RT Hyde. "Physical activity as an index of heart attack risk in college alumni." Am J Epidemiol 108, no. 3 (1978): 161-75.

Park, JH, and MS Tallman. "Managing acute promyelocytic leukemia without conventional chemotherapy: Is it possible?" Expert Rev Hematol 4, no. 4 (2011): 427-36.

Pauling, L. "Orthomolecular psychiatry. Varying the concentrations of substances normally present in the human body may control mental disease." Science 160, no. 825 (1968): 265-71.

Peled, T, E Landau, E Prus, AJ Treves, A Nagler, and E Fibach. "Cellular copper content modulates differentiation and self-renewal in cultures of cord blood-derived CD34+ cells." Br J Haematol 116, no. 3 (2002): 655-61.

Peled, T, E Glukhman, N Hasson, S Adi, H Assor, D Yudin, C Landor, J Mandel, E Landau, E Prus, A Nagler, and E Fibach. "Chelatable cellular copper modulates differentiation and self-renewal of cord blood-derived hematopoietic progenitor cells." Exp Hematol 33, no. 10 (2005): 1092-100.

Peled, T, E Fibach, and A Treves. "Methods of controlling proliferation and differentiation of stem and progenitor cells ". U.S. Patent 6,962,698: Gamida Cell Ltd. (Jerusalem, IL), Hadasit Medical Research Services and Development, Ltd. (Jerusalem, IL), filed Aug 17, 1999, and issued Nov 08, 2005.

Penland, JG, and JR Prohaska. "Abnormal motor function persists following recovery from perinatal copper deficiency in rats." J Nutr 134, no. 8 (2004): 1984-8.

Percival, SS. "Copper and immunity." Am J Clin Nutr 67, no. (5 Suppl) (1998): 1064S-68S.

Perez-Meza, D, M Leavitt, and R Trachy. "Clinical evaluation of graftcyte moist dressings on hair graft viability and quality of healing." Int J Cos Surg 6, no. 1 (1998): 80-84.

Pesakova, V, J Novotna, and M Adam. "Effect of the tripeptide glycyl-l-histidyl-l-lysine on the proliferation and synthetic activity of chick embryo chondrocytes." Biomaterials 16, no. 12 (1995): 911-5.

Pickart, L. "A tripeptide in human plasma that increases the survival of hepatocytes and the growth of hepatoma cells." University of California, San Francisco, 1973.

Pickart, L, and MM Thaler. "Tripeptide in human serum which prolongs survival of normal liver cells and stimulates growth in neoplastic liver." Nat New Biol 243, no. 124 (1973): 85-7.

Pickart, L, MM Thaler, and M Millard. "Effect of transition metals on recovery from plasma of the growth-modulating tripeptide glycylhistidyllysine." J Chromatogr 175, no. 1 (1979): 65-73.

Pickart, L, JH Freedman, WJ Loker, J Peisach, CM Perkins, RE Stenkamp, and B Weinstein. "Growth-modulating plasma tripeptide may function by facilitating copper uptake into cells." Nature 288, no. 5792 (1980): 715-7.

Pickart, L, WH Goodwin, W Burgua, TB Murphy, and DK Johnson. "Inhibition of the growth of cultured cells and an implanted fibrosarcoma by aroylhydrazone analogs of the gly-his-lys-Cu(II) complex." Biochem Pharmacol 32, no. 24 (1983): 3868-71.

Pickart, L. "Suppression of growth of a fibrosarcoma in mice with gly-his-lys: Cu 2+ and ascorbic acid." Unpublished, 1985.

Pickart, L, D Downey, S Lovejoy, and B Weinstein. "Gly-l-his-l-lys:Copper(II) - a human plasma factor with superoxide dismutase-like and wound-healing properties." In Superoxide and superoxide dismutase in chemistry, biology and medicine, edited by G Rotilio, 555-58: Elsevier Science, 1986.

Pickart, L, and S Lovejoy. "Biological activity of human plasma copper-binding growth factor glycyl-l-histidyl-l-lysine." Methods Enzymol 147 (1987): 314-28.

Pickart, L. "Chemical derivatives of GHL-Cu." U.S. Patent 4,665,054: Bioheal, Inc., filed Feb 08, 1985, and issued May 12, 1987.

———. "Iamin (Prezatide Copper Acetate): A human growth factor with multiple wound-healing properties." In Biology of copper complexes, edited by JR Sorenson, 273-85. Clifton, NJ: Humana Press, 1987.

———. A. "Methods and compositions for preventing ulcers ". U.S. Patent 4,767,753: Skin Biology, Inc., filed May 11, 1987, and issued Aug 30, 1988.

———. B. "Use of GHL-Cu as a wound-healing and anti-inflammatory agent." U.S. Patent 4,760,051: filed Jan 24,1985, and issued Jul 26, 1988.

———. "Method of healing wounds in horses." U.S. Patent 4,937,230: ProCyte Corporation, inc., filed Dec 04, 1987, and issued Jun 26, 1990.

———. A. "Methods and compositions for healing bone using gly his lys: Copper." U.S. Patent 5,059,588: ProCyte Corporation, Inc., filed Oct 13, 1989, and issued Oct 22, 1991.

———. B. "Methods and compositions for healing ulcers." U.S. Patent 5,023,237: ProCyte Corporation, Inc., filed Aug 30, 1989, and issued Jun 11, 1991.

———. A. "Cosmetic and skin treatment compositions." U.S. Patent 5,135,913: ProCyte Corporation, Inc., filed Jun 16, 1988, and issued Aug 04, 1992.

———. B. "Method of using copper(II) containing compounds to accelerate wound healing." U.S. Patent 5,164,367: ProCyte Corporation, Inc., filed Mar 26, 1990, and issued Nov 17, 1992.

———. C. "Methods and compositions for healing ulcers ". U.S. Patent 5,145,838: Skin Biology, Inc., filed Jun 10, 1991, and issued Sept 08, 1992.

———. "GHK-copper 2+ strongly lowers blood pressure in goats." Unpublished Safety Study, 1993.

———. "Method for stimulating hair growth using GHL-Cu complexes." U.S. Patent 5,177,061: ProCyte Corporation, filed Sept 22, 1989, and issued Jan 05, 1993.

———. "Cosmetic and skin treatment compositions." U.S. Patent 5,348,943: ProCyte Corporation, Inc., filed Aug 03, 1992, and issued Sept 20, 1994.

———. "Tissue protective and regenerative compositions." U.S. Patent 5,382,431: Skin Biology, Inc, filed Sept 29, 1992, and issued Jan 17, 1995.

———. A. "Metal-peptide compositions and methods for stimulating hair growth." U.S. Patent 5,550,183: ProCyte Corporation, Inc., filed Mar 07, 1995, and issued Aug 27, 1996.

———. D. "Tissue protective and regenerative compositions." U.S. Patent 5,554,375: Skin Biology, Inc., filed Jan 06, 1995, and issued Sept 10, 1996.

Pickart, L. . "Compositions and methods for skin tanning and protection." 5698184 (1997).

Pickart, L. "Formula of love." Cosmetics & Medicine (Russia) 2 (2005): 24-33.

———. "The human tri-peptide GHK and tissue remodeling." J Biomater Sci Polym Ed 19, no. 8 (2008): 969-88.

Pickart, L, and A Margolina. "GHK-copper peptide in skin remodeling and anti-aging." SOFW Journal 136 (2010): 10-20.

Pickart, L, and F Pickart. "A possible mechanism whereby skin remodeling may suppress cancer metastasis genes." In Society for the Advancement of Wound Care and the Wound Healing Society, A8-A62. Dallas, Texas: Wound Repair and Regeneration 2011. See also http://reverseskinaging.com/wound-healing-society-2011.html

Podda, M, MG Traber, C Weber, LJ Yan, and L Packer. "UV-irradiation depletes antioxidants and causes oxidative damage in a model of human skin." Free Radic Biol Med 24, no. 1 (1998): 55-65.

Pohunkova, H, J Stehlik, J Vachal, O Cech, and M Adam. "Morphological features of bone healing under the effect of collagen-graft-glycosaminoglycan copolymer supplemented with the tripeptide gly-his-lys." Biomaterials 17, no. 16 (1996): 1567-74.

Politis, MJ, and A Dmytrowich. "Promotion of second intention wound healing by emu oil lotion: Comparative results with furasin, polysporin, and cortisone." Plast Reconstr Surg 102, no. 7 (1998): 2404-7.

Pollard, JD, S Quan, T Kang, and RJ Koch. "Effects of copper tripeptide on the growth and expression of growth factors by normal and irradiated fibroblasts." Arch Facial Plast Surg 7, no. 1 (2005): 27-31.

Poole, TJ, and BR Zetter. "Stimulation of rat peritoneal mast cell migration by tumor-derived peptides." Cancer Res 43, no. 12 Pt 1 (1983): 5857-61.

Porter, RH, and J Winberg. "Unique salience of maternal breast odors for newborn infants." Neurosci Biobehav Rev 23, no. 3 (1999): 439-49.

Proxyte Corp. Press Release. Redmond, WA. (1997).

Prohaska, JR, and RG Hoffman. "Auditory startle response is diminished in rats after recovery from perinatal copper deficiency." J Nutr 126, no. 3 (1996): 618-27.

Purba, MB, A Kouris-Blazos, N Wattanapenpaiboon, W Lukito, E Rothenberg, B Steen, and ML Wahlqvist. A. "Can skin wrinkling in a site that has received limited sun exposure be used as a marker of health status and biological age?" Age Aging 30, no. 3 (2001): 227-34.

Purba, MB, A Kouris-Blazos, N Wattanapenpaiboon, W Lukito, EM Rothenberg, BC Steen, and ML Wahlqvist. B. "Skin wrinkling: Can food make a difference?" J Am Coll Nutr 20, no. 1 (2001): 71-80.

Pyo, HK, HO Yoo, OH Won, OH Lee, YU Kang, HO Eun, KH Cho, and KH Kim. "The effect of tripeptide-copper complex on human hair growth in vitro." Arch Pharm Res 30, no. 7 (2007): 834-9.

Rabenstein, DL, JM Robert, and S Hari. "Binding of the growth factor glycyl-l-histidyl-l-lysine by heparin." FEBS Lett 376, no. 2 (1995): 216-20.

Raju, KS, G Alessandri, M Ziche, and PM Gullino. "Ceruloplasmin, copper ions, and angiogenesis." J Natl Cancer Inst 69, no. 5 (1982): 1183-8.

Raju, KS, G Alessandri, and PM Gullino. "Characterization of a chemoattractant for endothelium induced by angiogenesis effectors." Cancer Res 44, no. 4 (1984): 1579-84.

Rao, MS, B Hattiangady, and AK Shetty. "The window and mechanisms of major age-related decline in the production of new neurons within the dentate gyrus of the hippocampus." Aging Cell 5, no. 6 (2006): 545-58.

Rittschof, D , and JH Cohen. "Crustacean peptide and peptide-like pheromones and kairomones." Peptides 25, no. 9 (2004): 1503-16.

Rock, E, A Mazur, JM O'Connor, MP Bonham, Y Rayssiguier, and JJ Strain. "The effect of copper supplementation on red blood cell oxidizability and plasma antioxidants in middle-aged healthy volunteers." Free Radic Biol Med 28, no. 3 (2000): 324-9.

Saari, JT, AM Bode, and GM Dahlen. "Defects of copper deficiency in rats are modified by dietary treatments that affect glycation." J Nutr 125, no. 12 (1995): 2925-34.

Sage, EH, and RB Vernon. "Regulation of angiogenesis by extracellular matrix: The growth and the glue." J Hypertens Suppl 12, no. 10 (1994): S145-52.

Saxen, L, PC Holmberg, M Nurminen, and E Kuosma. "Sauna and congenital defects." Teratology 25, no. 3 (1982): 309-13.

Schaal, B, G Coureaud, D Langlois, C Ginies, E Semon, and G Perrier. "Chemical and behavioural characterization of the rabbit mammary pheromone." Nature 424, no. 6944 (2003): 68-72.

Schagen, S, R Voegeli, D Imfeld, T Schreier, and CC Zouboulis. "Lipid regulation in SZ95 sebocytes by glycyl-histidyl-lysine." Presented at the 16th European Academy of Dermatology and Venereology Congress, Vienna, May 16-20 2007.

Scher, RK. "Foods which contain biotin." Prevention 46 (1994): 122.

Schlesinger, DH, L Pickart, and MM Thaler. "Growth-modulating serum tripeptide is glycyl-histidyl-lysine." Experientia 33, no. 3 (1977): 324-5.

Schlumpf, M, B Cotton, M Conscience, V Haller, B Steinmann, and W Lichtensteiger. "In vitro and in vivo estrogenicity of UV screens." Environ Health Perspect 109, no. 3 (2001): 239-44.

Schlumpf, M, K Kypke, M Wittassek, J Angerer, H Mascher, D Hascher, C Vokt, M Birchler, and W Lichtensteiger. "Exposure patterns of UV filters, fragrances, parabens, phthalates, organochlor peticides, PBDEs, and PCBs in human milk: Correlation of UV filters with use of cosmetics." Chemosphere 81, no. 10 (2010): 1171-83.

Schmidt, SP, JR Resser, RL Sims, DL Mullins, and DJ Smith. "The combined effects of glycyl-l-histidyl-l-lysine copper (II) and cell-tak on the healing of linear incision wounds." Wounds 6 (1994): 62-67.

Senoo, M, F Pinto, CP Crum, and F McKeon. "p63 is essential for the proliferative potential of stem cells in stratified epithelia." Cell 129, no. 3 (2007): 523-36.

Sensenbrenner, M, GG Jaros, G Moonen, and P Mandel. "Effects of synthetic tripeptide on the differentiation of dissociated cerebral hemisphere nerve cells in culture." Neurobiology 5, no. 4 (1975): 207-13.

Simeon, A, F Monier, H Emonard, P Gillery, P Birembaut, W Hornebeck, and FX Maquart. "Expression and activation of matrix metalloproteinases in wounds: Modulation by the tripeptide-copper complex glycyl-l-histidyl-l-lysine-Cu2+." J Invest Dermatol 112, no. 6 (1999): 957-64.

Simeon, A, Y Wegrowski, Y Bontemps, and FX Maquart. A. "Expression of glycosaminoglycans and small proteoglycans in wounds: Modulation by the tripeptide-copper complex glycyl-l-histidyl-l-lysine-Cu(2+)." J Invest Dermatol 115, no. 6 (2000): 962-8.

Simeon, A, H Emonard, W Hornebeck, and FX Maquart. B. "The tripeptide-copper complex glycyl-l-histidyl-l-lysine-Cu2+ stimulates matrix metalloproteinase-2 expression by fibroblast cultures." Life Sci 67, no. 18 (2000): 2257-61.

Smakhtin, MY, LA Sever'yanova, AI Konoplya, and IA Shveinov. "Tripeptide gly-his-lys is a hepatotropic immunosuppressor." Bull Exp Biol Med 133, no. 6 (2002): 586-7.

Smakhtin, MIu, AI Konoplia, LA Sever'ianova, and IA Shveinov. "[Pharmacological correction of immuno-metabolic disorders with the peptide gly-his-lys in hepatic damage induced by tetrachloromethane]." Patol Fiziol Eksp Ter (Russia), no. 2 (2003): 19-21.

Sobel, N, V Prabhakaran, CA Hartley, JE Desmond, GH Glover, EV Sullivan, and JD Gabrieli. "Blind smell: Brain activation induced by an undetected airborne chemical." Brain 122 (Pt 2) (1999): 209-17.

Sorenson, JR. "Evaluation of copper complexes as potential anti-arthritic drugs." J Pharm Pharmacol 29, no. 7 (1977): 450-2.

Sorenson, JR, and W Hangarter. "Treatment of rheumatoid and degenerative diseases with copper complexes: A review with emphasis on copper-salicylate." Inflammation 2, no. 3 (1977): 217-38.

Sorenson, JR, K Ramakrishna, and TM Rolniak. "Antiulcer activities of D-penicillamine copper complexes." Agents Actions 12, no. 3 (1982): 408-11.

Sorenson, JR. Inflammatory diseases and copper: The metabolic and therapeutic roles of copper and other essential metalloelements in humans, Experimental biology and medicine. Clifton, New Jersey: Humana Press, 1982.

———. "A role for copper in mediating oxidative damage associated with degenerative disease processes seems to be more imaginary than real." Med Biol 63, no. 1 (1985): 40-1.

———. "Biology of copper complexes." Experimental Biology and Medicine 16 (1987).

———. "Antiinflammatory, analgesic, and antiulcer activities of copper complexes suggest their use in a physiologic approach to treatment of arthritic diseases." Basic Life Sci 49 (1988): 591-4.

Sorenson, JR, LS Soderberg, MV Chidambaram, DT de la Rosa, H Salari, K Bond, G.L Kearns, RA Gray, CE Epperson, and ML Baker. "Bioavailable copper complexes offer a physiologic approach to treatment of chronic diseases." Adv Exp Med Biol 258 (1989): 229-34.

Sorenson, JR. "Copper complexes offer a physiological approach to treatment of chronic diseases." Prog Med Chem 26 (1989): 437-568.

Steenvoorden, DP, and G Beijersbergen van Henegouwen. "Protection against UV-induced systemic immunosuppression in mice by a single topical application of the antioxidant vitamins C and E." Int J Radiat Biol 75, no. 6 (1999): 747-55.

Stenn, KS, AG Messenger, and HP Baden, eds. The molecular and structural biology of hair, Annals of the new york academy of sciences. New York, NY: New York Academy of Sciences, 1991.

Stephens, TJ, ML Sigler, MB Finkley, and Y Appa. "Skin benefits of an SPF 20 copper peptide containing face cream." Presented at the 61st Annual American Academy of Dermatology Meeting, San Francisco, CA, 2003.

Stern, RS, and N Laird. "The carcinogenic risk of treatments for severe psoriasis. Photochemotherapy follow-up study." Cancer 73, no. 11 (1994): 2759-64.

Stolarz-Skrzypek, K, T Kuznetsova, L Thijs, V Tikhonoff, J Seidlerová, T Richart, Y Jin, A Olszanecka, S Malyutina, E Casiglia, J Filipovský, K Kawecka-Jaszcz, Y Nikitin, and Staessen JA; European Project on Genes in Hypertension (EPOGH) Investigators. "Fatal and nonfatal outcomes, incidence of hypertension, and blood pressure changes in relation to urinary sodium excretion." JAMA 305, no. 17 (2011): 1777-85.

Storm, HM, SY Oh, BF Kimler, and S Norton. "Radioprotection of mice by dietary squalene." Lipids (United States) 28, no. 6 (1993): 555-9.

Stromberg, BE, PB Khoury, and EJ Soulsby. "Development of larvae of ascaris suum from the third to the fourth stage in a chemically defined medium." Int J Parasitol 7, no. 2 (1977): 149-51.

Su, X, M Paris, YJ Gi, KY Tsai, MS Cho, YL Lin, JA Biernaskie, S Sinha, C Prives, LH Pevny, FD Miller, and ER Flores. "TAp63 prevents premature aging by promoting adult stem cell maintenance." Cell Stem Cell 5, no. 1 (2009): 64-75.

Sugimoto, Y, I Lopez-Solache, F Labrie, and V Luu-The. "Cations inhibit specifically type I 5 alpha-reductase found in human skin." J Invest Dermatol 104, no. 5 (1995): 775-8.

Swaim, SF, DM Bradley, JS Spano, and et al. "Evaluation of multipeptide copper complex medications on open wound healing in dogs." J Am Anim Hosp Assoc 29 (1993): 519-25.

Swaim, SF, DM Vaughn, SA Kincaid, NE Morrison, SS Murray, MA Woodhead, CE Hoffman, JC Wright, and JR Kammerman. "Effect of locally injected medications on healing of pad wounds in dogs." Am J Vet Res 57, no. 3 (1996): 394-9.

Tavera-Mendoza, LE, and JH White. "Cell defenses and the sunshine vitamin." Sci Am 297, no. 5 (2007): 62-5, 68-70, 72.

Taylor, RS, KE Ashton, T Moxham, L Hooper, and S Ebrahim. "Reduced dietary salt for the prevention of cardiovascular disease: A meta-analysis of randomized controlled trials (Cochrane review)." Am J Hypertens 24, no. 8 (2011): 843-53.

Thornfeldt, CR. "Chronic inflammation is etiology of extrinsic aging." J Cosmet Dermatol 7, no. 1 (2008): 78-82.

Timpe, ED, RE Trachy, and I Dumwiddle. "Evaluation of telogen hair follicle stimulation using an in vivo model: Results with peptide copper complexes." In Dermatologic research techniques, edited by HI Maibach, 241-54. Boca Raton: CRC Press, 1996.

Traber, MG, M Podda, C Weber, J Thiele, M Rallis, and L Packer. "Diet-derived and topically applied tocotrienols accumulate in skin and protect the tissue against ultraviolet light-induced oxidative stress." Asia Pacific J Clin Nutr 6, no. 1 (1997): 63-67.

Trachy, RE, TD Fors, L Pickart, and H Uno. "The hair follicle-stimulating properties of peptide copper complexes. Results in C3H mice." Ann N Y Acad Sci 642 (1991): 468-9.

Trachy, RE, L Patt, G Duncan, and B Kalis. A. "Phototrichogram analysis of hair follicle stimulation: A pilot clinical study with a peptide-copper complex." In Dermatologic research techniques, edited by H. I. Maibach, 217-26: CRC Press, 1996.

Trachy, RE, U Uno, S Packard, and L Patt. B. "Quantitative assessment of peptide-copper complex-induced hair follicle stimulation using the fuzzy rat." In Dermatologic research techniques, edited by HI Maibach, 227-39. Boca Raton: CRC Press, 1996.

Trumbo, P, AA Yates, S Schlicker, and M Poos. "Dietary reference intakes for vitamin A, vitamin K, boron, chromium, copper, iodine, iron, manganese, molybdenum, nickel, silicon, vanadium, and zinc." J Am Diet Assoc 101, no. 3 (2001): 294-301.

Turnlund, JR, WR Keyes, SK Kim, and JM Domek. "Long-term high copper intake: Effects on copper absorption, retention, and homeostasis in men." Am J Clin Nutr 81, no. 4 (2005): 822-8.

Uauy, R, M Olivares, and M Gonzalez. "Essentiality of copper in humans." Am J Clin Nutr 67, no. 5 Suppl (1998): 952S-59S.

Uğurlu, T, M Türkoğlu, and T Ozaydın. "In vitro evaluation of compression-coated glycyl-l-histidyl-l-lysine-Cu(II) (GHK-Cu(2+))-loaded microparticles for colonic drug delivery." Drug Dev Ind Pharm 37, no. 11 (2011): 1282-9.

Uno, H. The histopathology of hair loss. Kalamazoo, MI: The Upjohn Company, 1988.

Uno, H, and S Kurata. "Chemical agents and peptides affect hair growth." J Invest Dermatol 101, no. 1 Suppl (1993): 143S-47S.

Vinci, C, V Caltabiano, AM Santoro, AM Rabuazzo, M Buscema, R Purrello, E Rizzarelli, R Vigneri, and F Purrello. "Copper addition prevents the inhibitory effects of interleukin 1-beta on rat pancreatic islets." Diabetologia 38, no. 1 (1995): 39-45.

Viossat, B, FT Greenaway, G Morgant, JC Daran, NH Dung, and JR Sorenson. "Low-temperature (180 K) crystal structures of tetrakis-mu-(niflumato) di(aqua)dicopper(II) N,N-dimethylformamide and N,N-dimethylacetamide solvates, their EPR properties, and anticonvulsant activities of these and other ternary binuclear copper(II)niflumate complexes." J Inorg Biochem 99, no. 2 (2005): 355-67.

Wegrowski, Y, FX Maquart, and JP Borel. "Stimulation of sulfated glycosaminoglycan synthesis by the tripeptide-copper complex glycyl-l-histidyl-l-lysine-Cu2+." Life Sci 51, no. 13 (1992): 1049-56.

Williams, RJ. Biochemical individuality. The basis for the genetotrophic concept New York: Wiley, 1956.

Williams, DM. "Copper deficiency in humans." Semin Hematol 20, no. 2 (1983): 118-28.

Winberg, J, and RH Porter. "Olfaction and human neonatal behaviour: Clinical implications." Acta Paediatr 87, no. 1 (1998): 6-10.

Wise, JA, RJ Morin, R Sanderson, and K Blum. "Changes in plasma carotenoid, alpha-tocopherol, and lipid peroxide levels in response to supplementation with concentrated fruit and vegetable extracts: A pilot study." Current Therapeutic Research 57, no. 6 (1996): 445-61.

Zemtsov, A, M Gaddis, and VM Montalvo-Lugo. "Moisturizing and cosmetic properties of emu oil: A pilot double blind study." Australas J Dermatol 37, no. 3 (1996): 159-61.

Zetter, BR, N Rasmussen, and L Brown. "Methods of laboratory investigation: An in vivo assay for chemoattractant activity." Lab Invest 53, no. 3 (1985): 362-8.

Zhai, H, YH Leow, and HI Maibach. A. "Human barrier recovery after acute acetone perturbation: An irritant dermatitis model." Clin Exp Dermatol 23, no. 1 (1998): 11-3.

Zhai, H, N Poblete, and HI Maibach. B. "Sodium lauryl sulfate damaged skin in vivo in man: A water barrier repair model." Skin Res Tech 4, no. 1 (1998): 24-27.

———. C. "Stripped skin model to predict irritation potential of topical agents in vivo in humans." Int J Dermatol 37, no. 5 (1998): 386-9.

Zhai, H, YC Chang, M Singh, and HI Maibach. "In vivo nickel allergic contact dermatitis: Human model for topical therapeutics." Contact Dermatitis 40, no. 4 (1999): 205-8.

Ziegler, TA, and RB Forward, Jr. "Larval release behaviors in the caribbean spiny lobster, panulirus argus: Role of peptide pheromones." J Chem Ecol 33, no. 9 (2007): 1795-805.

INDEX
ALPHABETICAL GUIDE TO WORDS FREQUENTLY USED

A

Abrasion 83
Acid mantle 116
Acne 125
Acne scars 85
Age spots 96
Aging reversal 13
Alien chemicals 16
Alpha hydroxy acids 42
Alpha lipoic acid 15
Anti-inflammatory 206, 220
Antioxidants 47
Arginine/ornithine 202
Artificial implants 22
Artificial methods 21, 23
Ascorbic acid 46
Astringents 120
Attraction 166

B

Baby fat 135
Bath, bathing 118
Beard growth 143
Beauty 270
Bedsores 106
Beta hydroxy acids 36
Biological Healing Oils 43, 122
Blackheads 125
Blemish removal 84
Blond hair, green out 141
Blood circulation 114
Body perfumes 175
Bonding 169
Bone healing 233
Botulinum toxin 56
Bovine collagen 23
Breast lift 72
Burns, radiation 104
Burns, thermal 104

C

Calcium 202
Cancer metastasis 237
Chemical peels 89
Chemoattraction 223
Choline / inositol 202
Chondroitin sulfate 202
Clarifying shampoos 147
Clinically proven 19
Coenzyme Q10, CoQ-10 47
Collagen 70
Color cosmetics 17
Comedones 125
Conditioners 148
Contact dermatitis 111
Copper and disease 260
Copper, daily 257
Copper, healing 257
Copper, love 268
Cortisol 130
Cortisone 110
Cosmetic moisturizers 122, 127

D

Dermatitis 104
Dermabrasion 88
DHEA 268
DHT, Dihydrotestosterone
     133,134
Diabetes 109
Diet 198
Dietary fiber 208
DMAE 78
DNA 17
Dry skin 108

E

Eczema 108
Elastin 28

Emu oil 113
Exercise 129
Exfoliating Hydroxy Acids 52
Expensive perfumes 170
Eye area 60
Eyebrows 156
Eyelashes 156
Eyelids 62

F

Fiber 208
Fibroblasts 70
Folic acid 202
Fragile, sensitive skin 104
Free radicals 185

G

Gamma-linolenic acid (GLA) 206
GHK-Cu 216
Ginkgo biloba 141
Glow 30
Glucosamine 202
Glycosaminoglycans 28
Glycyl-histidyl-lysine 217
GraftCyte 139
Grape seed extract 202

H

Hair, brushing 150
    color 145
    damage 147
    follicles 235
    gray 146
    growth 149
    hormone shifts 136
    length 149
    loss 134
    permanents 151
    relaxers 152
    removal 153
    straightening 151
    thinning 136
    transplantation 232
Hands 128
Heating lights 22
HIV/AIDS skin problems 111
Hyaluronic acid 53
Hydrogen peroxide 107
Hyperpigmentation 91
Hypopigmentation 91

I

Immune-compromised 111
Immune deficient 262
Inflammation 220
Infra-red machines 23
Intestinal healing 233

J

Jewelry 271
Junk Science 19, 20

K

Keratin 145

L

Lactic acid 43
Laser resurfacing 90
Lasers 74
Lipids 115
Lips 130
Liver, restore 232
Long Hair Clinics 133
Loose, sagging skin 69
Lutein 47
Lycopene 47

M

Magnesium 202
Make-up 99
Melanin 138
Melatonin 202
Methods of Skin Renewal 18
Microdermabrasion cloths 88
Microwaves 74
Minoxidil 140
Models and Actors 99
Moisturizers 122
Moles 88
Moral need 270
MSM (methylsulfonylmethane) 162

N

N-acetyl-carnitine 202
Needling, skin 92
Nerve outgrowth 224
Nerve paralyzers 56
Neuropeptides 22

O

Omega fatty acids 200, 205

P

Pheromones 166
Photodamage 97
Phytonutrients 206
Pitted scars 85
Plant extracts, toxic 17
Pore cleansing 75
Pore size 75
Pores, tighten 75
Pregnant, pregnancy 265
Propecia 132
Psoriasis 112
Puff up skin 21

R

Remodeling, skin 39
Retinoic acid 45
Retinol 45
Reverse aging 13
Rosacea 91

S

Sagging skin 69
Salicylic acid 43
Saunas 119
Saw palmetto oil 141
Scalp damage 138
Scars 79
Second-generation SRCPs 228
Shampoo 147
Shaving 153
Shower 118
Silicone injections 22
Sjorgren's Syndrome 109
Skin allergies 110
Skin barrier damage 104
Skin firmness 70
Skin products 49
Skin remodeling copper peptides
     (SRCPs) 36
Skin tags 86
Skin ulcers 106
Soap pH 118
Soy isoflavones 140, 141
Stem cells 236
Stepford Wives 22

Strength of SRCPs in Skin Biology
     products 51
Stress 130
Stretch marks 86
Subcutaneous fat 29
Sulfur donor 135
Sunblockers 186
Sun damage 87
Sunlight health 181
Sunscreens, chemical 186
Suntanning 183
Supplements 202

T

Terminal hair follicles 140
TGF-beta-1
     (transforming growth factor)
     137, 267
Tighten skin 69
Tissue repair 243
Titanium dioxide 186
Tocotrienols 124, 202
Toners 120
Toothpick trick for scars 85
Trans-fats 200
Tricomin 139

U

Unnatural methods 23

V

Vegetable extracts 207
Vellus hair follicles 29
Vitamin C 46
Vitamins 209

W

Wheelchairs 106
Whiteheads 125
Wound Healing 38
Wrinkles 59
Wine 212, 267

X

X-ray, acne 22

Z

Zinc 202
Zinc oxide 186